R.D. Rubens and I. Fogelman (Eds.)

BONE METASTASES

Diagnosis and Treatment

With 82 Figures

Springer-Verlag
London Berlin Heidelberg New York
Paris Tokyo Hong Kong

R.D. Rubens, BSc, MD, FRCP
Imperial Cancer Research Fund Clinical Oncology Unit, United
Medical and Dental Schools of Guy's and St. Thomas's Hospitals,
London SE1 9RT

I. Fogelman, BSc, MD, FRCP
Department of Nuclear Medicine, Guy's Hospital, London SE1 9RT

ISBN 3-540-19619-6   Springer-Verlag Berlin Heidelberg New York
ISBN 0-387-19619-6   Springer-Verlag New York Berlin Heidelberg

British Library Cataloguing in Publication Data
Bone metastases.
1. Man. Bones. Cancer. Metastasis
I. Rubens, Robert D. *1943–*   II. Fogelman, Ignac
616.99471
ISBN 3-540-19619-6 v, West Germany

Library of Congress Cataloging-in-Publication Data
Bone metastases: diagnosis and treatment/Robert D. Rubens and
Ignac Fogelman (eds.).
p.   cm.
Includes index.
ISBN 0-387-19619-6. – ISBN 3-540-19619-6
1. Bone metastasis.   I. Rubens, R.D. (Robert David)   II. Fogelman, Ignac, 1948–   .
[DNLM: 1. Bone Neoplasms–secondary.   WE 258 B7105]   RC280. B6B668   1991
616.99'471–dc20
DNLM/DLC   90-10095
for Library of Congress   CIP

Typeset by Best-Set Typesetters, Ltd, Hong Kong
Printed by Henry Ling Ltd, The Dorset Press, Dorchester, UK
2128/3916-543210 Printed on acid-free paper

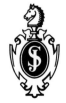

Dr. S. AL-Ismail

Preface

The subject of this book is the secondary involvement of the skeleton by a primary cancer arising elsewhere. It does not deal with the less common primary tumours of bone or bone marrow.

The morbidity from bone metastases is extensive – pain, fracture, hypercalcaemia, neurological complications, marrow suppression – yet patients so affected can live for many years. Breast cancer, in which over 70% of patients with advanced disease have skeletal involvement, often has a particularly long clinical course. Considering the high prevalence of this disease, the resulting problem for the health service is enormous. Although breast cancer accounts for the largest proportion of patients with malignant bone disease, skeletal metastases are an important complication of other carcinomas, particularly those arising in the prostate, lung, kidney and thyroid.

Patients with bone metastases often require palliative and supportive treatment for many months, sometimes years. While our understanding of the biology of cancer and the pathogenesis of bone metastases has advanced considerably, improvements in treatment have been slow to follow. Nevertheless, important progress has been made. Approaches to the endocrine treatment of cancer have undergone remarkable changes over a decade in which anti-oestrogens, anti-androgens, aromatase inhibitors and LH–RH agonists have replaced older hormonal treatments and ablative operations. More effective chemotherapy has become established and radiotherapeutic and orthopaedic surgical techniques have improved. Our increasing realisation of the importance of osteoclast activation in mediating the skeletal damage caused by metastatic cells has led to the use of bisphosphonates for the treatment of both osteolysis and hypercalcaemia. It is likely that this innovation will prove to have made a major contribution to a reduction in the suffering of patients with bone metastases. Further developments can confidently be expected from other new approaches.

With advances in treatment, diagnostic tests for both the identification of bone metastases and monitoring response to treatment assume greater importance. Radionuclide scanning remains the most sensitive test for detecting lesions, whilst radiological imaging is needed for assessing structural damage. In both these areas, important developments have been made. Further promise comes from the application of nuclear magnetic resonance, which also provides the possibility to study biochemical processes in vivo by spectroscopy. This could become an important guide for both the selection and monitoring of treatment. Meanwhile, progress has been made in the identification of biochemical indices for assessing response to treatment using more conventional methods.

The purpose of this book is to bring together these exciting developments which are gradually improving the prospects for patients with bone metastases. We hope that all those involved in the care of patients with cancer will find it useful.

London   Robert Rubens
July 1990   Ignac Fogelman

Contents

Contributors

B.F. Boyce, MB ChB, MRCPath
Associate Professor, Department of Pathology, University of
Texas Health Science Center at San Antonio, TX 78284-7750,
USA

Susan E.M. Clarke, MSc, MRCP
Consultant Physician, Department of Nuclear Medicine, Guy's
Hospital, London SE1 9RT

R.E. Coleman, MD, MRCP
Senior Registrar in Medical Oncology, ICRF Medical Oncology
Unit, Western General Hospital, Edinburgh EH4 2AX

D.J. Dodwell, BSc, MB ChB, MRCP
Registrar in Medical Oncology, University of Manchester,
Christie Hospital and Holt Radium Institute, Manchester M20
9BX

I. Fogelman, BSc, MD, FRCP
Consultant Physician, Department of Nuclear Medicine, Guy's
Hospital, London SE1 9RT

C.S.B. Galasko, ChM, FRCS(Eng), FRCS(Ed)
Professor of Orthopaedic Surgery, University of Manchester and
Consultant Orthopaedic Surgeon, Salford Health Authority,
Department of Orthopaedic Surgery, Clinical Sciences Building,
Hope Hospital, Salford M6 8HD

P.J. Hoskin, BSc, MB BS, MRCP, FRCR
Senior Registrar in Radiotherapy and Oncology, The Royal
Marsden Hospital, London SW3 6JJ

A. Howell, MB BS, FRCP
Senior Lecturer and Consultant in Medical Oncology, Christie
Hospital, Manchester M20 9BX

J.H. McKillop, BSc, PhD, FRCP
Professor of Medicine, Muirhead Chair of Medicine, University
Department of Medicine, Royal Infirmary, Glasgow G4 0SF

S.H. Ralston, MD, MRCP
Wellcome Senior Research Fellow and Honorary Consultant
Physician, University Department of Orthopaedic Surgery,
Western Infirmary, Glasgow G11 6NT

Sheila Rankin, FRCR
Consultant Radiologist, Department of Radiology, Guy's
Hospital, London SE1 9RT

M.A. Richards, MA, MD, MRCP
Senior Lecturer and Honorary Consultant, Clinical Oncology
Unit, Guy's Hospital, London SE1 9RT

R.D. Rubens, BSc, MD, FRCP
Imperial Cancer Research Fund, Professor of Clinical Oncology,
United Medical and Dental Schools of Guy's and St Thomas's
Hospitals, Guy's Hospital, London SE1 9RT

Clare Terrell, FRCR
Medical Director, St. Elizabeth Hospice, Ipswich, Suffolk IP3
8LX

J. Wedley, MB ChB, FFARCS
Consultant Anaesthetist, Guy's Hospital London and Pain Relief
Clinic, Guy's Hospital, London SE1 9RT

1   The Nature of Metastatic Bone Disease

R.D. Rubens

Biology of Bone Metastases

Metastases in bone are common, yet malignant tumours rarely arise in the skeleton. Primary cancers in other tissues, notably the breast and colon, are common but seldom do metastases become established in these structures. The lungs, however, frequently give rise to cancer and secondary tumour growth in them is often seen. This variability in the patterns of primary tumour growth in different tissues and their susceptibility to metastatic disease is as intriguing as it is poorly understood. Before addressing bone metastases specifically, some general aspects of tumour biology will be considered briefly.

Cancers arise from a disturbance of cell regulation which results in the abnormal proliferation of cells to the detriment of the host. They are characterised by the constituent malignant cells having the ability to invade into surrounding structures and to detach from the tissue of origin to lead to secondary growths elsewhere. The mechanisms involved in the evolution of cancer have been obscure, but recently substantial progress has been made in unravelling the nature of the complex underlying molecular and cellular processes.

The development and behaviour of cancer must ultimately be determined by the genetic control of cell regulation, but permissive factors in the environment of malignant cells are clearly important additional determinants for full expression of clinical disease. The initiating factors for malignant growth may reside in an individual's genotype, as in hereditary cancers such as carcinoma of the colon in patients with polyposis coli, or be external as for ionising radiation causing genetic damage ultimately expressed as, for example, acute leukaemia or breast cancer.

Once the malignant process has been initiated, a complex series of mechanisms needs to take place in order for the cancer to become established and manifested as clinical disease. Although the primary tumour itself can give rise to serious problems, it is usually the establishment of distant metastases that is responsible for the gravity of cancer and presents the most difficulties for treatment. Secondary spread can occur in a variety of ways including through lymphatic vessels, across serous cavities or along nerves, but blood-borne spread is the most important. The processes involved from the initiation of cancer growth to the destructive effects of metastatic disease are illustrated in Fig. 1.1.

After a cell has acquired a malignant phenotype, it proliferates at the primary site. Initially, nutrients for cellular growth will be provided by simple diffusion, but soon this becomes inadequate and a tumour vasculature develops. This is by extension of the blood supply from surrounding tissues. Endothelial cells of tumour blood vessels differ from those of normal tissues. Experiments with tritiated thymidine labelling and autoradiography have shown that tumour endothelial cells multiply with a doubling time of a few days, while endothelial cells of normal tissues divide only rarely. Much evidence points to the malignant cells as the source of the stimulus for endothelial cell growth which is known as tumour angiogenesis factor. Tumour cell blood vessels require the continual presence of this factor for growth and maintenance (D'Amore 1986).

Next, cancer cells begin to invade into local structures including their own blood vessels. This process is facilitated by proteolytic enzymes. Once access to the circulation has been gained, tumour emboli can travel throughout the body. It seems likely that, in the bloodstream, tumour cells are susceptible to a variety of host defence mechanisms including lysis by lymphocytes, monocytes and natural killer cells (Hanna and Fidler 1980) in addition to mechanical damage from blood turbulence and trapping in capillaries. Studies with injected radio-labelled tumour cells suggest that fewer than one in a thousand entering the circulation actually survive to develop into metastases (Fidler 1970).

Which cells ultimately form metastases seems to be determined by a cellular phenotype acquired in the primary tumour rather than from the random survival of a minority of cells (Fidler and Hart 1982). By the time of clinical diagnosis,

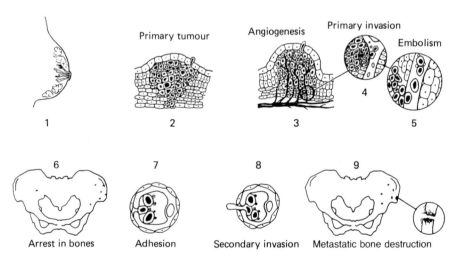

Fig. 1.1.   The pathogenesis of cancer metastasis. 1, Primary tumour develops in epithelial tissue; 2, sub-epithelial invasion occurs; 3, tumour vasculature develops; 4, malignant cells invade tumour blood vessels; 5, tumour emboli disseminate in the circulation; 6, metastatic cells are arrested in distant organs; 7, metastatic cells adhere to blood vessels of distant organs; 8, metastatic cells invade into distant tissues; 9, metastatic proliferation and subsequent destructive effects.

most malignant tumours contain a heterogeneous population of cells with a variety of phenotypes including metastatic capacity. This may be the result of a multicellular origin of the neoplasm or continuous evolution in tumours of a unicellular origin. These mechanisms of diversification are likely to operate in both the primary tumour and metastatic tissue. Cells which metastasise appear to be genetically less stable than non-metastatic cells. It is likely that, within this process, selection rather than randomness determines which cells from a heterogeneous primary tumour will evolve into metastases. Some metastases may be clonal in origin, while others may arise from different progenitor cells from the same primary.

When "pre-metastatic" cells have arrived at the site of secondary growth, they adhere either to capillary endothelial cells or to exposed basement membrane (Kramer et al. 1980). Extravasation then follows, presumably by a process similar to invasion at the primary site. Growth of metastases again requires vascularisation. Destructive effects in the host tissue then follow which, in the case of bone metastases, are mediated by osteoclasts stimulated by paracrine factors from the cancer cells (Galasko 1976). These factors include prostaglandin E2 (Tsao et al. 1983), osteoclast activating factor (Durie et al. 1981), transforming growth factor alpha (Ibbotson et al. 1985), parathormone-like substances (Hirshorn et al. 1979) and tumour necrosis factor (Bertolini et al. 1986); intermediary tissue macrophages producing interleukin-1 are also involved (Gowen et al. 1983). In the late stages of metastatic disease, further damage is probably caused by ischaemia.

We are rapidly understanding more about the genetic basis of cancer. Genes have been identified which have clear associations with malignant growth. Many of these oncogenes encode for either physiological growth factors or normal growth factor receptors, but abnormal or amplified expression can result in cancerous proliferation. Homologues of these oncogenes have been found in the transforming genes of many carcinogenic retroviruses. Other genes function to regulate or inhibit cell division. Loss of the function of these genes can also lead to uncontrolled growth and they have been termed tumour suppressor genes or anti-oncogenes. The protein products of anti-oncogenes can function within the nucleus or be involved in extranuclear activity concerned with growth and differentiation. For example, a gene has been identified on chromosome 18 which is found to be deleted in some human colorectal cancers. Interestingly, this gene shows significant homology to cell adhesion molecules and other cell surface glycoproteins (Fearon et al. 1990). Further work in this field may provide an explanation of how alteration of cell–cell adhesion could lead to detachment of malignant cells from primary tumours to produce metastases.

Patterns of Bone Metastases

Autopsy studies show that bone metastases are particularly common in patients dying from advanced cancer arising in the breast, bronchus, prostate, kidneys and thyroid (Table 1.1). As a result of sampling errors at post mortem examinations, there is probably a considerable underestimate of the true incidence of metastases in the skeleton. Given the high prevalence of carcinoma

Table 1.1.   Incidence of skeletal metastases in autopsy studies. (Galasko 1981)

| | | Incidence (%) of bone metastases | |
Primary tumour site	Number of studies	Median	Range
Breast	5	73	47–85
Prostate	6	68	33–85
Thyroid	4	42	28–60
Kidney	3	35	33–40
Bronchus	4	36	30–55
Oesophagus	3	6	5– 7
Gastro-intestinal tract	4	5	3–11
Rectum	3	11	8–13

of the breast, bronchus and prostate, these cancers probably account for over 80% of patients with metastatic bone disease. By contrast, the common cancers arising in the alimentary tract give an incidence of recognisable metastases in well under 10% of such patients.

Irrespective of the tissue of origin of the cancer, the distribution of bone metastases is predominantly in the axial skeleton, particularly the spine and pelvis, and ribs, rather than the appendicular skeleton, although lesions in the humeri and femora are not uncommon (Galasko 1981). This distribution is similar to the red bone marrow in which slow blood flow possibly assists attachment of metastatic cells. In 1889, Stephen Paget remarked on the disparate pattern of bone metastases: "The evidence seems to me irresistible that in cancer of the breast the bones suffer in a special way, which cannot be explained by any theory of embolism alone" (Paget 1889). He suggested that the properties of the tissues in which metastases developed were determinants of this process. While this may well be a factor in metastasis development, some elegant anatomical studies a half century later made an important contribution to our understanding of the patterns of metastatic distribution in the skeleton.

The high incidence of bone metastases without pulmonary lesions raised questions about the route of cancer cells from the primary tumours to the skeleton. The absence of lung deposits makes it unlikely that malignant cells pass through the pulmonary into the systemic circulation. Even if lung tissue is not receptive as a site for metastatic disease to become established, tumour cells are unlikely to pass through its narrow capillaries, particularly as aggregates in tumour emboli. Batson's work demonstrating the existence of the vertebral-venous plexus provided the explanation. He clearly demonstrated in human cadaver and animal experiments how venous blood in both the pelvis and from the breast flowed, not only into the venae cavae, but also directly into the vertebral-venous plexus. Moreover, the flow into the vertebral veins predominated when intrathoracic or intra-abdominal pressure was elevated as for example during Valsalva's manoeuvre and so presumably its clinical counterparts such as coughing (Batson 1940).

These experiments explained the predilection of prostatic and breast cancer to produce metastases in the axial skeleton and limb girdles. Further studies demonstrated the extent of this remarkable network of valveless vessels which involve the epidural veins, perivertebral veins, veins of the thoraco-abdominal wall, and veins of the head and neck all carrying blood under low pressure

(Batson 1942). In this system, blood is continually subject to arrest and reversal of the direction of flow. This vertebral-venous system parallels, connects with, and provides by-passes for the portal, pulmonary and caval system of veins and so provides a pathway for the spread of disease between distant organs. Primary lung tumours can invade directly into the pulmonary venous system to disseminate through the arterial circulation.

Breast Cancer

Carcinoma of the breast is the cancer most commonly associated with metastatic bone disease. It is the most prevalent cancer in women of Western Europe and North America; in the United Kingdom there are 24 000 new cases each year and 15 000 deaths from this cause. It has a variable and often long clinical course and morbidity from bone metastases is a major health-care problem. The lesions are often of a mixed sclerotic/lytic variety. There are no powerful predictors of which patients are at risk of skeletal disease, but the incidence of bone metastases is significantly higher with steroid-receptor-positive and well-differentiated tumours (Coleman and Rubens 1987).

A study from the Breast Unit at Guy's Hospital showed the skeleton to be the most common site of metastatic disease in 587 patients dying from breast cancer, of whom 69% had radiological evidence of skeletal metastases before death compared to 27% each for lung and liver metastases (Coleman and Rubens 1987). Over a 10-year period, in 2240 patients presenting with primary breast cancer, 681 (30%) had relapsed after a median follow-up of 5 years of whom 395 (58%) had distant metastases. One hundred and eighty four had first relapse in bone representing 47% of all those with first distant relapse, 24% of the total with any relapse and 8% of the total study population. Patients with first relapse in the skeleton did not differ from those with first relapse in the liver either in terms of age, menstrual status or median post-operative disease-free interval.

Nevertheless, survival experience was markedly different in these two metastatic groups. Median survival of 498 patients with first relapse in bone was 20 months compared to a survival of only 3 months after first relapse in liver (Fig. 1.2). In 253 patients with metastatic disease apparently remaining confined to the skeleton, the median duration of survival was 24 months. Hence, bone metastases can be a protracted problem for many patients with this disease.

One hundred and forty-five (29%) of the patients with first relapse in bone developed one or more of the principal complications of bone destruction. Hypercalcaemia developed in 86 patients, 17% of those with first relapse in bone, pathological fracture in 78(16%) and spinal cord compression in 13 (3%). While hypercalcaemia in advanced breast cancer is usually associated with demonstrable bone metastases, this is not always found to be the case. In a review of 147 patients with hypercalcaemia in advanced breast cancer, 125 (85%) had definite radiographic evidence of bone metastases, but in 22 (15%) there was no such evidence of skeletal involvement. In the latter group, there was a significantly higher incidence of liver metastases and inappropriately high renal tubular reabsorption of calcium suggesting that liver involvement may be associated with a humoral component in the pathogenesis of hypercalcaemia under these circumstances (Coleman et al. 1988a).

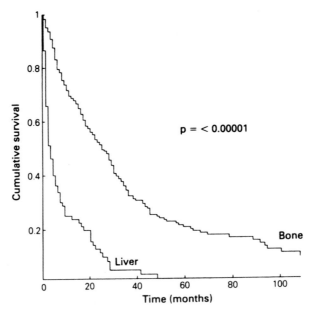

Fig. 1.2. Survival of patients with breast cancer after first relapse in bone compared to survival after first relapse in the liver (Coleman and Rubens 1987).

Lung Cancer

Lung cancer is the commonest cancer in the UK where it accounts for nearly one-fifth of all new cases of cancer and is responsible for more than 40 000 deaths a year. There has been a steady increase in the incidence of this cancer throughout this century, closely related to tobacco smoking habits, but in the last few years a decrease of deaths from this cause has been noted. The incidence of bone metastases identified at the time of primary diagnosis is highest in the small cell variety and lowest with squamous cell tumours, but at autopsy the incidence of bone metastases is similar for the four main histological types of lung cancer (squamous cell, small cell, large cell and adenocarcinoma) at about one-third (Muggia and Chervu 1974). Survival from primary diagnosis of lung cancer is poor and fewer than 10% of patients are alive at 5 years. Once metastatic disease is evident, most patients will be dead within a few months. Bone metastases from lung cancer are usually of the osteolytic type but, because of the poor survival prospects, morbidity from these metastases is much less of a long-term health care problem than in breast cancer.

Prostatic Cancer

Carcinoma of the prostate has an annual incidence of about 11 000 and causes some 7500 deaths in the UK each year. The skeleton is by far the most common site of metastatic disease and the majority of lesions are typically osteoblastic on plain radiography. Nevertheless, computed tomography (CT) scanning often identifies lytic areas within predominantly sclerotic lesions. Moreover, histological studies have demonstrated increased bone resorption in metastatic prostatic cancer (Urwin et al. 1985). Unexpectedly, markers of increased bone resorption are also seen at osseous sites unaffected by metastatic disease. This suggests that generalised trabecular bone loss occurs in prostatic cancer, a factor which could contribute to morbidity in these patients who still have a median survival prospect of about 17 months after the diagnosis of bone metastases (Clain 1965).

Morbidity from Bone Metastases

Several important complications give rise to the morbidity from bone metastases. They include pain, impaired mobility, pathological fracture, spinal cord compression, hypercalcaemia (Chap. 8) and suppression of bone-marrow function.

Pain is frequently the presenting symptom of metastatic bone disease. A variety of mechanisms may be involved. The cytokines mediating osteoclastic destruction of bone, such as prostaglandins, probably also activate pain receptors. Possibly this is the reason for the transient exacerbation of bone pain in some patients shortly after the start of systemic treatments destined ultimately to lead to bone healing. Compression or infiltration of nerve roots and reflex muscle spasm are also factors likely to contribute to pain.

The precise incidence of pathological fracture in patients with metastatic bone disease is uncertain. In a series from the Memorial Sloan Kettering Cancer Center, 150 (8%) of 1800 patients with metastatic bone disease had pathological fractures of either the femur (90%) or humerus (10%) (Higinbotham and Marcove 1965). The inclusion of rib and vertebral fractures would give an incidence of pathological fracture affecting a much higher proportion of patients with bone metastases. In this series, breast cancer was responsible for 53% of pathological fractures, renal carcinoma for 11%, lung for 8%, thyroid and lymphoma each for 5% and prostatic cancer for 3%; a variety of cancers accounted for the remainder. Radiological assessment of long bones suggests that with metastatic destruction of over 50% of cortical thickness the risk of fracture is very high and this acts as a useful guide for prophylactic surgery (Fidler 1973). In a recent series of 498 patients with metastatic bone disease from breast cancer, 78 (16%) sustained a pathological fracture of a long bone after which the median duration of survival was 12 months (range 0–66 months) (Coleman and Rubens 1987).

Compression of the spinal cord or cauda equina in patients with metastatic disease of the spine is a medical emergency necessitating prompt diagnosis and treatment. Its causes include pressure from an enlarging extradural mass, spinal angulation following vertebral collapse, vertebral dislocation following pathological fracture or, rarely, pressure from intradural metastases. The standard diagnostic test is myelography, which often reveals multiple levels of compression; similar information can be obtained from magnetic resonance imaging. Pain is the most common initial symptom and affected 125 of 130 (96%) patients in one series (Gilbert et al. 1978). Two types of pain occur, local spinal and radicular. Radicular pain varies with the location of the tumour, being more common in the cervical (79%) and lumbo-sacral (90%) regions and less so with thoracic lesions (55%). Both local spinal and radicular pain are experienced close to the site of the lesion identified at myelography. Motor weakness, sensory loss and autonomic dysfunction are all commonly present at diagnosis of spinal cord or cauda equina compression each affecting more than half of patients. The most common primary tumours producing this complication in decreasing order of frequency are carcinoma of the breast, lung cancer, prostatic cancer, lymphoma and renal carcinoma.

Extensive infiltration of the bone marrow by metastatic disease leads to leucoerythroblastic anaemia and pancytopenia with consequent predisposition to infection and haemorrhage. Radiotherapy, often needed in the treatment of metastatic bone disease, can exacerbate this problem and compromises the ability to give effective chemotherapy. Animal experiments have shown that cytotoxic drugs can interfere with osteoblastic function and new bone formation (Friedlaender et al. 1984), but the clinical significance of these findings is unknown. Other iatrogenic factors can also aggravate the morbidity from bone metastases. For example, ovarian ablation and corticosteroids predispose to osteoporosis. In elderly patients, it can sometimes be difficult to distinguish between osteoporotic and metastatic vertebral collapse while in such patients arthritic and degenerative disease can further exacerbate disability.

Assessment of Skeletal Disease

Assessment of metastatic disease in the skeleton has been and remains a difficult problem. It has relied on plain radiography to give structural information on the damage from malignant disease. However, the sensitivity of this technique is relatively low and substantial damage has to occur before radiographs become abnormal. CT scanning is a more sensitive radiographic technique, but is more readily applied to elucidate specific lesions rather than for more regular use in assessing the skeleton.

Radionuclide bone scanning gives functional information on osteoblastic activity in the skeleton. It is far more sensitive than plain radiography for detecting lesions, but is less specific as increased osteoblast activity occurs in association with various benign disorders. Consequently, isotope scanning is used as a screening test for skeletal lesions, selected radiographs being performed of areas of abnormal uptake to study further the structural nature of the problem. Isotope scanning is also used in the initial staging of primary cancers which commonly metastasise to the skeleton in order to determine whether or not radical treatment is appropriate. The frequency of positive scans under these circumstances is low and the cost-effectiveness of this approach has been questioned (Coleman et al. 1988c).

Assessing response to treatment in the skeleton is also difficult as it is not possible directly to observe regression of cancer in bone. Plain radiography can only detect recalcification in sites of previous lytic disease and ability to identify this process is usually delayed for many months. CT scanning of selected lesions can improve on this and also enables healing to be observed in small lytic areas in predominantly osteoblastic lesions, a process not normally visible by plain radiography. Radionuclide scanning is of little value in monitoring response as abnormal uptake on the scan is frequently exaggerated in the early stages of a response to treatment, no doubt as the result of enhanced osteoblastic activity (Coleman et al. 1988b). Nevertheless, many months after a response to treatment has been established, a bone scan can be expected to revert towards normal. Because of the difficulties in assessing response to treatment in the skeleton, other methods have been evaluated. Symptomatic assessment and biochemical indices can give early information on whether or not bone metastases are responding to treatment (Chap. 6).

Our perception of metastatic bone disease will change with time as a result of developments in treatment and diagnostic techniques. Improvements in treatment should lessen the incidence of metastatic disease and alter the clinical course of cancer, while improvements in diagnostic techniques, both in specificity and sensitivity, will modify our recognition of the behaviour of metastases.

References

Batson OV (1940) The function of the vertebral veins and their role in the spread of metastases. Ann Surg 112:138–149

Batson OV (1942) The role of the vertebral veins in metastatic processes. Ann Intern Med 16:38–45

Bertolini DR, Nedwin GE, Bringman TS, Smith DD, Mundy GR (1986) Stimulation of bone resorption and inhibition of bone formation in vitro by human tumour necrosis factors. Nature 319:516–518

Clain A (1965) Secondary malignant disease of bone. Br J Cancer 19:15–29

Coleman RE, Rubens RD (1987) The clinical course of bone metastases from breast cancer. Br J Cancer 55:61–66

Coleman RE, Fogelman I, Rubens RD (1988a) Hypercalcaemia and breast cancer – an increased humoral component in patients with liver metastases. Eur J Surg Oncol 14:423–428

Coleman RE, Mashiter G, Whitaker KB, Moss DW, Rubens RD (1988b) Bone scan flare predicts successful systemic therapy for bone metastases. J Nucl Med 29:1354–1359

Coleman RE, Rubens RD, Fogelman I (1988c) Reappraisal of the baseline bone scan in breast cancer. J Nucl Med 29:1045–1049

D 'Amore PA (1986) Growth factors, angiogenesis and metastasis. In: Welch DR, Bhuyahn BK, Liotta LA (Eds). Cancer metastasis: experimental and clinical strategies, Alan R Liss Inc, New York pp 269–283 (Progress in clinical and biological research, vol 212)

Durie BGM, Salmon SE, Mundy GR (1981) Relation of osteoclast activating factor production to extent of bone disease in multiple myeloma. Br J Haematol 477:21–30

Fearon ER, Cho KR, Nigro JM, Kern SE, Simons JW, Ruppert JM, Hamilton SR, Preisinger AC, Thomas G, Kinzler KW, Vogelstein B (1990) Identification of a chromosome 18q gene that is altered in colorectal cancers. Science 247:49–56

Fidler IJ (1970) Metastasis: quantitative analysis of distribution and fate of tumour emboli labelled with ^{125}I-5-iodo-2'-deoxyuridine. J Natl Cancer Inst, 45:773–782

Fidler IJ, Hart IR (1982) Biological diversity in metastatic neoplasms: origins and implications. Science 217:998–1003

Fidler M (1973) Prophylactic internal fixation of secondary neoplastic deposits in long bones. Br Med J i:341–343

Friedlaender GE, Tross RB, Doganis AC, Kirkwood JM, Baron R (1984). Effects of chemotherapeutic agents on bone. I. Short-term methotrexate and doxorubicin (Adriamycin) treatment in a rat model. J Bone Joint Surg [Am] 66:602–607

Galasko CSB (1976) Mechanism of bone destruction in the development of skeletal metastases. Nature 263:507–508

Galasko CSB (1981) The anatomy and pathways of skeletal metastases. In: Weiss L, Gilbert AH, (Eds) Bone metastasis. GK Hall, Boston, pp 49–63

Gilbert RW, Kim J-H, Posner JB (1978) Epidural spinal cord compression from metastatic tumor: diagnosis and treatment. Ann Neurol 3:40–51

Gowen M, Wood DD, Ihrie EJ, McGuire MKB, Graham R, Russel GG (1983) An interleukin 1-like factor stimulates bone resorption in vitro. Nature 306:378–380

Hanna N, Fidler IJ (1980) Role of natural killer cells in the destruction of circulating tumour emboli. J Natl Cancer Inst 65:801–809

Higinbotham NL, Marcove RC (1965) The management of pathological fractures. J Trauma 5:792–798

Hirshorn JE, Vrhovsek E, Posen S (1979) Carcinoma of the breast associated with hypercalcaemia and the presence of parathyroid-hormone-like substances in tumor. J Clin Endocrinol Metab 48:217–221

Ibbotson KJ, Twardzik DR, D'Souza SM, Hargreaves WR, Todaro GJ, Mundy GR (1985) Stimulation of bone resorption in vitro by synthetic transforming growth factor-alpha, Science 228:1007–1009

Kramer RH, Gonzalez R, Nicolson GL (1980) Metastatic tumour cells adhere preferentially to the extracellular matrix underlying vascular endothelial cells. Int J Cancer 26:639–645

Muggia FM, Chervu LR (1974) Lung cancer: diagnosis in metastatic sites. Semin Oncol 1:217–228

Paget S (1889) The distribution of secondary growths in cancer of the breast. Lancet i:571–573

Tsao SW, Burman JF, Pittam MR, Carter RL (1983) Further observations on the mechanisms of bone destruction by squamous carcinomas of the head and neck: the role of host stroma. Br J Cancer 48:697–704

Urwin GH, Percival RC, Harris S, Beneton MNC, Williams JL, Kanis JA (1985) Generalised increase in bone resorption in carcinoma of the prostate. Br J Urol 57:721–723

2　Normal Bone Remodelling and Its Disruption in Metastatic Bone Disease

B.F. Boyce

Introduction

Bone is a metabolically active tissue which is continually being remodelled by a process involving the removal of microscopic packets of calcified matrix and their subsequent replacement at the same site by new bone. This normal physiological process can be disturbed by the direct local and/or the distant systemic effects of tumour cell products released by neoplastic cells. Recent research has indicated that many of the factors that may be involved in the regulation of bone remodelling and are produced by normal cells in the bone micro-environment can also be produced in excessive amounts by neoplastic cells. Thus metastatic malignant cells could directly interfere with the function of normal bone cells and so disrupt the bone micro-architecture.

In this chapter the process of bone remodelling will be outlined along with a review of our present understanding of the paracrine/autocrine controlling mechanisms involved. In addition, the local effects of neoplastic cells on bone cells. Thus, metastatic malignant cells could directly interfere with the function of tumours on normal skeletal activity.

Normal Bone Structure

Bone is composed of a collagenous matrix (predominantly type 1 collagen) which is laid down by osteoblasts in closely-packed parallel sheets or lamellae along with a variety of extracellular proteins, such as osteocalcin and growth factors, glycosaminoglycans, proteoglycans and lipids. The matrix is calcified by means of the deposition of hydroxyapatite crystals along the collagen fibres and as a result more than 99% of the body's calcium resides within bone.

There are two main types of bone: compact and cancellous. Compact or cortical bone is solid and composed of numerous microscopic cylindrical structures called haversian systems. These consist of a small central channel containing nutrient blood vessels and surrounded by concentric lamellae of collagen. Compact bone is a major constituent of long bones and of the outer shell of predominantly cancellous bones such as vertebral bodies. The haversian systems within cortical bone run parallel to the lines of stress and if there is an alteration in the direction of stress within a bone their orientation may be changed through remodelling.

Cancellous (spongy or trabecular) bone is composed of a network of interconnected plates or trabeculae surrounded by bone marrow (Fig. 2.1). Although this type of bone is much less dense than cortical bone it is still able to provide considerable structural support when present in normal amounts. As a result of its larger surface area and probably also because of its greater exposure to haemopoietic cells, cancellous bone is metabolically more active than compact bone. These differences are likely to account in part for the observation that metastatic deposits are encountered more frequently within cancellous than within cortical bone (Berrettoni and Carter 1986).

Normal Bone Modelling

Bone formation (or modelling) which begins in utero consists of two main types of ossification: endochondral and membranous. In endochondral bone formation, which gives rise to long bones, cartilage is laid down and calcified at epiphyseal plates. It is removed subsequently by chondroclasts and replaced in the metaphysis by bone matrix which is laid down as trabeculae and calcified by osteoblasts. The new bone formed at the metaphysis is soon removed by multinucleate osteoclasts as the long bone lengthens, leaving the medullary cavity of the larger long bones virtually free of trabecular bone. Simultaneously, new compact bone is laid down upon the periosteal bone surfaces of the growing bones to increase the thickness of the shafts while older bone is removed from the internal (endosteal) surface to increase the size of the medullary cavity.

Normal osteoclast function is an important aspect of this process. A primary abnormality in osteoclast function occurs in osteopetrosis (Mills et al. 1988) and results in the persistence of thick cortical bone which nevertheless is structurally weak and prone to fracture. Furthermore, the failure to remove bone from endosteal surfaces means that the medullary cavities remain narrow and of insufficient size to accommodate the volume of red bone marrow required to maintain normal haemopoiesis. Bone marrow transplantation, by providing effective osteoclast precursors, offers hope of a cure for this debilitating and often fatal condition (Fischer et al. 1986).

In contrast to endochondral bone formation, membranous ossification does not go through an intermediate cartilaginous stage. In this process, which gives rise for example to the flat bones of the skull and to the vetebral bodies, bone matrix is produced by osteoblasts that proliferate in ossification centres as spindle-shaped fibroblast-like cells. The matrix initially is highly cellular and has a woven (or basket weave) configuration. It is later removed by osteoclasts but subsequently is replaced by lamellar matrix to give rise to the bone trabeculae (or plates) that characterise the interior of vertebral bodies or to the compact bone of the vault of the skull.

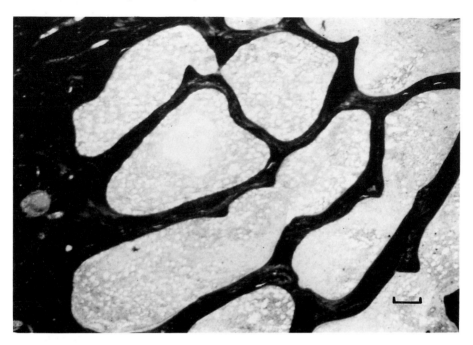

Fig. 2.1. Undecalcified section of iliac bone. Haversian canals can be seen as pale circular or oval shapes in the dense cortical bone on the left of the micrograph. In the normal young adult skeleton trabeculae are interconnected, as illustrated, and surrounded by bone marrow. With age, and particularly after the menopause, osteoclastic resorption through the full thickness of the plates destroys the connectivity and weakens the bone. 1% aqueous toluidine blue. The bar represents 320 μm.

The difference between membranous and endochondral ossification is manifested vividly in achondroplasia by the physical appearance of the circus dwarf. He typically has short limbs due to defective endochondral ossification but because membranous bone formation is unaffected has a normal size head and a trunk of near normal length. The process of membranous ossification will be touched upon later in this chapter when osteoblastic metastases are discussed.

Normal Bone Remodelling

Once formed, bones provide support for soft tissues and protection for vital organs. Like other supporting materials, such as metal in aircraft or asphalt on roads, bones suffer from fatigue damage due to wear and tear. Bone remodelling is the process which facilitates the removal of effete or damaged microscopic foci of bone on bone surfaces and their replacement by new bone matrix. It is generally considered to begin after bone growth or modelling has ceased and thus will begin at different times in different bones depending, for example, on when the various epiphyses close.

Three main bone cell types are involved: the osteoclast, a multinucleate cell of the mononuclear phagocyte lineage; the osteoblast, a mononuclear cell of the stromal cell series in marrow; and the osteocyte, a mononuclear cell of the osteoblast lineage that becomes incorporated within bone matrix during its synthesis (Owen 1980). The recent increase in our knowledge of the biology of osteoclasts and osteoblasts has led to a better understanding of the derangements that occur in bone in patients with neoplastic and metabolic bone disease.

Remodelling of Cortical Bone

Remodelling of cortical bone begins on the inner surface of the haversian canal. Osteoclasts tunnel into the bone, often along lines of stress, causing cylindrical defects behind the leading edge of resorption (the cutting cone) or may resorb through several pre-existing haversian systems. Sheets of osteoblasts appear behind the advancing front of osteoclasts on the bone surface and lay down concentric layers of new matrix to fill in the cylindrical defects. Some of the osteoblasts become incorporated within the matrix as osteocytes where they reside until their release during the next phase of resorption at that site.

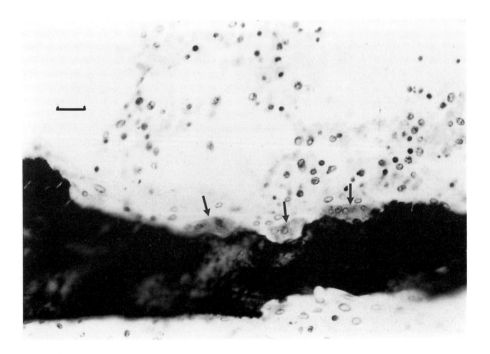

Fig. 2.2. Howship's resorption lacunae. A resorption lacuna is present on each side of the trabecula. Multinucleate osteoclasts (*arrow*) are resorbing the matrix in close association with mononuclear haemopoietic cells. 1% aqueous toluidine blue. The bar represents 20 µm.

Remodelling of Cancellous Bone

Remodelling of cancellous bone begins on the marrow surface of the trabecular plates which are covered by a layer of flattened cells (bone lining cells) that are probably in the osteoblast lineage. Osteoclasts resorb down into the bone to a mean depth of 60 μm (Eriksen 1986) and then dig a trench parallel to the bone surface (Fig. 2.2). A team of osteoblasts is attracted to these sites and they lay down osteoid matrix in the defect in thin parallel sheets or lamellae until the original contour of the bone surface is restored (Fig. 2.3). As in cortical bone, some of the osteoblasts become incorporated within the bone as osteocytes which communicate with one another by means of thin cytoplasmic processes (dendrites) that run within microscopic canaliculi (Fig. 2.4). One possible function of these cells is the detection of areas of microdamage to bone and communication of this information to bone lining cells on the bone surface.

The osteoblasts are also responsible for calcification of the osteoid and during this process they release large amounts of alkaline phosphatase. Calcification starts in the base of the resorption bay (Howship's lacuna) along the cement or reversal line and there is usually a delay of 10–15 days between the deposition of osteoid and the initiation of its mineralisation. Mineralisation of osteoid can be observed in undecalcified sections of bone stained with toluidine blue as a dark blue line (mineralisation front) at the interface between osteoid and calcified

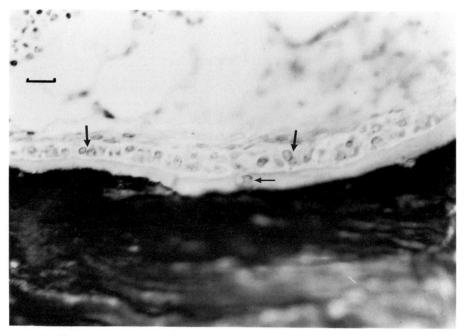

Fig. 2.3. New bone formation. Osteoblasts (*large arrows*) are present on the surface of a layer of newly synthesised osteoid (pale) as they fill in a resorption lacuna. During matrix synthesis the cells are plump and some become incorporated into the osteoid as osteocytes (*small arrow*). 1% aqueous toluidine blue. The bar represents 20 μm.

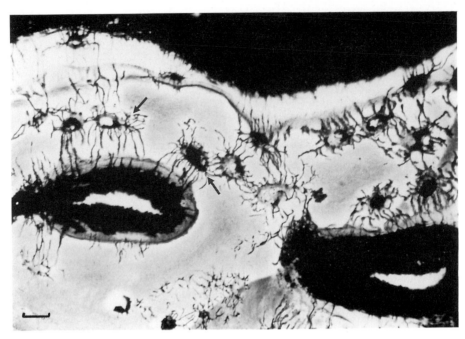

Fig. 2.4. Osteocytes within bone. The dendritic processes (*arrows*) of osteocytes can be seen communicating with one another in this decalcified section which has been prepared using the method of Tripp and McKay and counterstained with Van Geisen. The bar represents 12 µm.

bone (Fig. 2.5). Normally it is present on more than 60% of this interface and its extent is reduced in osteomalacia. Mineralisation can also be observed under fluorescent microscopy by means of the technique known as double tetracycline labelling (Frost 1969) and rates of mineralisation and of bone formation can be calculated using the techniques of histomorphometry (Boyce 1990).

Each remodelling site has been referred to as a basic multicellular unit (BMU) of bone turnover (Frost 1973) and it has been estimated that there are between one and two million of these along the bone surfaces of the normal adult skeleton. The total number of BMUs increases in conditions such as hyperparathyroidism, due to the osteoclast stimulating activity of parathyroid hormone, and leads to the increase in the extent of resorption and formation surfaces typical of osteitis fibrosa.

In bone remodelling units, resorption is always followed by formation rather than vice versa, a phenomenon that has been called "coupling" (Frost 1973). The process has many similarities to the system used to repair damaged sections of motorways which, of course, also undergo fatigue damage due to the wear and tear caused by traffic.

Many aspects of the remodelling process remain poorly understood. For example, it is not known what factors other than microdamage determine the sites on bone surfaces to which osteoclasts are attracted. The factors that determine the depth and length of resorption bays or that tell osteoblasts that they have synthesised enough matrix to fill in a Howship's lacuna are also unknown. However, it is likely that these processes are controlled locally by the

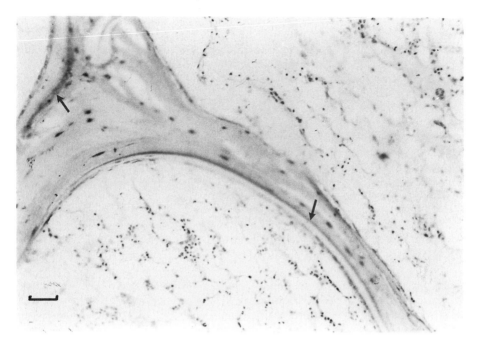

Fig. 2.5. Normal mineralisation fronts. Normal mineralisation fronts (*arrows*) are present as dark lines (*arrows*) at the interface between osteoid and calcified bone. 1% aqueous toluidine blue; 5% EDTA. The bar represents 50 μm.

generation of chemical signals. Study of the exaggerated effects of neoplastic cells on bone should lead to an increase in our understanding of the signalling mechanisms and of their roles in normal bone remodelling.

Regulation of Bone Remodelling

How Do Osteoclasts Resorb Bone?

The osteoclast is a highly specialised cell with complex functions for the removal of the organic (matrix) and inorganic (mineral) components of bone. It is formed from a precursor cell which is probably in the mononuclear phagocyte lineage (Nijweide et al. 1986) by means of cytoplasmic fusion of committed mononuclear cells to give rise to the typical multinucleate appearance. In remodelling sites in normal subjects the cells typically have 2–6 nuclei. However, this number may increase dramatically in conditions such as hyperparathyroidism, Paget's disease or malignancy where there is a greater than normal stimulus to their formation.

Once formed, the osteoclast binds to the bone surface by means of specialised cytoplasmic extensions which have a characteristic villus-like ruffled border. Here the cell secretes the proteases (Delaisse et al. 1987) necessary for the removal of the organic matrix and generates H^+ ions through the action of carbonic anhydrase (Gay et al. 1984) and a proton pump (Baron et al. 1986) for the dissolution of the hydroxyapatite crystals. A sealing zone is formed around the periphery of these cytoplasmic extensions for the maintenance of the acidic environment and for the protection of adjacent cells. Thus, both matrix and mineral are removed simultaneously.

Recent studies of osteoclasts isolated from bone have shown that they are able to form resorption pits in slices of mineralised bone (Chambers 1980, 1985). However, they do not appear to be able to initiate resorption on the surface of normal bone because of the presence of a thin layer of unmineralised matrix that covers the mineralised bone (Chambers and Fuller 1985) and is situated beneath the bone-lining cells (Fig. 2.6). As will be seen below these bone-lining osteoblasts are thought to play a major role in the process of bone resorption.

Factors Which Stimulate Bone Resorption: Osteoblasts Play a Paracrine Role

Many factors are known to stimulate bone resorption in vitro (Table 2.1). Some of these, e.g., parathyroid hormone (PTH) act systemically, but nevertheless may stimulate the production locally of another bone resorbing substance e.g., granulocyte – monocyte colony-stimulating factor (GM-CSF) (Horowitz et al. 1989a) or interleukin-6 (Feyen et al. 1989). Many of the others such as the

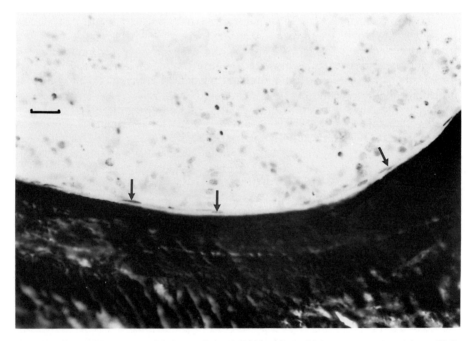

Fig. 2.6. Bone lining cells. A thin layer of uncalcified matrix (pale) is present on the surface of fully mineralised matrix (dark) which is covered by a layer of flattened bone lining cells (*arrow*). 1% aqueous toluidine blue. The bar represents 20 μm.

Table 2.1. Agents known to stimulate bone resorption in vitro

Systemic factors	Local factors
Parathyroid hormone (PTH)	Interleukin-1 (IL-1)
1,25(OH)$_2$ vitamin D$_3$	Tumour necrosis factor α (TNFα)
Thyroid hormone	Tumour necrosis factor β (lymphotoxin) (TNFβ)
Corticosteroids	Transforming growth factors
Parathyroid hormone-related protein (PTH-rP)	α and β (TGFα, TGFβ)
	Epidermal growth factor (EGF)
	Platelet-derived growth factor (PDGF)
	Prostaglandins (PGS)
	Oxygen-derived free radicals (ODFR)
	Colony stimulating factors (GM-CSF)

cytokines (interleukin-1 (IL-1) and tumour-necrosis factor (TNF)) and the growth factors are likely to act predominantly as local stimulators of resorption (Tashjian et al. 1982, 1985, 1987; Gowen et al. 1983; Ibbotson et al. 1986; Boyce et al. 1989) although systemic administration of some can cause hypercalcaemia and bone resorption (Tashjian et al. 1986; Garrett et al. 1987; Sabatini et al. 1988).

Surprisingly, none of these factors appears to act directly on osteoclasts. The receptors for them are expressed on osteoblasts rather than osteoclasts and it is now widely believed that osteoblasts control bone resorption by their effects on osteoclasts. This regulatory role for osteoblasts was postulated more than 10 years ago (Martin et al. 1979; Chambers 1980; Rodan and Martin 1981) and the elegant studies of Chambers and his co-workers since then have supported the hypothesis.

In vitro studies of isolated avian or mammalian osteoclasts have shown that the activity of these cells is not stimulated when they are exposed to any of the known osteoclast stimulating factors alone (Chambers et al. 1985). Indeed prostaglandins have a direct transient (1–2 h) inhibitory effect on osteoclast motility (Chambers and Ali 1983) unlike the prolonged inhibitory effect of calcitonin. However, osteoclast activity is increased when the cells are exposed to known osteoclast-stimulating factors in the presence of osteoblasts (Thompson et al. 1986, 1987) either through direct cell–cell contact (Chambers 1982) or through the local release of an osteoblast-derived osteoclast-stimulating factor (McSheehy and Chambers 1986, 1987). The existence of a diffusible factor is supported by the observation that separation of osteoclasts and osteoblasts by a semi-permeable membrane does not prevent osteoclast activation. Furthermore, the conditioned medium of osteoblasts that have been exposed to known osteoclast activating factors can stimulate osteoclasts in the absence of osteoblasts. To date, attempts to purify this factor have been unsuccessful.

In addition to these effects on osteoclasts, the osteoblast appears to have other complex functions that are involved in the initiation of bone resorption. As stated earlier, quiescent bone surfaces appear to be covered by a thin layer of uncalcified matrix and this in turn is covered by the extensive cytoplasm of bone lining cells. It has been proposed that these two layers form an effective barrier to bone resorption by osteoclasts (Chambers and Fuller 1985) and that their removal is essential for bone resorption to be initiated.

Rodent osteoblasts have been shown to secrete metalloproteinases and latent collagenase which can degrade the bone matrix (Sakamoto and Sakamoto 1986). Collagenase can be activated by the simultaneous release by osteoblasts of tissue plasminogen activator whose production can be stimulated by many of the agents that stimulate bone resorption (Hamilton et al. 1985). Furthermore, osteoblasts can produce tissue inhibitors of collagenase and other metalloproteinases (Cawston et al. 1981; Heath et al. 1984; Partridge et al. 1987). Thus, it appears that osteoblasts may exercise a considerable degree of fine control over the stimulation or inhibition of bone resorption.

In addition to the removal of the collagenous covering on bone surfaces, contraction of the bone-lining cell cytoplasm has to take place to allow resorption to proceed. This could be mediated by prostaglandin (Shen et al. 1986) either as a result of mechanical stress or as a consequence of the local release of factors such as IL-1 or TNF whose bone resorbing activity is mediated, in part at least, by prostaglandins (Tashjian et al. 1987; Boyce et al. 1989).

Growth Factors Within Bone may Play a Role in Bone Remodelling

In addition to the removal of bone matrix and mineral, osteoclasts release non-collagenous proteins from bone during resorption. These include transforming growth factor β(TGFβ), insulin-like growth factor-1(IGF-1), skeletal growth factor (SGF; IGF-II) and platelet-derived growth factor (PDGF). These factors can stimulate DNA synthesis and replication of osteoblasts (Canalis 1980, 1986, 1987; Centrella et al. 1986, 1987; Pfeilschifter et al. 1987) and thus may have a regulatory role in the proliferation of osteoblasts at sites of bone resorption (for reviews see Hauschka et al. 1986 and Canalis et al. 1988).

Bone matrix and platelets are the most abundant sources of TGFβ and PDGF in the body. Thus, it is possible that these factors have a stimulatory effect on the rapid bone formation that occurs during fracture repair. In most circumstances TGFβ exists in a latent form as an inactive large-molecular-weight complex with its binding protein. Recent studies have shown that osteoblasts produce TGFβ (Gehron-Robey et al. 1987) and that organ cultures of bone release TGFβ in inactive form (Pfeilschifter et al. 1990). The inactive TGFβ can be activated by acid (Pfeilschifter et al. 1990) and by isolated osteoclasts (Oreffo et al. 1989). This has led to speculation that activation of TGFβ may take place in the acidic environment under the ruffled border of the osteoclast during bone resorption. Release of activated TGFβ and other growth factors at resorption sites could thus account for a local proliferative effect on osteoblast precursors and, at least in part, explain the attraction of osteoblasts to sites of bone resorption.

Activated TGFβ has been shown to inhibit bone resorption (Pfeilschifter et al. 1988) and to inhibit the activity of isolated osteoclasts (Oreffo et al. 1990). Thus it may be that this protein not only stimulates osteoblasts at sites of bone remodelling but also plays a role in limiting the amount of resorption carried out by individual osteoclasts.

Osteoblasts May Have an Autocrine Role in Bone Remodelling

Osteoblasts not only respond to most of the growth factors/cytokines by producing a local osteoclast stimulating factor they also produce many of them

(Centrella and Canalis 1985, 1987; Heldin et al. 1986; Wergedal et al. 1986, Gehron-Robey et al. 1987). This has led to speculation that, once stimulated by an osteotropic factor, osteoblasts may promote the coupling of formation to resorption by secreting factors such as IL-1, IGF-I, SGF, TGFβ or PDGF that stimulate their own proliferation and activity (Wergedal et al. 1990). In vitro studies have indicated that these agents can stimulate proliferation of osteoblasts and increase collagen, alkaline phosphatase and osteocalcin production, indices of activity of differentiated osteoblasts. (For reviews see Hauschka et al. 1986 and Canalis et al. 1988).

The availability of many of these factors as recombinant or highly purified molecules has led to the design of studies to examine their local effects on bone in vivo. Thus the injection of IL-1 into the subcutaneous tissues overlying the calvariae of normal mice has been shown to cause increased bone resorption locally, which is followed by increased new bone formation at the sites of resorption (Boyce et al. 1989). Furthermore, this local injection model was used subsequently to show that TGFβ can cause increased new bone formation in the calvariae of neonatal rats (Noda and Camilliere 1989). Since the effects of IL-1 on bone formation were observed after its administration had been stopped, it is likely that the increased new bone formation was maintained by the local production of IL-1 or other factors by osteoblasts or by other cells in the bone micro-environment. Thus, studies to date support a local role for growth factors to increase bone resorption and/or formation in conditions where they may be produced locally in large concentrations.

Macrophages May Also Be Involved in Bone Remodelling

The complex events that occur during bone remodelling are likely to involve cells other than osteoblasts and osteoclasts. Macrophages in particular can produce many of the factors known to stimulate bone resorption and some that can also stimulate bone formation (Table 2.2) (Nathan 1987). Although conclusive proof is awaited, one popular belief is that macrophages are present in Howship's lacunae where they may play a role in the final phase of resorption, perhaps by smoothing out the resorbed surface in preparation for matrix synthesis by osteoblasts (Baron et al. 1983; Eriksen 1986). Since macrophages can release osteoblast-stimulating factors it is possible that they also function as modulators of osteoblastic activity. As will be seen later, it is possible that macrophages associated with metastatic tumour deposits (McBride 1986) may be responsible for mediating the bone loss or perhaps the increased bone formation seen in affected bones.

Effects of Tumours on Bone

Metastatic Tumour Deposits; Most Cause Osteolysis

Bone is a common metastatic site for many epithelial (carcinomas) and some mesenchymal (sarcomas) tumours (Fig. 2.7). The reasons for the preferential metastasis to bone marrow in comparison, for example, to the kidneys which

Table 2.2.   Factors which stimulate indices of bone formation in vitro

Transforming growth factor β (TGFβ)
Insulin-like growth factor I (IGF-I)
Fibroblast growth factors (FGF acidic and basic)
Bone morphogenetic protein (BMP)
Platelet-derived growth factor (PDGF)
Skeletal growth factor (SGF, IGF-II)
Bone-derived growth factor (BDGF, β$_2$ microglobulin)
Prostaglandins (PGS)
Interleukin-1 (IL-1)
Tumour necrosis factor α (TNFα)
Tumour necrosis factor β (Lymphotoxin)
Macrophage-derived growth factor (MDGF)

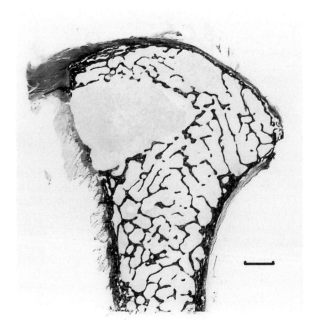

Fig. 2.7.   Osteolytic metastases. Two osteolytic deposits of tumour are present near the top of the iliac crest. At these sites the bone trabeculae have been destroyed completely by tumour-mediated osteoclastic resorption. 1% aqueous toluidine blue. The bar represents 2 mm.

receive 25% of the cardiac output are not entirely understood. It is likely that the sinusoidal system within marrow is more conducive to the establishment of metastatic deposits than is a simple arterial-venous capillary bed. This could also explain the ready growth of metastases in the liver. Interestingly the spleen, which also has a sinusoidal system, is an infrequent site of growth of metastases. Here, however, the enviroment for malignant cells may be more hostile since one function of this organ is the destruction of cells such as effete red blood cells.

There is abundant evidence that stromal cells within bone marrow (Metcalf 1986) and indeed osteoblasts (Felix et al. 1988; Horowitz et al. 1989b) secrete growth factors for haemopoietic cells. Recent studies have indicated that stromal cells can also secrete a factor which promotes the proliferation of prostatic cancer cells in vitro (Chackal-Roy et al. 1989). Thus, it is possible that the growth of metastases in marrow is actually promoted by some of the resident cells.

Do Malignant Cells Resorb Bone?

In osteolytic metastases malignant cells can often be seen in resorption bays on bone surfaces. This led to speculation that the neoplastic cells were directly responsible for the bone resorption at these sites. The suggestion was supported by the observation that human breast cancer cells appeared to be able to resorb bone particles directly in vitro (Eilon and Mundy 1978). However, it is now generally considered that tumour-associated osteolysis is carried out by osteoclasts and that the effects of malignant cells are indirect (Mundy 1988). The mere presence of malignant cells within a resorption site on a bone surface need not imply that these cells removed the bone matrix any more than the presence of children playing with shovels in a trench in a road would indicate that the children had dug the hole rather than workmen.

Numerous studies have demonstrated that malignant cells secrete many of the factors known to stimulate the proliferation and activity (indirectly) of osteoclasts (for review see Mundy (1988)). These include prostaglandins, cytokines and growth factors such as epidermal growth factor (EGF), transforming growth factors α and β and PDGF. Their local release in bone marrow by metastatic deposits is likely to account for the increased numbers of osteoclasts that are responsible for the osteolysis (Fig. 2.8). Recently, squamous carcinoma cells have been shown to produce IL-1 (Sato et al. 1988), the most powerful known stimulator of bone resorption in vitro. Interestingly, many of these factors such as EGF, TGFα, TGFβ, PDGF, TNF and IL-1 appear to have their bone resorbing effects mediated at least in part through prostaglandins (Tashjian et al. 1982, 1985, 1986, 1987; Boyce et al. 1989). Disappointingly, however, inhibitors of prostaglandin synthesis, such as indomethacin, only rarely suppress bone resorption in malignancy (Brenner et al. 1982).

Are Tumour-Associated Immune Cells Involved in Bone Resorption?

Malignant cells could also stimulate bone resorption by producing a factor(s) that stimulates tumour-associated immune cells to release osteoclast-activating factors. Macrophages can account for up to 20%–30% of the cells in a mass of tumour (McBride 1986) and, as was stated earlier, can produce osteoclast and osteoblast-stimulating factors. Recent preliminary findings indicate that human melanoma cells produce a factor which stimulates macrophages to release increased amounts of TNF and IL-1 in vitro (Sabatini et al. 1989). The increased TNF and IL-1 production by non-tumour cells could account in part for the

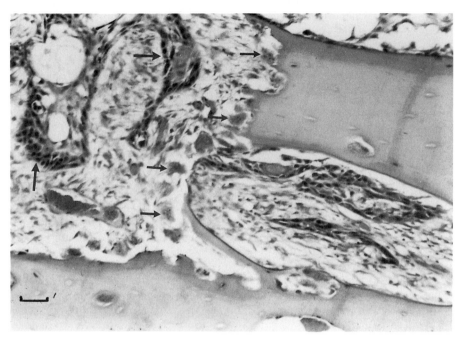

Fig. 2.8. Tumour-mediated bone resorption. Numerous multinucleated osteoclasts (*small arrows*) are resorbing bone adjacent to a deposit of secondary squamous carcinoma (*large arrows*). Haematoxylin and eosin, decalcified section. The bar represents 50 μm.

hypercalcaemia, increased bone resorption and cachexia seen in malignancy. Studies to purify the cytokine-releasing factor from the melanoma cell conditioned medium have shown that it is granulocyte – monocyte colony-stimulating factor (GM-CSF) (Sabatini et al. 1990), an agent that also stimulates bone resorption by promoting the proliferation of osteoclast precursors.

Osteosclerosis

Prostatic cancer accounts for the majority of osteosclerotic metastatic tumour deposits in men, but this effect is not invariable. Some prostatic cancers can cause osteolysis while others have a dimorphic effect causing both osteolysis and osteosclerosis. A similar picture can be seen with some breast and lung cancers.

Recent studies have indicated that prostatic cancer cells can produce osteoblast stimulating factors in culture (Jacobs et al. 1979) and that the mRNA extracted from the tumour cells codes for a factor with osteoblast stimulating activity (Simpson et al. 1985). Furthermore, cell extracts from malignant, hyperplastic and normal post-pubertal but not normal pre-pubertal prostate glands produce osteoblast stimulating activity in vitro (Koutsilieris et al. 1987). These observations led the authors to suggest that the production of osteoblast stimulating factors by post-pubertal prostate might account in part for the larger bones in men than in women.

The increased bone mass in metastatic deposits appears to be produced by mechanisms independent of the remodelling process, i.e., the bone formation is not preceded by bone resorption (Valentin Opran et al. 1980). New bone is formed predominantly by two mechanisms: the production of new matrix on the surface of existing trabeculae, presumably by direct stimulation of the bone-lining cells to start producing matrix again; and the production of new bone within the marrow cavity between existing trabeculae by means of membranous ossification. Both forms of new bone formation are seen typically in metastatic deposits (Fig. 2.9).

The osteoblast stimulating factor(s) produced by prostatic cancer cells have yet to be purified to homogeneity and sequenced (Koutsilieris et al. 1987). However, growth factors with osteoblast stimulating activity such as TGFβ and PDGF have been purified from some malignant tumours. Their actions appear to be localised to the metastatic sites and indeed the bone adjacent to them may be osteopenic as a result of age-related bone loss. Despite this localised effect there is hope that identification and purification of osteoblast stimulating factors from tumours may allow their production for therapeutic use in osteoporosis, particularly if they can be targeted to bone.

Osteosclerosis is also seen in myelofibrosis, in which there is proliferation of both haemopoietic and stromal cells which suggests that the proliferating marrow cells can produce osteoblast stimulating activity.

The breast cancer cell line MCF7 produces TGFβ which can stimulate osteoblasts to increase their production of collagen, osteocalcin and alkaline

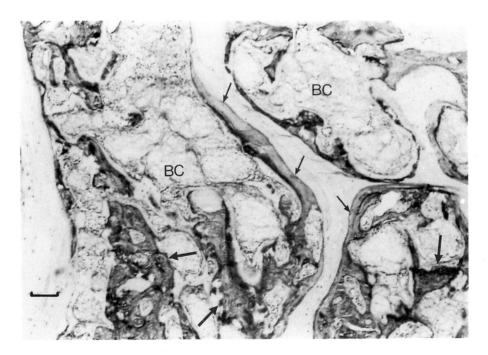

Fig. 2.9. Osteoblastic metastasis. Metastatic breast carcinoma (BC) is present within the bone marrow cavity and is stimulating the formation of new bone (dark staining; *small arrows*) on the surface of pale-staining existing trabeculae and de novo within the medullary cavity (*large arrows*). 1% aqueous toluidine blue; 5% EDTA. The bar represents 125 μm.

phosphatase in vitro. As mentioned earlier, TGFβ has been shown to stimulate the local production of new bone formation when injected over the calvariae of neonatal rats. Thus, the osteosclerosis seen in association with some metastatic breast cancer deposits could be due in part at least to the local release of TGFβ.

Effects of Some Specific Tumour Cell Types in Bone

Breast Cancer

Breast cancer is one of the most common examples of osteolytic metastatic disease. Several human breast cancer cell lines, including MCF7, have been shown to secrete a number of osteotropic factors that could account for the increased bone destruction around tumour deposits. These include TGFα, TGFβ, EGF, parathyroid hormone-related protein (PTH-rP) and prostaglandins (Travers et al. 1988). More recently, studies have indicated that another breast cancer cell product, procathepsin D, may also have osteoclast stimulating effects (Wo et al. 1990). The normally lysosomal enzyme is secreted in large quantities by MCF7 cells (Cavailles et al. 1989) under the regulatory control of oestrogens. Its active form stimulates bone resorption in vitro and is associated with the proteolysis of collagen chains and with the activation of TGFβ. Procathepsin D is taken up by osteoclasts through receptor-mediated endocytosis and thus may play a major role in the local stimulation of bone resorption around metastatic breast cancer deposits.

Haematological Malignancies

Detailed consideration of the effects of leukaemias and lymphomas on bone is beyond the scope of this book on metastatic bone disease. However, the effects of haematological malignancies are worthy of brief mention since study of these is likely to increase our understanding of normal bone cell function. Recent studies have indicated that much of the osteoclast stimulating activity of myeloma cells resides in lymphotoxin (TNFβ) (Garrett et al. 1987), a product of

Table 2.3.   Agents produced by macrophages and their effects on bone

Increased bone resorption	Increased bone formation
IL-1	IL-1
TNF	TNF
TGFβ	TGFβ
PDGF	PDGF
Prostaglandins	Prostaglandins
1,25(OH)$_2$ Vitamin D$_3$	Macrophage-derived growth factor
GM-CSF	
Oxygen-derived free radicals	

B lymphocytes. The in vitro bone-resorbing effects of lymphotoxin are equipotent with TNFα (cachexin), the agent responsible for the cachexia associated with malignancy and severe illness. Recent preliminary data have suggested that myeloma cells may also produce IL-1 and IL-6. Thus a number of cytokines released by myeloma cells could be responsible for the characteristic localised osteolytic defects.

Deposits of malignant lymphoma in bone rarely lead to radiologically identifiable osteolytic defects. However, localised bone resorption is often seen microscopically on bone surfaces adjacent to deposits of non-Hodgkin lymphomas in bone marrow, which suggests that neoplastic lymphoid cells as well as plasma cells may be able to elaborate osteoclast stimulating factors.

Osteoblastic stimulation is seen most frequently in myelofibrosis and other myelodysplasias. Here, it is likely that the proliferating haemopoietic cells secrete a factor(s) responsible for the marrow fibrosis and for osteoblast stimulation. Typically new bone is laid down on the surface of existing trabeculae in myelofibrosis without previous bone resorption. Interestingly, some cases of myeloma have been associated with osteosclerosis at affected sites (Blaguiere et al. 1982). However, the factors responsible for this effect have not yet been identified.

Summary

Bone is a metabolically dynamic tissue which continually renews itself by the process of bone remodelling, whereby osteoclasts remove discrete microscopic packets of bone from bone surfaces and osteoblasts fill in the defects by laying down new bone matrix. Our understanding of bone cell biology has advanced rapidly in recent years, in part due to study of the effects on bone of malignant cells and their secretory products. Because malignant cells can produce excessive quantities of agents that may be produced at low concentration locally by normal cells, it has been possible to purify many of the factors that are likely to be involved in the control of normal bone remodelling. The subsequent application of the techniques of molecular biology to produce large quantities of many of these factors as recombinant molecules has facilitated the widespread use of these agents in both in vitro and in vivo studies.

Thus, we now have convincing evidence that metastatic tumour deposits cause bone resorption by the local release of cytokines and growth factors to stimulate osteoclastic bone resorption. Osteosclerosis results from the local release by malignant cells of osteoblast stimulating factors which are not yet as well characterised as osteoclast stimulating factors. There is also persuasive evidence that the normal control of bone remodelling is mediated through the osteoblast rather than the osteoclast since the former rather than the latter cells have the cell surface receptors for most of the known osteotropic factors and respond to them.

Many questions concerning the control of normal bone turnover remain unanswered. The study of the effects of malignant cells and their cell products is likely to continue to yield new insights into our understanding of bone cell biology and to answer many of these questions.

References

Baron R, Vignery A, Horowitz M (1983) Lymphocytes, macrophages and the regulation of bone remodelling. In: Peck WA (ed) Bone and mineral research, Annual 2. Elsevier, New York, pp 175–246

Baron R, Neff L, Roy C, Boivert A, Caplan M (1986) Evidence of a high and specific concentration of (Na^+, K^+)ATPase in the plasma membrane of the osteoclast. Cell 46:311–316

Berrettoni BA, Carter JR (1986) Mechanisms of cancer metastasis to bone. J Bone Joint Surg [Am] 68:308–312

Blaguiere RM, Guyer DM, Buchanan RB, Gallagher PJ (1982) Sclerotic bone deposits in myeloma. Br J Radiol 55:591–593

Boyce BF (1990) Bone biopsy and histomorphometry in metabolic bone disease. In: Stevenson JC (ed) New techniques in metabolic bone disease. Wright, London, pp 110–131

Boyce BF, Aufdemorte TB, Garrett IR, Yates AJP, Mundy GR (1989) Effects of interleukin-1 on bone turnover in normal mice. Endocrinology 125:1142–1150

Brenner DE, Harvey HA, Lipton A, Demers L (1982) A study of prostaglandin E_2, parathormone and response to indomethacin in patients with hypercalcemia of malignancy. Cancer 49:556–561

Canalis E (1980) Effect of insulin-like growth factor I on DNA and protein synthesis in cultured rat calvaria. J Clin Invest 66:709–719

Canalis E (1986) Interleukin-1 has independent effects on DNA and collagen synthesis in culture of rat calvariae. Endocrinology 118:74–81

Canalis E (1987) Effects of tumor necrosis factor on bone formation in vitro. Endocrinology 121:1596–1604

Canalis E, McCarthy T, Centrella M (1988) Growth factors and the regulation of bone remodelling. J Clin Invest 81:277–281

Cavailles V, Garcia M, Rochefort H (1989) Regulation of cathepsin D and P52 gene expression by growth factors in MCF-7 human breast cancer cells. Mol Endocrinol 3:552–558

Cawston TE, Galloway WA, Mercer A, Murphy G, Reynolds JJ (1981) Purification of rabbit bone inhibitor of collagenase. Biochem J 195:159–165

Centrella M, Canalis E (1985) Transforming and non-transforming growth factors are present in medium conditioned by fetal rat calvariae. Proc Natl Acad Sci USA 82:7335–7339

Centrella M, Canalis A (1987) Isolation of EGF-dependent transforming growth factor (TGF-β-like) activity from culture medium conditioned by fetal rat calvariae. J Bone Mineral Res 2:29–36

Centrella M, Massagué J, Canalis E (1986) Human platelet-derived transforming growth factor-β stimulates parameters of bone growth in fetal rat calvariae. Endocrinology 119:2306–2312

Centrella M, McCarthy T, Canalis E (1987) Transforming growth factor β is a bifunctional regulator of replication and collagen synthesis in osteoblast enriched cell cultures from fetal rat bone. J Biol Chem 262:2869–2874

Chackal-Roy M, Niemeyer C, Moore M, Zetter BR (1989) Stimulation of human prostatic carcinoma cell growth by factors present in human bone marrow. J Clin Invest 84:43–50

Chambers TJ (1980) The cellular basis of bone resorption. Clin Orthop Rel Res 151:283–293

Chambers TJ (1982) Osteoblasts release osteoclasts from calcitonin-induced quiescence. J Cell Sci 57:247–260

Chambers TJ (1985) The pathobiology of the osteoclast. J Clin Pathol 38:241–252

Chambers TJ, Ali N (1983) Inhibition of osteoclastic motility by prostaglandins I_2, E_1, E_2 and 6-oxo-E_1. J Pathol 139:383–397

Chambers TJ, Fuller K (1985) Bone cells predispose endosteal surfaces to resorption by exposure of bone mineral to osteoclastic contact. J Cell Sci 76:155–163

Chambers TJ, McSheehy PMJ, Thomson BM, Fuller K (1985) The effect of calcium-regulating hormones and prostaglandins on bone resorption by osteoclasts disaggregated from neonatal rabbit bones. Endocrinology 116:234–239

Delaisse JM, Boyde A, McConnachie E et al. (1987) The effects of inhibitors of cysteine-proteinases and collagenase on the resorptive activity of isolated osteoclasts. Bone 8:305–313

Eilon G, Mundy GR (1978) Direct resorption of bone by human breast cancer cells in vitro. Nature 276:726–728

Eriksen EF (1986) Normal and pathological remodelling of human trabecular bone: Three dimensional reconstruction of the remodelling sequence in normals and in metabolic bone disease. Endocr Rev 7:379–408

Felix R, Elford PR, Stoercklé C et al. (1988) Production of haemopoietic growth factors by bone tissue and bone cells in culture. J Bone Mineral Res 3:27–36

Feyen JHM, Elford P, Di Padova FE, Trechsel U (1989) Interleukin-6 is produced by bone and modulated by parathyroid hormone. J Bone Miner Res 4:633–638

Fischer A, Giscelli C, Friedrich W et al. (1986) Bone marrow transplantation for immunodeficiencies and osteopetrosis: European survey (1968–85). Lancet ii:1080–1084

Frost HM (1969) Tetracycline-based histological analysis of bone remodelling. Calcif Tissue Res 3:211–237

Frost HM (1973) The origin and nature of transients in human bone remodelling dynamics. In: Frame B, Parfitt AM, Duncan H (eds) Clinical aspects of metabolic bone disease. Excerpta Medica; Amsterdam, pp 124–137

Garrett IR, Durie BGM, Nedwin GE et al. (1987) Production of lymphotoxin, a bone-resorbing cytokine, by cultured human myeloma cells. N Engl J Med 317:526–532

Gay CV, Ito MB, Schraer H (1984) Carbonic anhydrase activity in isolated osteoclasts. Metab Bone Dis Relat Res 5:33–39

Gehron-Robey PG, Young MF, Flanders KC et al. (1987) Osteoblasts synthesize and respond to transforming growth factor-type β(TGF-β) in vitro. J Cell Biol 105:457–463

Gowen M, Wood DD, Ihrie EJ, McGuire NKB, Russell RGG (1983) An interleukin-I-like factor stimulates bone resorption in vitro. Nature 306:378–380

Hamilton JA, Lingelbach SR, Partridge NC, Martin TJ (1985) Regulation of plasminogen activator production by bone-resorbing hormones in normal and malignant osteoblasts. Endocrinology 116:2186–2191

Hauschka PV, Maurakos AE, Lafrati MD, Doleman SE, Klagsbrun M (1986) Growth factors in bone matrix. J Biol Chem 261:12665–12674

Heath JK, Atkinson SJ, Meikle MC, Reynolds JJ (1984) Mouse osteoblasts synthesize collagenase in response to bone resorbing agents. Biochim Biophys Acta 802:151–154

Heldin C-H, Johnsson A, Wennergren S, Wernstedt C, Bedsholtz C, Westermark B (1986) A human osteosarcoma cell line secretes a growth factor structurally related to a homodimer of PDGF A-chains. Nature 319:511–514

Horowitz MC, Coleman DL, Flood PM, Kupper TS, Jilka RS (1989a) Parathyroid hormone and lipopolysaccharide induce murine osteoblast-like cells to secrete a cytokine indistinguishable from granulocyte-macrophage colony-stimulating factor. J Clin Invest 83:149–157

Horowitz MC, Coleman DL, Ryaby JT, Einhorn TA (1989b) Osteotropic agents induce the differential secretion of granulocyte-macrophage colony-stimulating factor by the osteoblast cell line MC3T3-El. J Bone Miner Res 4:911–921

Ibbotson KJ, Harrod J, Gowen M et al. (1986) Human recombinant transforming growth factor alpha stimulates bone resorption and inhibits formation in vitro. Proc Natl Acad Sci USA 83:2228–2232

Jacobs SC, Pikna D, Lawson RK (1979) Prostatic osteoblastic factor. Invest Urol 17:195–198

Koutsilieris M, Rabbini SA, Bennett HPJ, Goltzman D (1987) Characteristics of prostate-derived growth factors for cells of the osteoblast phenotype. J Clin Invest 80:941–946

Martin TJ, Partridge NC, Greaves M, Atkins D, Ibbotson KJ (1979) Prostaglandin effects on bone and role in cancer hypercalcaemia. In: MacIntyre I, Szelke M (eds) Molecular Endocrinology Elsevier, North-Holland, Amsterdam, pp 251–264

McBride WH (1986) Phenotype and functions of intratumoral macrophages. Biochim Biophys Acta 865:27–41

McSheehy PMJ, Chambers TJ (1986) Osteoblast-like cells in the presence of parathyroid hormone release soluble factors that stimulate osteoclastic bone resorption. Endocrinology 119:1654–1659

McSheehy PMJ, Chambers TJ (1987) 1,25-dihydroxy vitamin D3 stimulates rat osteoblastic cells to release a soluble factor that increases osteoclastic bone resorption. J Clin Invest 80:425–429

Metcalf D (1986) The molecular biology and functions of the granulocyte-macrophage colony-stimulating factors. Blood 67:257–267

Mills BG, Yabe H, Singer FR (1988) Osteoclasts in human osteopetrosis contain viral-nucleocapsid-like nuclear inclusions. J Bone Miner Res 3:101–106

Mundy GR (1988) Hypercalcemia of malignancy revisited. J Clin Invest 82:1–6

Nathan CF (1987) Secretory products of macrophages J Clin Invest 79:319–326

Nijweide PJ, Burger EH, Feyen JM (1986) Cells of bone: proliferation, differentiation and hormonal regulation. Physiol Rev 66:855–886

Noda M, Camilliere JJ (1989) In vivo stimulation of bone formation by transforming growth factor-β. Endocrinology 124:2991–2994

Oreffo ROC, Mundy GR, Seyedin SM, Bonewald LF (1989) Activation of the bone-derived TGFβ complex by isolated osteoclasts. Biochem Biophys Res Commun 158:817–823

Oreffo ROC, Bonewald L, Kukita A et al. (1990) Inhibitory effects of the bone-derived growth factors, osteoinductive factors and TGFβ on isolated osteoclasts. Endocrinology 126:3067–3075

Owen M (1980) The origin of bone cells in the postnatal organism. Arthritis Rheum 23:1073–1080

Partridge NC, Jeffrey JJ, Ehlick LS et al. (1987) Hormonal regulation of the production of collagenase and a collagenase inhibitor activity by rat osteogenic sarcoma cells. Endocrinology 120:1956–1962

Pfeilschifter J, D'Souza SM, Mundy GR (1987) Effects of transforming growth factor-β on osteoblastic osteosarcoma cells. Endocrinology 121:212–218

Pfeilschifter JP, Seyedin SM, Mundy GR (1988) Transforming growth factor beta inhibits bone resorption in fetal rat long bone cultures. J Clin Invest 82:680–685

Pfeilschifter J, Bonewald L, Mundy GR (1990) Characterization of the latent transforming growth factor β complex in bone. J Bone Miner Res 5:49–58

Rodan GA Martin TJ (1981) Role of osteoblasts in hormonal control of bone resorption – a hypothesis. Calcif Tissue Int 33:349–351

Sabatini M, Boyce B, Aufdemorte T, Bonewald L, Mundy G (1988) Infusions of recombinant human interleukins 1-α and 1-β cause hypercalcemia in normal mice. Proc Natl Acad Sci USA 85:5235–5239

Sabatini M, Bonewald L, Chavez J, Mundy GR (1989) Production of GM-CSF by a human tumour associated with leukocytosis and hypercalcemia induces cytokine production by host cells. J Bone Miner Res [Suppl 1] 4:S155 (abstr)

Sabatini M, Chavez J, Mundy GR, Bonewald LF (1990) Stimulation of tumour necrosis factor release from monocytic cells by the A375 human melanoma via granulocyte-macrophage colony stimulating factor. Cancer Res 50:2673–2678

Sakamoto S, Sakamoto M (1986) Bone collagenase, osteoblasts and cell-mediated bone resorption. In: Peck WA (Ed) Bone and mineral research vol 4 Elsevier, Amsterdam, pp 49–102

Sato K, Fujii Y, Kasano K, Tsushima T, Shizume K (1988) Production of interleukin-1 alpha and a parathyroid hormone-like factor by a squamous cell carcinoma of oesophagus (EC-G1) derived from a patient with hypercalcemia. J Clin Endocrinol Metab 67:592–621

Shen V, Rifas L, Kohler G, Peck WA (1986) Prostaglandins change cell shape and increase intercellular gap junctions in osteoblasts cultured from rat fetal calvaria. J Bone Miner Res 1:243–249

Simpson E, Harrod J, Eilan G et al. (1985) Identification of a messenger ribonucleic acid fraction in human prostatic cancer cells coding for a novel osteoblast-stimulating factor. Endocrinology 117:1615–1620

Tashjian Jr AH, Hohmann EL, Antonaides HN et al. (1982) Platelet-derived growth factor stimulates bone resorption via a prostaglandin-mediated mechanism. Endocrinology 111: 118–124

Tashjian Jr AH, Voelkel EF, Lazzaro M et al. (1985) α and β transforming growth factors stimulate prostaglandin production and bone resorption in cultured mouse calvaria. Proc Natl Acad Sci USA 82:4535–4538

Tashjian Jr AH, Voelkel EF, Lloyd W, Derynck R, Winkler ME, Levine L (1986) Actions of growth factors on plasma calcium: epidermal growth factor and human transforming growth factor-alpha cause elevation of plasma calcium in mice. J Clin Invest 78:1405–1409

Tashjian Jr AH, Voelkel EF, Lazzaro M et al. (1987) Tumour necrosis factor-α (cachectin) stimulates bone resorption in mouse calvaria via a prostaglandin-mediated mechanism. Endocrinology 120:2029–2036

Thomson BM, Saklatvala J, Chambers TJ (1986) Osteoblasts mediate interleukin-I responsiveness of bone resorption by rat osteoclasts. J Exp Med 164:104–112

Thomson BM, Mundy GR, Chambers TJ (1987) Tumour necrosis factors α and β induce osteoblastic cells to stimulate osteoclastic bone resorption. J Immunol 138:775–779

Travers MT, Barrett-Lee PJ, Berger U et al. (1988) Growth factor expression in normal, benign and malignant breast tissue. Br Med J 296:1621–1624

Valentin Opran A, Edouard C, Charhon S, Meunier PJ (1980) Histomorphometic analysis of iliac bone metastases of prostatic origin. In: Donath A, Huber H (eds) Bone and tumours. Médicine et hygiène, Genève, pp 24–28

Wergedal JE, Mohan S, Taylor AK et al. (1986) Human skeletal growth factor is produced by human osteoblast-like cells in culture. Biochim Biophys Acta 889:163–170

Wergedal JE, Mohan S, Lundy M et al. (1990) Skeletal growth factor and other growth factors known to be present in bone matrix stimulate proliferation and protein synthesis in human bone cells. J Bone Miner Res 5:179–186

Wo Z, Bonewald LF, Oreffo ROC et al. (1990) The potential role of procathepsin D secreted by breast cancer cells in bone resorption. In: Cohn DV, Glorieux FH, Martin TJ (eds) Calcium regulation and bone metabolism. Elsevier, North-Holland, Amsterdam, pp 304–310

3   The Bone Scan in Metastatic Disease

I. Fogelman and J.H. McKillop

Introduction

In recent years there have been dramatic advances in all the imaging specialities, with growth of the use of ultrasound and computed tomography (CT) scanning and the introduction of magnetic resonance imaging (MRI). An integrated imaging approach to a specific problem is required for optimal results and the use of these newer modalities is discussed elsewhere in this book. Nevertheless, despite these changes the radionuclide bone scan remains unchallenged in its role of investigating skeletal pathology, because of its exquisite sensitivity for lesion detection and its ability rapidly to evaluate the whole skeleton. In contrast to routine radiology, sites such as ribs, sternum and scapula are clearly seen. The early experience of bone scanning was almost exclusively in patients with known malignancy and, while the role of bone scanning has now expanded to many benign situations, the identification of metastases still remains the most important indication for a bone scan. In this review we shall attempt to define the role of bone scanning in the detection and monitoring of skeletal metastases.

Pathophysiology of Skeletal Uptake of Diphosphonate

A skeletal radiograph indicates the net result of bone resorption and repair. For a destructive lesion in trabecular bone to be recognised on x-ray examination, it must be greater than 1–1.5 cm in diameter, with loss of approximately 50% of bone mineral content (Edelstyn et al. 1967). The bone scan, which is almost exclusively performed using a technetium-99m labelled diphosphonate, provides quite different information, which reflects skeletal metabolic activity. While the exact mechanism of uptake of bone-seeking radiopharmaceuticals is incompletely understood, it is thought most likely that they react through the phosphorus group by chemisorption onto the calcium of hydroxyapatite in bone, i.e., the diphosphonate molecule is adsorbed onto the surface of bone (Fig. 3.1) (Francis and Fogelman 1987). The major factors which affect this adsorption are believed to be osteoblastic activity and skeletal vascularity, and there is preferential uptake of tracer at sites of active bone formation. The bone scan, therefore, reflects the metabolic reaction of bone to a disease process, whether neoplastic, traumatic or inflammatory. When bone resorption occurs, there may not be sufficient bone destruction to be identified on x-ray examination, although the bone scan may be strongly positive. This ability to detect functional change, which occurs earlier than structural change, is the explanation of why the bone scan is more sensitive than conventional radiology. Bone scan findings are, however, non-specific, because virtually all disease processes result in an alteration in osteoblastic activity and blood flow. Thus to obtain optimal information, the bone scan will often require to be correlated with corresponding radiographs or other investigations.

Bone Scan Imaging

A bone scan is generally performed by acquiring multiple images of the skeleton 3–4 h after the intravenous injection of 550 MBq of technetium-99m (^{99m}Tc) methylene diphosphonate (MDP). To be able adequately to evaluate an abnormal bone scan one must be familiar not only with the normal bone scan, but also with the commonly found variants. If a lesion is identified, particularly

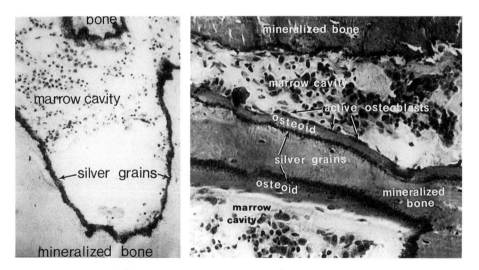

Fig. 3.1. Micro-autoradiographs of the endosteal surface of rabbit bone in which ^{3}H-HEDP was administered intraperitoneally. The concentration of silver grains indicating the adsorption of ^{3}H-HEDP on the bone surface is seen totally lining the resorption cavity on the left. From the image on the right it is apparent that the heavy concentration of silver grains appear below the osteoid layers on either side of the spicule of bone and below the osteoblasts lining the surface of the osteoid. (From Francis and Fogelman (1987.)

when solitary, further investigation will be required. A suggested pathway for investigation of a bone scan abnormality is shown in Fig. 3.2. Appropriate plain radiographs of a focal lesion should be obtained in the first instance (Fig. 3.3.). If these are normal and clinically a metastasis is likely then CT or MRI of the area may be diagnostic. If clinically relevant a bone biopsy may be necessary to resolve the issue.

While bone scan appearances are non-specific, recognisable patterns of bone scan abnormalities are commonly seen which may strongly suggest a specific diagnosis. Metastases usually are seen as multiple, irregularly distributed foci of

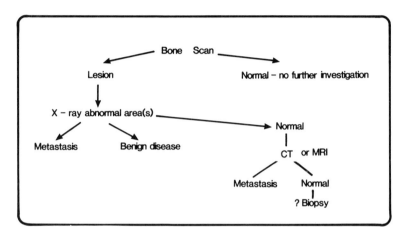

Fig. 3.2. Recommended protocol for the investigation of a lesion detected on a bone scan.

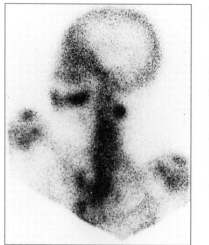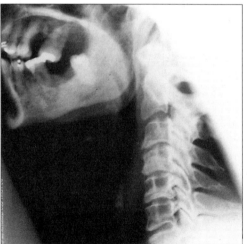

a   b

Fig. 3.3.a,b. A patient with known carcinoma of the breast. **a** The only abnormalities seen in the bone scan are demonstrated on the lateral view of the skull where focal lesions are present in the mandible and upper cervical spine. **b** X-ray, however, reveals that the lesions are due to local dental disease and degenerative change.

increased tracer uptake which do not correspond to any single anatomical structure (Goris and Bretille 1985) (Fig. 3.4). Generally they affect the axial skeleton, but metastatic disease may involve the distal skeleton in approximately 7% of cases (Corcoran et al. 1976; Rappaport et al. 1978; Brown 1983). Because of this it is recommended that the entire skeleton be imaged.

As stated, imaging a lesion depends upon a local osteoblastic reaction and if a lesion does not induce this then a false negative study may occur. This has best been documented in multiple myeloma where there may be purely lytic lesions with little osteoblastic reaction (Fig. 3.5). Nevertheless, even here a completely

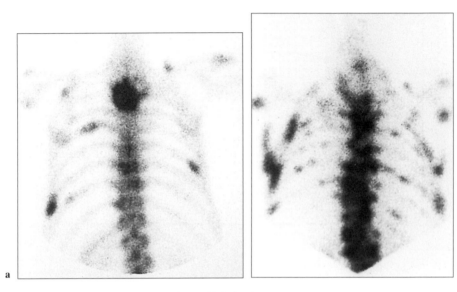

Fig. 3.4.a,b. Two cases demonstrating multiple focal lesions in the spine and ribs due to metastatic involvement.

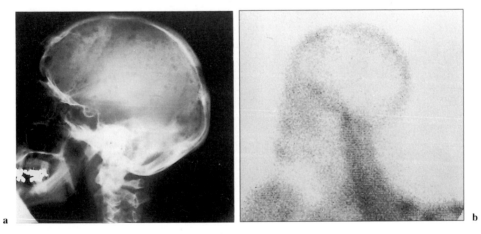

Fig. 3.5. **a** Lateral skull x-ray. **b** Corresponding bone scan image. This patient with multiple myeloma had extensive skeletal involvement as is apparent on the x-ray films. However, the bone scan image is essentially normal.

negative bone scan is unusual, although often bone scan findings are less dramatic than corresponding x-ray examination (Wahner et al. 1980; Waxman et al. 1981; Wolfenden et al. 1980). This situation may also arise with other tumours where there are rapidly growing lytic lesions. In extreme cases where there has been significant bony destruction a photon-deficient area may develop (cold spot) (Fig. 3.6). When seen on the bone scan this is an ominous sign although cold lesions may also arise from other pathologies such as avascular necrosis or infection. It should also be remembered that an apparent photon-deficient lesion may be an artefact due to the presence of metal such as a medallion, coins in the pockets or a pacemaker. Approximately 2% of metastases are reported to produce cold lesions (Kober et al. 1979). Sclerotic metastases, on the other hand, are clearly visualised on the bone scan, but very occasionally a lesion may be so slow-growing in its evolution that the alteration in metabolic activity is such that a focal increase in uptake cannot be distinguished from normal background activity.

Where there are extensive skeletal metastases the focal lesions may coalesce to produce diffusely increased uptake – the so-called super scan of malignancy

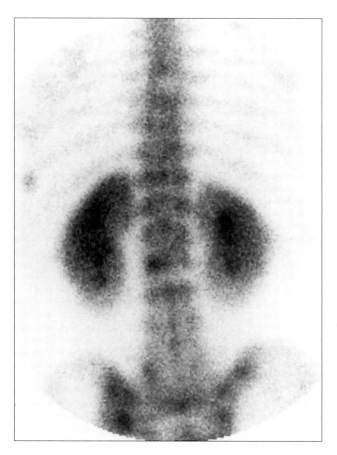

Fig. 3.6.   A patient with carcinoma of the breast. Bone scan reveals focal areas of increased tracer uptake, representing metastases in lumbar spine, pelvis and left 10th rib posteriorly. Note, however, that there is a photon-deficient lesion (cold spot) at T8.

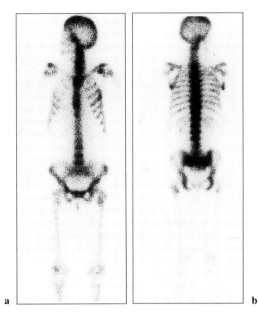

Fig. 3.7.a,b. Whole body bone scan: **a** anterior and **b** posterior views. There is high uptake of tracer throughout the skeleton with relative non-homogeneity, particularly in the ribs. Some more discrete abnormalities are seen in the left 4th rib anteriorly and the left anterior superior iliac spine. There is also abnormal tracer accumulation in the skull. Renal images are not visualised. This is a patient with carcinoma of the breast and scan findings were due to disseminated metastatic disease throughtout the skeleton. This is a "super scan" of malignancy.

(Fig. 3.7, 3.8). This occurs most often in prostatic cancer, but is seen with other tumours such as breast cancer. The initial impression upon viewing such a study is that the quality of the scan is extremely good because of the very high uptake of tracer in the skeleton with increased contrast between bone and background

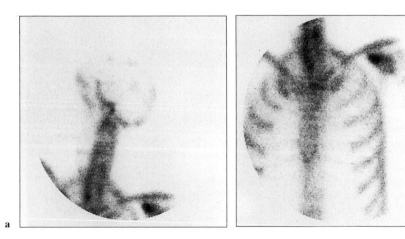

Fig. 3.8.a-g. Bone scan views. **a** Lateral skull. **b** Anterior chest.

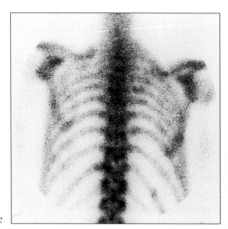

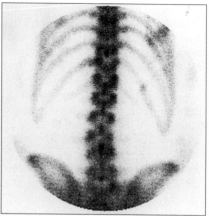

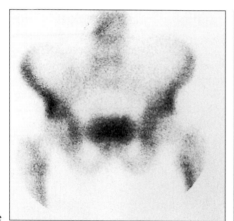

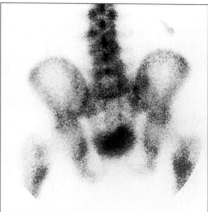

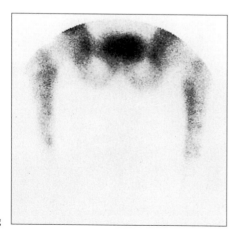

Fig. 3.8.(*continued*) **c** Posterior thoracic spine. **d** Posterior lumbar spine. **e** Anterior pelvis. **f** Posterior pelvis. **g** Anterior femora. This is a further case of the "super scan" of malignancy in a 79-year-old male with carcinoma of the prostate. Once again, note the high uptake of tracer throughout the skeleton with heightened contrast between bone and soft tissue with renal images not visualised. Also there is non-homogeneity of tracer uptake apparent in ribs, skull and upper femora.

soft tissue. This can lead, on occasions, to the presence of metastases being misread (Constable and Cranage 1981). The renal images are invariably faint or absent and provide an important diagnostic feature. Generally, the peripheral skeleton is not particularly well visualised in contrast to the "super scan" found in metabolic bone disease. Furthermore, there is usually some focal disease and in addition non-homogeneity of tracer uptake, especially in the ribs (Fogelman et al. 1977). It is rare for any real doubt to exist as to whether a bone scan is normal or represents a super scan of malignancy, but in such cases a single radiograph of the pelvis will be diagnostic. If quantitative studies of skeletal uptake of tracer are performed, then this too will provide further diagnostic information.

While treatment of metastatic disease can lead to clinical improvement, it is often difficult to obtain an objective measure of this (Fig. 3.9). It has been suggested that bone metastases may be less responsive than other metastases (Marsoni et al. 1985). This may be a true phenomenon if metastases in bone were selectively biologically different, but it seems more likely that any differences reflect the insensitivity of assessment methods (Coleman and Rubens 1985). On standard radiographs, sclerosis of lytic metastases constitute tumour regression, but in some cases patients will have evidence of sclerosis before starting therapy. It is not possible to assess response in patients with sclerotic lesions. Further, even when x-ray evidence of response to successful therapy is obtained, it is generally not evident for 6 months and on occasion for more than a year. Complete remission with return of the normal trabecular pattern is rare.

The use of serial bone scans to assess response to therapy is also difficult. Findings associated with healing may be confused with progression of disease, and complete resolution of scan abnormalities is uncommon. After successful therapy, the increased skeletal metabolism reflecting formation of immature new bone eventually ceases and tracer uptake correspondingly falls. However,

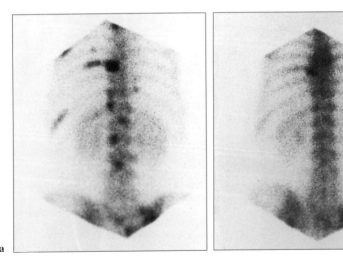

a   b

Fig. 3.9. **a** A patient with carcinoma of breast with extensive skeletal metastases as demonstrated by bone scan. **b** Following chemotherapy, a repeat study shows significant resolution of disease.

healing causes an inital increase in tracer uptake which may be mistaken for progressive disease – the so-called "flare phenomenon" (Greenberg et al. 1972; Rossleigh et al. 1984; Alexander et al. 1982) (Fig. 3.10). It should be noted that a reduction in tracer uptake may be seen in rapidly progressive disease which is so aggressive that there is little chance for new bone formation, although this situation is rare (Hayward et al. 1977).

It is apparent that bone scans obtained early during the course of therapy may be misleading unless the possibility of a flare response is kept in mind. New lesions appearing after 6 months of therapy indicate progressive disease. The flare phenomenon is not a new observation (Gillespie et al. 1975; Greenberg et al. 1972; Rossleigh et al. 1984; Alexander et al. 1982), although it has not previously been appreciated as a common finding when the bone scan is performed early on, following successful response to therapy (Coleman et al. 1988a) (see Chap. 6).

The bone scan may also have a role to play in assessing patients with pathological fracture. Assessment of risk of fracture cannot be obtained from a bone scan, but if a patient has particularly heavy tumour involvement in the limbs then this should be commented upon and radiographs obtained for further evaluation. Even if the prognosis is poor and perhaps only a matter of some months, it may still be worthwhile carrying out prophylactic insertion of a prosthesis in appropriate cases to remove the risk of the patient being confined to bed by a pathological fracture. In a review of 29 patients with pathological fracture of long bone secondary to metastatic breast cancer, there were 22 fractures of the femora and 12 of the humeri (Fogelman and Coleman 1988). The disease was predominantly lytic in 28 of these 29 patients and 27 had widespread radiological evidence of bone involvement. Fracture is generally a late manifestation of skeletal metastatic involvement with the median time to fracture 2 years (0–8 years). In that study 25 patients had a bone scan performed in the previous 3 months with a focal abnormality seen at the site of subsequent fracture in 23 (92%) of cases. The radiological features which have been

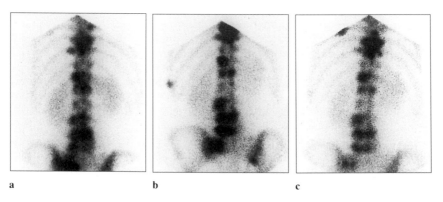

a   b   c

Fig. 3.10. **a** Bone scan from a woman with multiple metastases from carcinoma of the breast. **b** Scan 3 months later, after introduction of systemic chemotherapy shows increased tracer uptake in previously noted lesions and a new area of increased uptake in left posterior rib. **c** At 6 months, after introduction of therapy, the uptake in lesions is less and fewer lesions are visualised than on the immediate post treatment scan. This series of scans demonstrates the flare phenomenon.

suggested to predict fractures include lytic lesions larger than 2.5 cm in diameter, involvement of more than 50% of the diameter and erosion of the cortex (Beals et al. 1971). There are no specific scan features to suggest imminent fracture although in 16 patients the tracer uptake was intense and the dominant abnormality was in the long bones (Fogelman and Coleman 1988). The role of the bone scan in identifying potential sites of fracture has not been systematically assessed. Routine bone scans at regular intervals are unlikely to be cost effective although a policy of scanning patients prior to a change in systemic therapy and obtaining plain films of abnormal foci in long bones would be expected to identify most sites of major structural damage.

In hypercalcaemia of malignancy the bone scan findings may range from normal to extensive metastatic disease. In general the bone scan findings correlate poorly with the degree of hypercalcaemia (Ralston et al. 1982), but this varies from tumour to tumour. In breast cancer, for example, the bone scan findings in hypercalcaemia are typically those of widespread bone metastases and it is uncommon to have a normal bone scan. In carcinoma of the lung this would be a much more common finding explained by the presence of a humoral factor (a parathyroid hormone-like substance) of malignancy which, in addition to altering skeletal metabolism, also has a direct effect on the renal tubules leading to increased reabsorption of calcium (Bourgeois et al. 1989).

Recently, it had become apparent that diffuse marrow involvement by tumour can provide characteristic appearances on the bone scan. In this situation, increased tracer uptake is found at the ends of long bones with striking changes present in the knees and a typical globular appearance at the ends of the long bones, which is often most pronounced in the humeri. While bone metastases arise from malignant cells in the bone marrow, usually the skeleton is severely affected before diffuse bone marrow infiltration occurs. Nevertheless, on occasions diffuse bone marrow infiltration can occur with little or no radiological evidence of bone involvement. When bone scan appearances are suggestive of this a marrow scan may be diagnostic. There has been some suggestion that marrow imaging in itself may provide a sensitive means of detecting early metastatic involvement of the skeleton but, while logical, this has not as yet been found to be of clinical value in practice (Bourgeois et al. 1989; Sven et al. 1989).

Uptake of ^{99m}Tc diphosphonate may on occasion be seen in extra-osseous tissues such as damaged muscle or metastases, particularly in the liver, but has been reported in a wide variety of situations (Fig. 3.11, 3.12) (Gray 1987). The mechanism of this uptake is not known, but the common factor appears to be the presence of micro-calcification. Diffusely increased uptake throughout the lungs or, less commonly, stomach uptake is found in severe hypercalcaemia. Diffusely increased tracer uptake throughout the renal parenchyma may on occasion be seen in association with hypercalcaemia, but is most often found in patients who have received chemotherapy and is thought to reflect microtubular damage (Koizumi et al. 1981) (Fig 3.13). This must be differentiated from abnormal retention of tracer in the renal collecting system, which may be indicative of renal obstruction (Fig. 3.14). This is a relatively common finding in patients with pelvic tumours where there is obstructive uropathy. It has also been reported in metastatic infiltrating lobular carcinoma of the breast in which post-mortem investigation showed diffuse retroperitoneal and ureteric infiltration (Wilkinson et al. 1985).

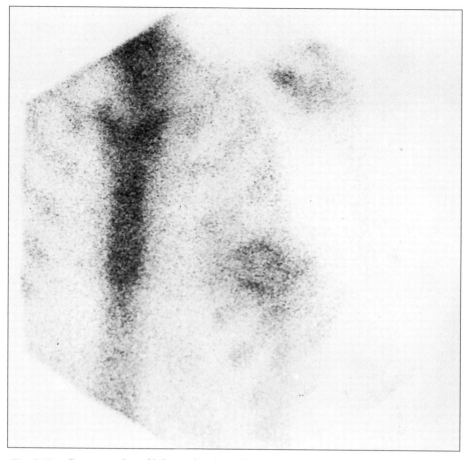

Fig. 3.11.   Bone scan view of left anterior chest. There is diphosphonate uptake associated with a primary breast neoplasm.

New Bone Scanning Agents

While the current sensitivity of the bone scan with ^{99m}Tc-MDP is extremely high for the identification of metastases, further improvement may be possible. A desirable goal should always be to identify a lesion at an earlier point in its evolution. It is well recognised that different diphosphonates have different affinities for the skeleton and, even among those compounds which have been used for routine imaging, this may be as much as fourfold (Fogelman 1987). Clearly contrast between bone and soft tissue (B/ST) is necessary for visualisation of the skeleton itself. But a scanning agent with a high B/ST ratio may not be the ideal agent for lesion detection. Identification of a focal lesion depends upon the contrast between the lesion itself and surrounding bone that is the ratio of counts in the lesion to those of background bone (L/B) (Fig. 3.15). There have been many studies comparing the ability of different diphosphonates

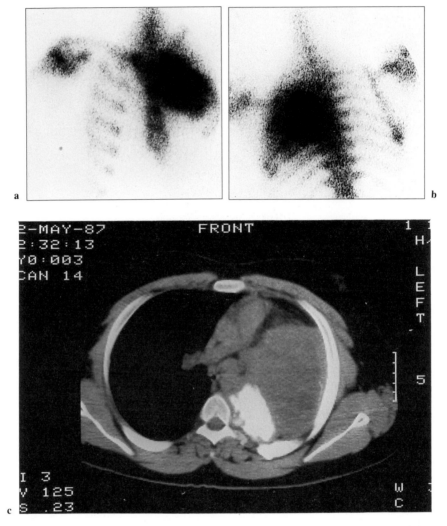

Fig. 3.12.a–c.   Bone scan views: **a** anterior and **b** posterior chest. **c** CT of thorax. There is intense abnormal tracer accumulation in left hemi-thorax in association with pulmonary metastases from osteogenic sarcoma which are clearly shown on CT image (**c**).

to identify metastases and this topic has been reviewed elsewhere (Fogelman 1982). In general, there has been little difference in sensitivity with no compound consistently identifying lesions that were not visualised with another. A further ^{99m}Tc diphosphonate has recently been evaluated – dimethylamino diphosphonate (DMAD). This is an experimental agent with low affinity for normal bone (approximately 10%, compared to 30% 24-h whole-body retention with MDP). However, the uptake in lesions is relatively intense, giving rise to higher L/B ratios. There are now three reports of the use of this compound

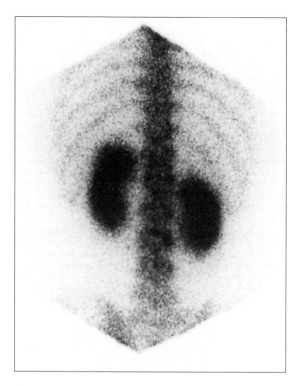

Fig. 3.13. Note intense increased tracer uptake in both kidneys. This is diffusely present throughout the renal parenchyma and is not associated with collecting systems.

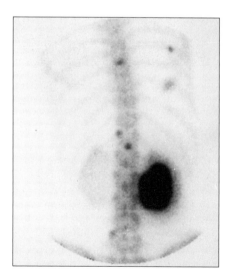

Fig. 3.14. Note the markedly increased tracer uptake associated with the right kidney (dilated collecting system) due to urinary tract outflow obstruction. There are metastases present in spine and ribs.

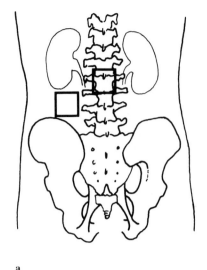

a

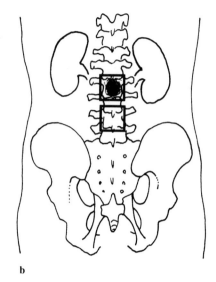

b

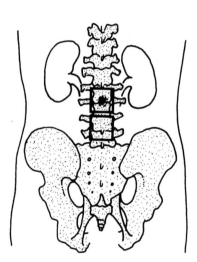

c

Fig. 3.15. **a** Regions of interest (*ROI*) selected over bone and soft tissue. B/ST ratio will reflect skeletal contrast. **b** ROI over normal bone and vertebra with lesion (*L/B* ratio). **c** As in **b** but there is higher skeletal affinity for tracer and while B/ST ratio will be higher, lesion contrast (*L/B*)ratio is lower.

which have all found that additional lesions were identified when compared with the standard MDP scan (Rosenthall et al. 1982; Smith et al. 1984; Coleman et al. 1987). These additional lesions have been in patients with widespread metastatic disease and have not altered management (Fig. 3.16). To date it has not been shown that DMAD can identify disease earlier than MDP. While DMAD has increased sensitivity for lesion detection it is unlikely that it will ever find a routine role in clinical practice. This is because the normal images appear of poor quality with low resolution of anatomical detail, for example ribs may not individually be visualised. Such a scan is unacceptable to most physicians.

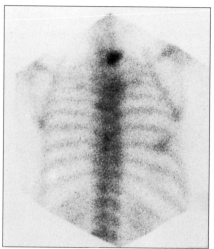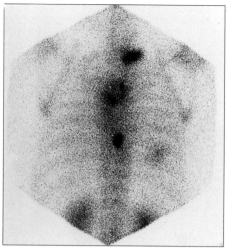

a   b

Fig. 3.16.a,b. A patient with carcinoma of the breast, bone scan image, **a** obtained with MDP and **b** with DMAD. Metastatic involvement of the thoracic spine is seen on MDP study but individual lesions are more obvious with DMAD and it is apparent that there is a lesion at T8 which may well have been missed on MDP scan.

Breast Cancer

There have been a large number of publications relating to the role of bone scanning in carcinoma of the breast. In clinically early breast cancer, the bone scan has been investigated both for pre-treatment staging (Sklaroff and Sklaroff 1976; El Domeiri and Shroff 1976) and for the early detection of metastatic disease during follow-up after treatment of the primary tumour (Citrin et al. 1976; Gerber et al. 1977; Kunkler et al. 1985; Khansur et al. 1987; Bishop et al. 1979; Furnival et al, 1980; Chaudary et al. 1983; Moneypenny et al. 1984; Wickerham et al. 1984; Thomsen et al. 1987). As discussed previously the bone scan and radiographs provide different information about the skeleton and findings from these investigations do not necessarily correlate. Several studies have addressed the relative sensitivity of these imaging techniques and results are summarised in Table 3.1. The majority of studies have found the bone scan to be more sensitive.

For many years there was considerable disagreement on the true incidence of a positive bone scan in early breast cancer (clinical stages I and II). This arose as the numerous reports provided inexplicably varied results, although it is fair to comment that the more recent studies have been in general agreement. In clinical stage one disease, the percentage of abnormal scans has ranged from 0% to 18%; in stage two, the range was from 0% to 41%. In general, earlier studies found a much higher incidence with a result that bone scanning became a routine pre-operative staging procedure in breast cancer. The more recent studies have shown a much lower detection rate and the value of a routine staging scan has therefore been questioned. This topic has recently been reviewed (Fogelman and Coleman 1988). One can speculate on the reasons for the wide variation in

Table 3.1. Comparison between bone scanning and plain radiography in the detection of skeletal metastases. Patients with a variety of advanced cancers are included. All studies were performed with ^{99m}Tc-labelled phosphate, polyphosphate, or diphosphonate. (From Fogelman and Coleman 1988)

Author	Year	Number of patients	Scan more accurate (%)	x-ray more accurate (%)	No difference (%)
Yeates et al.	1972	53	11	13	75
Shearer et al.	1974	67	12	1	87
Citrin et al.	1977	372	31	0	69
Nordman et al.	1977	142	3	5	92
Donato et al.	1979	60	23	7	70
Joo et al.	1979	170	34	2	64
Wahner et al.	1980	100	65	8	27
Total		964	28	3	69

reported incidence and, while it may in part reflect scanning technique, equipment or methods of staging (British Breast Group 1978), it is probable that the most important variables are differences in the reporting of scans and the subsequent investigation of abnormalities. Over the years we have learnt that certain "hot spots" are normal variants, for example, focally increased uptake at the pterion (the confluence of suture lines) in the skull (Merrick 1987a). Some workers have chosen to report any hot spot as positive on the bone scan (Perez et al. 1983). It is apparent that lesions due to degenerative disease are extremely common in the lower lumbar spine, shoulders and knees and would not be reported as suspicious of metastases by an experienced observer. Radiological confirmation of a metastasis is easier when radiographs are viewed in conjunction with a bone scan (Kunkler et al. 1985). Some departments may undertake more detailed investigation and when a CT scan is performed this may confirm a metastasis when plain films are negative. Nevertheless, because of the superior sensitivity of bone scanning, confirmation of some lesions will not initially be possible, but yet will become apparent with time as the metastasis grows and bone destruction increases. Galasko (1975) has reported a median lead time of 12–18 months for bone scans over radiographs whereas Moneypenny et al. (1984) found that most patients had simultaneous bone scan and radiographic confirmation. This differs from our experience where in serial 6-monthly follow-up scans in 560 patients followed for a median of 3½ years lead-time over radiographs ranged from 0 to 18 months (median 4 months) (Coleman et al. 1986).

Considerable controversy, however, does persist on how best to use the bone scan in breast cancer. Clearly some consider the low frequency of a positive bone scan in stage one and two breast cancer a poor return for the time and cost involved (Gerber et al. 1977; Bishop et al. 1979; Moneypenny et al. 1984; Spencer et al. 1981; Pauwels et al. 1982; Baker 1978) and they would recommend that base-line scans be restricted to stage three or four disease. Others consider it to be an important base-line for future comparison which in addition, when positive for metastatic disease, will influence clinical management (McNeil et al. 1978; Furnival et al. 1980; Wickerham et al. 1984). This debate is important as the bone scan is a commonly requested investigation and breast cancer is a common and extremely important clinical condition. At Guy's Hospital, the results of base-line bone scans performed in 1155 consecutive cases presenting between 1980 and 1986 have recently been reviewed (Coleman et al. 1988b). All of the patients were carefully staged by experienced breast surgeons and all the scans were performed using modern equipment and with the single agent ^{99m}TcMDP. All scans were reported by a Nuclear Medicine consultant and all identified lesions were investigated by the appropriate radiological tests with at least one year of follow-up data available for each patient. The results are shown in Table 3.2. The number of positive base-line scans is shown in relation to tumour size and 46 of these patients (4%) had a positive base-line scan and developed radiological evidence of metastases within 1 year. The frequency of a positive scan was less than quoted in many early studies, but was similar to several more recent studies (McNeil et al. 1978; Nomura et al. 1978; Ciatto et al. 1985; Khansur et al. 1987).

Although the incidence of skeletal metastases is low in patients with apparently operable breast cancer, the value to those patients in whom mastectomy cannot be curative and may be avoided should not be underestimated. Confirmation of metastatic disease in 20 of 28 patients with potentially operative tumours and a positive base-line scan resulted in alternative treatments being selected. As in other studies, the positive scan rate was higher in those with inoperable locally advanced disease. However, here the influence of a bone scan on initial management was paradoxically less. The ultimate treatment of these patients is radiotherapy for local control of the tumour and systemic treatment for the almost inevitable metastatic or micro-metastatic disease. A positive scan did not usually influence this, although it did indicate specific bony sites for observation with follow-up radiographs and was of value for direct palliative radiotherapy. It also helped to pre-empt pathological fractures or spinal cord compressions. It is apparent that a positive bone scan is a dire prognostic factor (Kunkler et al. 1985; Furnival et al. 1980), although this has been questioned in the past due to reported high false-positive and/or false-negative rates (Moneypenny et al. 1984; Perez et al. 1983). The Guy's experience of a positive bone scan indicates a poor prognosis with a median survival of 24 months (Coleman and Rubens 1987).

The reported false-positive rates for base-line bone scanning also vary greatly. In the Guy's review the incidence was 1.6%, but Perez et al. (1983) reported a

Table 3.2. Frequency of positive base-line scan and subsequent relapse in relation to tumour size. (From Fogelman and Coleman 1988)

Tumour size (T)	Number of patients	Bone relapse within 1 year	Bone relapse at any time	Positive base-line scan
T0	57	2[4][a]	3[5]	0[0]
T1	251	3[1]	23[9]	1[0.3]
T2	582	27[5]	106[18]	17[3]
T3	122	11[9]	36[30]	10[8]
T4	143	21[15]	52[36]	18[13]
Total	1 155	64[6]	220[19]	46[4]

[a] Numbers in square brackets denote the percentage of the number of patients.

70% false-positive rate. In that study, however, there was no attempt made to exclude benign causes for lesions and all hot spots were reported as positive whether they were due to trauma or osteoarthritis. It is apparent that the false-positive rate in the context of bone scanning must be dependent on the experience of the observer and on the subsequent investigation of focal lesions. Nevertheless, in most studies the reported false-positive rate has been between 1% and 3% (Gerber et al. 1977; McNeil et al. 1978; Kunkler et al. 1985). In general the exquisite sensitivity of the bone scan for lesion detection is well accepted and the false-negative rate is correspondingly low (Bishop et al. 1979). At Guy's the development of metastatic bone disease was missed in 1 out of 46 (2%) of cases. This is in marked contrast to Moneypenny et al. (1984) who reported 12 out of 45 (27%) cases with positive radiographs and negative bone scan. In our experience no patient with radiologically confirmed bone metastases from breast cancer has had an entirely normal bone scan, and in the case "missed" the bone scan was considered to be abnormal upon review.

The cost effectiveness of an investigation is often difficult to define in financial terms. In breast cancer premature death from metastatic disease may be accepted as inevitable in the light of present knowledge and with the presently available treatment. However adjuvant chemotherapy for patients with axillary lymph node involvement does prolong survival (Padmanabhan et al. 1986) and as the prognosis of undetectable micro-metastatic disease becomes increasingly influenced by new therapies then it may be correspondingly important to identify early metastatic disease and the use of sensitive imaging tests may increase proportionally. However, we would agree that patients with tumours less than 2 cm are most unlikely to have a positive scan; here scans are only of value as a base-line reference and for identifying other bone pathologies. It is recognised that routine bone scanning in this population may be inappropriate for many centres. However, the pick-up rate in larger tumours is significant, and it is probably worth trying to identify the 5% of patients with tumours that are 2–5 cm in size that will recur in bone within one year.

Prostatic Cancer

The skeleton is the major site of distant metastases in prostatic cancer with approximately 70% of patients eventually developing skeletal involvement (Vest 1954). There has, therefore, been considerable interest in the use of bone scanning in patients with prostatic cancer, both at the time of diagnosis and during subsequent follow-up. Prostatic metastases typically appear as foci of increased uptake on the bone scan. Diffuse skeletal involvement with prostatic cancer is relatively common, giving rise to the so-called "metastatic super scan" as noted above. Cold metastases occur infrequently in prostatic cancer. It should be remembered that lesions may change their scintigraphic appearance as they evolve, depending on the local balance of bone destruction and osteoblastic reaction (Shih et al. 1986).

A number of investigators have carried out bone scans at presentation and found an overall positivity rate which ranges from 30% to more than 50% (Shafer and Reinke 1977; O'Donoghue et al. 1978; McGregor et al. 1978;

Paulson et al. 1979; Biersack et al. 1980; Lund et al. 1984; Merrick et al. 1985). As might be expected the frequency of positive scans varies according to the stage of disease at presentation. Paulson et al. (1979) found that the rate of positive scans was 9% in clinical stage I, 20% in stage II, 24% in stage III and 60% in stage IV, while McNeil and Polak (1981) quoted a rate of 5% in stage I and 10% in stage II and 20% in stage III. Biersack et al. (1980) also reported positivity rates in different stages and found figures of 7% in T1, 19% in T2, 49% in T3 and 65% in T4. In a recent review article, Merrick (1989) has suggested rather higher figures ranging from 10% in T0 to 80% in T4.

The rate of positivity at presentation also varies according to the tumour type. Langhammer et al. (1980) found that in adenocarcinomas the frequency of bone scan metastases increased as the primary tumour became less differentiated. Merrick et al. (1985) reported positive bone scans in 31% of patients with well differentiated tumours and 57% of those with poorly differentiated tumours.

The ability of the bone scan to detect prostatic metastases was reviewed by McNeil (1984). She concluded that if the bone scan had a sensitivity of 100%, the relative sensitivities of other non-invasive investigations was: x-ray skeletal survey, 68%; serum alkaline phosphatase, 75%; and serum acid phosphatase, 60%.

The role of the bone scan in comparison to lymphangiography or node biopsy has been examined. Paulson et al. (1979) concluded that no non-invasive test alone or in combination with others provided "sufficient accuracy to exclude staging pelvic node dissection as a segment of the pre-treatment evaluation". In a more recent study, Hayward et al. (1987) found that 10 of 100 patients studied had a positive lymphangiogram and a negative bone scan, and concluded that the lymphangiogram should be obtained as part of the staging procedure if the bone scan is negative.

A recent modification has been suggested to the bone scan protocol for prostatic cancer patients with a view to identifying renal outflow obstruction. Narayam et al. (1988) performed standard bone scans with the addition of early dynamic renal images in 79 patients with prostatic cancer, all of whom had at least one other study of the kidneys (IVU, ultrasound or CT). The scintigraphic study identified all 5 acutely obstructed kidneys and 8 of 12 chronically obstructed kidneys. The remaining 4 chronically obstructed kidneys were correctly identified as non functional, but the destructive aetiology was not. The false-positive rate for obstruction was 24%. The authors concluded that early dynamic images were cost-effective for screening as no significant abnormalities were missed.

The finding of a positive bone scan in prostatic cancer has prognostic value. Lund et al. (1984) found that patients with an abnormal scan at presentation had a mortality of 45% in the first 2 years compared to a mortality of 20% in those with a normal initial scan. Merrick et al. (1985) have reported that, in patients studied before institution of systemic therapy, those with metastases on bone scan had a markedly worse prognosis than those without such abnormalities. This, however, was less predictive than the serum alkaline phosphatase. Developing this further, Soloway et al. (1988) have recently reported that the 2-year survival was inversely proportional to the extent of bone metastases on the initial scan and concluded that patients entered into trials of therapy for prostatic bone metastases should be stratified according to the extent of disease on the scan. George (1988) has prospectively studied the natural history of localised prostatic cancer, managed conservatively, over a 7-year period. He concluded that the likelihood of prostatic cancer causing death within 7 years is indicated primarily by the scintigraphic findings at diagnosis.

From the data presented so far, it can be concluded that a bone scan should be performed in all patients at the time of presentation with prostatic cancer for staging and prognostic purposes.

The place of the bone scan in the follow-up of patients with prostatic cancer is less clearly delineated. Lund et al. (1984) carried out serial bone scans and found that of patients with a negative initial scan around 10% had a positive study by 1 year and 20% by 2 years. They concluded that annual follow-up scans were justifiable as they could identify patients who would require hormonal therapy. Merrick et al. (1985) reported that scintigraphic change preceded elevation of the serum prostatic acid phosphatase in 81% of the patients in whom the initial bone scan and acid phosphatase were normal, but who developed evidence of distant metastases on follow-up. The mean interval between scintigraphic conversion and overt symptoms was 5.8 months. As a result they concluded that, if the alkaline phosphatase is normal, regular follow-up scans are necessary to identify patients who are likely soon to develop symptoms.

From these results it appears that bone scans are justifiable during follow-up if the patient has symptoms, signs or biochemical evidence of metastases or if systemic therapy is instituted. Regular bone scans in asymptomatic patients are difficult to justify and would only have a role if it is ever decided that systemic therapy is beneficial in patients with asymptomatic bone metastases.

Hetherington et al. (1988) have compared serial measurements of serum prostatic acid phosphatase (PAP) and serum prostatic specific antigen (PSA) to changes in serial bone scans in 120 patients with prostatic cancer. Ten patients with negative scans at presentation developed skeletal metastases during follow-up. The PAP and PSA were rising at the time of scan conversion in 5 and 9 of these patients respectively. Local progression of disease occurred in an additional 9 patients, in whom PAP was rising in 8 and PSA in all 9. In 66 patients with previously documented bone metastases, evidence of progression was seen on the bone scan in 36. At the time of first scan progression PAP was rising in 20 and PSA rising in 26. In 4 patients both serum markers were normal at the time of first evidence of progression.

Other studies have concluded that there is no role for routine follow-up bone scans in prostatic cancer. Huben and Schellhammer (1982) followed patients for a mean period of 47 months, during which time 19 of 100 patients with a normal initial scan developed abnormalities. They felt, however, that this did not alter management and concluded that repeat bone scans should be reserved for patients who were symptomatic. Corrie et al. (1988) reported that true positive scans developed during follow-up in only 7 of 107 patients, the majority of whom had bone pain either at the time the scan was positive or shortly after. A further 6 patients had false-positive scans. They concluded that routine scans during follow-up are not cost effective.

The bone scan appears to be of value in the assessment of the response to systemic therapy for metastases. Pollen et al. (1981) have stressed the importance of constancy of technique in sequential scans. In a series of patients followed for 12 months, they observed that in those who had disease progression on the scan in spite of systemic therapy the mortality was 93% whereas in patients who did not show worsening of the scan findings the mortality was 40%.

Levenson et al. (1983) also concluded that the bone scan used in conjunction with bone radiographs was useful in following the response of metastases to systemic therapy. Drelichman et al. (1984) used sequential scans with measurement of tumour to normal bone activity ratios and found that the changes observed generally correlated well with the subsequent clinical response. Sundkvist et al. (1988) adopted a similar approach, measuring lumbar spine uptake in patients with disseminated disease undergoing orchidectomy. Patients who showed an initial increase in activity then a fall, a flare phenomenon, had a good clinical response whereas patients who showed steadily increasing activity had progressive metastases.

Other Genito-urinary Tract Tumours

The skeleton is recognised as one of the more common sites for metastases from renal cell carcinoma. A number of studies have been undertaken to assess the value of routine bone scintigraphy at the time of presentation. Clyne et al. (1983) performed bone scans in 32 consecutive patients presenting with renal carcinoma. Nine patients (28%) had abnormal scans of which 2 were shown to be false-positive. Of the 7 (22%) who had true-positive scans, 5 had bone pain at the time. Rosen and Murphy (1984) found abnormal scans in 3 of 40 (7.5%) patients at presentation. Blacher et al. (1985) reported a higher rate of positivity: 27/85 patients (32%) had an abnormal scan at presentation. In all of these patients there was evidence of bone metastases either from bone pain, an elevated serum alkaline phosphatase or routine x-rays (chest x-ray, IVU or angiogram). There were 2 false-negative bone scans and 8 false-positive studies (sensitivity 93%; specificity 86%).

From the above results it appears that the bone scan does not have a place as a routine staging investigation in renal carcinoma and should be reserved for patients with clinical or biochemical evidence of bone metastases. The bone scan is valuable in this subgroup in confirming the presence of bone metastases and establishing their extent. A similar situation exists during follow-up. Clyne et al. (1983) followed up 23 patients with a normal initial scan. Eight developed a true positive scan of whom 6 had bone pain at the time of the scan becoming abnormal.

Two studies have stressed the importance of looking for "cold" (photopenic) bone metastases in renal carcinoma. Reddy and Merrick (1983) found bone scans to be falsely negative in 4 of 12 patients with renal carcinoma bone metastases because of failure to report cold lesions. Kim et al. (1983) also reported the relatively high incidence of "cold" metastases in renal carcinoma.

Around 25% of patients with bladder carcinoma have bone metastases at autopsy (Babaian et al. 1980; Kishi et al. 1981). In a retrospective study, Parsarathy et al. (1978) found positive bone scans in 13 of 26 patients studied. Prospective studies have suggested a much lower incidence of positive bone scans at presentation with figures of 1 in 52 and 2 in 114 being reported by Berger et al. (1981) and Lindner and Dekernion (1982) respectively. Davey et al. (1985) studied 221 patients with bladder cancer, with bone scans being undertaken as part of tumour staging. Ten patients (4.5%) had true-positive scans at presen-

tation and a further 4 had false-positive scans. Ten patients with negative scan
at presentation had evidence of bone metastases within 1 year. Brismar and
Gustafson (1988) found no true-positive scans in 68 patients with 1 false-positive
result. Reviewing the literature they concluded that the true positive rate for
bone scans at presentation is around 3% with a false-positive rate of 2%. They
also conclude from the literature that surgery was avoided in only 4 of 458
patients (0.9%) because of bone scintigraphy results.

It thus appears that bone scanning has no role in the routine pre-operative
staging of patients with bladder carcinoma. It should be reserved for patients
with clinical or other evidence of bone metastases, both at presentation and
during follow-up.

The role of bone scanning has been examined in various tumours of the female
genital tract. Katz et al. (1979) reviewed the findings of bone scans at
presentation in 100 women with carcinoma of the cervix. All 79 patients with
stage 0, I or II disease had negative scans, but metastases were found in 4
patients with advanced or recurrent disease. They concluded that bone scanning
was not warranted in asymptomatic patients with stage 0, I or II disease. They
observed a high frequency of urinary tract abnormalities on the bone scan in
patients with cervical carcinoma and commented on the need to assess carefully
any bone scans performed for their presence. Kamath et al. (1983) also found a
low incidence of positive bone scans in clinically early carcinoma of cervix.

Du Toit and Grove (1987) retrospectively reviewed the bone scan results in
540 patients with carcinoma of the cervix. None of the 210 patients with stage I
or II disease had true-positive scans. Eleven of the 340 with stage III or IV
disease on clinical grounds had true-positive scans (3.2%). The result of the
bone scan changed the staging in 6 (1.1%) patients who moved from stage III
to stage IV because of the scintigraphic findings. In this study, false-positive
bone scans were obtained in 43 (7.9%) of patients. Bassan and Glaser (1982)
suggested that tumour type was more important than clinical stage. In a series
of 88 patients, 14 had positive bone scans (6 stage I, 6 stage II and 2 stage IV).
Of the 19 patients with poorly differentiated turmours on histology, 13 had
positive bone scans. Bassan and Glaser therefore concluded that bone scans
were required in all patients with poorly differentiated tumours whatever the
clinical stage.

In summary, therefore, it appears that there is no place for routine bone
scanning in asymptomatic patients with clinically early and well differentiated
carcinoma of the uterine cervix. There may be a need for routine bone scanning
in patients with poorly differentiated tumours or locally advanced tumours, but
even this is questionable.

In endometrial carcinoma, only 1 of 111 patients in 3 series had bone scan
evidence of metastases at presentation (Mettler et al. 1981; Kamath et al. 1982;
Harbert et al. 1982). In patients with recurrent disease the frequency of bone
metatases was higher at 14 of 77 (Harbert et al. 1982).

Patients with early ovarian cancer also have a low incidence of bone
metastases, with none of 49 having abnormalities in 2 series (Mettler et al.
1981; Harbert et al. 1982). In stage III ovarian cancer the incidence was 3
of 40 (Mettler et al. 1981).

Thus at presentation with endometrial cancer and ovarian cancer the bone
scan should be reserved for symptomatic patients.

Merrick (1987b) has assessed the role of bone scintigraphy in 61 patients with
testicular cancer. Bone metastases were found at presentation in 2 of 26 patients

with seminoma and 1 of 29 with teratoma. Three patients developed positive bone scans 5 to 18 months later despite normal initial scans, and a further patient had autopsy evidence of disseminated skeletal metastases 1 month after a normal scan. Merrick concludes that the bone scan is not required in the initial evaluation of patients with clinically early testicular tumours, but may be of value in patients presenting with stage IV seminoma. Bone scintigraphy is prognostically useful in patients with recurrence after radical treatment for seminoma (Merrick 1987b).

Lung Cancer

The skeleton is one of the commonest sites of extrathoracic spread in lung cancer (Gilbert and Kagan 1976; Komaki et al. 1977). In unselected patients studied at presentation, the rate of positive bone scans is high, with figures between 30% (Donato et al. 1979; Operchal et al. 1976) and 50% being reported (Kelly et al. 1979; Merrick and Merrick 1986). Many of these unselected patients either have symptoms of bone metastases or have evidence of spread of disease to extra-skeletal metastatic sites. The bone scan is much more pivotal in patients who are asymptomatic or who have potentially resectable tumours. In asymptomatic patients, Hooper et al. (1978) found a positive bone scan rate at presentation of 8% while Kies et al. (1978) reported a rate of 19% and Kelly et al. (1979) a rate of 14%. Ramsdell et al. (1977) found a true-positive rate of only 2% in patients with potentially resectable tumours. Turner and Haggith (1981) found abnormal bone scans in 4 of 57 patients with potentially operable tumours. In 3 the abnormality indicated local rib involvement which did not preclude thoracotomy.

Small cell or anaplastic lung cancer has been reported to have a high rate of positive bone scans at presentation by both Bitran et al. (1981) and Levenson et al. (1983) though Merrick and Merrick (1986) found no difference in positivity rates between different histological types of lung cancer.

The ominous prognosis of an abnormal bone scan in lung cancer has been shown by Gravenstein et al. (1979) and Levenson et al. (1981).Merrick and Merrick (1986) found that survival was unrelated to age, sex or cell type, but that bone pain and abnormal bone scintigraphy were both independently associated with significantly reduced survival.

A bone scan should be obtained in all patients with lung cancer and clinical or biochemical evidence of bone metastases. It has recently been suggested that patients with clinical evidence of non-skeletal metastases should also be studied by bone scanning and CT of the brain as clinical abnormalities were not specific for the organ in which metastases were subsequently detected (Quinn et al. 1986). A bone scan is also indicated in all patients with potentially resectable tumours, even if asymptomatic for bone metastases in view of the poor prognosis associated with metastases and the significant morbidity and mortality associated with surgery which has no possibility of success in the presence of distant metastases.

The bone scan will be abnormal in patients with hypertrophic pulmonary osteoarthropathy (HPOA), with findings ranging from localised bracelet-like activity to generalised uptake in the long bones (Lopez-Majano and Sobti 1984).

The long bones may show intense pericortical activity, the so-called double stripe or tramline sign (Terry et al. 1975) (Fig. 3.17). The scan evidence of HPOA may resolve quickly after treatment of the primary tumour and normalisation within 1 month of radiation therapy and surgical resection has been reported, although radiographs showed no change (Freeman and Tonkin 1976).

Neuroblastoma

The bone scan plays an important role in the evaluation of children with neuroblastoma. Howman-Giles et al. (1979) found abnormal bone scans in 29 of 63 patients and Podarsky et al. (1983) abnormalities in 21 of 42 scans. It is not clear from these studies what proportion of the children were studied at presentation and how many during follow-up. They reported that some false-positive results occur and that there are also false negatives, due in some cases to symmetrical metastases in the metaphyses of the long bones. Both studies also recorded a high frequency of tracer uptake in the primary tumours. The primary tumour uptake does not correlate with tumour calcification (Podarsky et al. 1983; Smith et al. 1980). Daubenton et al. (1987) have recently considered the prognostic value of bone scintigraphy in neuroblastoma. They concluded the scintigraphic evidence of bone metastases has a very poor prognosis irrespective of the results of other investigations.

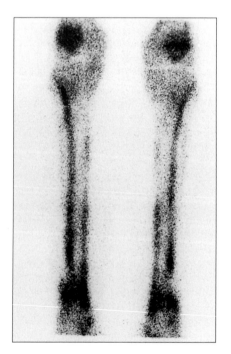

Fig. 3.17. Bone scan view of the tibiae showing increased tracer uptake along cortical borders (double stripe sign). The appearances are characteristic of HPOA.

The full assessment of patients presenting with neuroblastoma should include a bone scan in addition to a whole body study using [123]I- or ^{131}I-labelled metaiodobenzylguanidine (mIBG), specific uptake of which images metastatic disease elsewhere.

Other Tumours

A number of studies have been performed on the role of bone scanning in melanoma. In clinically early disease, Roth et al. (1975) reported an incidence of positive scans at presentation of 1 of 51 patients, Thomas et al. (1979) none of 74 and Aranha et al. (1979) none of 50. Au et al. (1984) found abnormalities in 5 of 112 patients with early disease, but all were false-positive scans. In more advanced disease Roth et al. (1975) had a positive scan rate of 2 of 15 and Thomas et al. (1979) 10 of 57. Fon et al. (1981) studied 50 patients who were mainly "symptomatic or stage III" and found a positive scan rate of 26 in 50, confirmed in "most cases" to be metastases by bone biopsy. Fon et al. (1981) also commented on osteolytic lesions on radiology giving rise to false-negative bone scans. Muss et al. (1979) carried out bone scans in patients with advanced melanoma. True-positive results were found in 14 of 49 patients, with a further false-positive. All patients with an abnormal scan had bone pain. None of the 13 patients with bone pain but negative scans developed evidence of metastases on follow-up.

Routine bone scanning is not justifiable for asymptomatic patients presenting with stage I or II melanoma, but is a reasonable part of the initial evaluation of patients with more advanced disease. Radiographs should be obtained of all sites which are symptomatic, but normal on bone scan, to ensure that osteolytic lesions are not missed.

Bone metastases are common in thyroid cancer. In the case of well-differentiated tumours the metastases may remain functional and can be detected by whole body ^{131}I scanning. Hoefnagel et al. (1986) have suggested that the potassium analogue thallium-201 is superior to ^{131}I for whole-body imaging in thyroid cancer. DeGroot and Reilly (1984) have compared various investigations (including bone scanning) in 108 patients with thyroid cancer. They concluded that bone scans were useful in patients who were complaining of bone pain or had known metastases elsewhere but were of no value in the routine follow-up of asymptomatic patients previously treated for thyroid cancer.

In medullary carcinoma of the thyroid, Johnson et al. (1984) found bone scanning to be of value in locating skeletal metastases in patients with elevated serum calcium.

Alimentary tumours rarely metastasise to bone, except in advanced disease, and the little evidence in the literature suggests that bone scanning should be performed only when the patient has clinical evidence of bone metastases (Antoniades et al. 1976; Hatfield et al. 1976; Vider et al. 1977). In head and neck tumours a similar conclusion has been reached (Wolfe et al. 1979; Belson et al. 1980).

References

Alexander JL, Gillespie PJ, Edelstyn GA (1982) Serial bone scanning using technetium 99m diphosphonate in patients undergoing cyclical combination chemotherapy for advanced breast cancer. Clin Nucl Med 7:397–402

Antoniades J, Croll MN, Walner RJ, Brady LW, McKhann CB (1976) Bone scanning in carcinoma of the colon and rectum. Dis Colon Rectum 19:139–143

Aranha GV, Simmons RL, Gunnarsson A, Grage TB (1979) The value of preoperative screening procedures in stage I and II malignant melanoma. J Surg Oncol 11:1–6

Au FC, Maier WP, Malmud LS, Goldman LI, Clark WH (1984) Preoperative nuclear scans in patients with melanoma. Cancer 53:2095–2097

Babaian RJ, Johnson DE, Llamas L, Ayala AG (1980) Metastases from transitional cell carcinoma of urinary bladder. Urology 16:142–144

Baker RR (1978) Preoperative assessment of the patient with breast cancer. Surg Clin North Am 64:1039–1050.

Bassan JS, Glaser MG (1982) Bony metastases in carcinoma of the uterine cervix. Clin Radiol 33:623–625

Beals RK, Lawton GD, Swell WE (1971) Prophylactic internal fixation of the femur in metastatic breast cancer. Cancer 28:1350–1354

Belson TP, Lehman RH, Chobanian DL, Malin TC (1980) Bone and liver scans in patients with head and neck carcinoma. Laryngoscope 90:1291–1296

Berger GL, Sadlowski RW, Sharpe JR, Finney RP (1981) Lack of value of routine preoperative bone and liver scans in cystectomy candidates. J Urol 125:637–639

Biersack HJ, Wegner G, Distelmaier W, Krause U (1980) Ossare Metastasierung des Prostatakerzinoms in Abhangigkeit von Tumorgrosse und Geschwulstdifferenzienung. Nuklearmedizin 19:29–32

Bishop HM, Blamey RW, Morris AH, Rose DH, Preston B, Lane J, Doyle PJ (1979) Bone scanning: its lack of value in the follow-up of patients with breast cancer. Br J Surg 66:752–754

Bitran LD, Beukerman C, Pinsky S (1981) Sequential scintigraphic staging of small cell carcinoma. Cancer 47:1971–1975

Bourgeois P, Gassavelis C, Malarme M, Feremans W, Fruhling J (1989) Bone marrow scintigraphy in breast cancer. Nucl Med Commun 10:389–400

Brismar J, Gustafson T (1988) Bone scintigraphy in staging of bladder carcinoma. Acta Radiologica 29:251–252

British Breast Group (1978) Bone scanning in breast cancer. Br Med J ii:180–181

Brown ML (1983) Significance of the solitary lesion in pediatric bone scanning. J Nucl Med 24:114–115

Ciatto S, Pacini P, Bravetti P, Cataliotta L, Cardona G, Crescioli R, Pupi A (1985) Staging breast cancer – screening for occult metastases. Tumori 71:339–344

Citrin DL, Bessent RG, Greig WR (1977) A comparison of the sensitivity and accuracy of the Tc^{99m} phosphate bone scan and skeletal radiograph in the diagnosis of bone metastases. Clin Radiol 28:107–117

Citrin DL, Furnival CM, Bessent RG, Greig WR, Bell G, Blumgart LH (1976) Radioactive technetium phosphate bone scanning in preoperative assessment and follow-up study of patients with primary carcinoma of the breast. Surg Gynecol Obstet 143:360–364

Chaudary MA, Maisey MN, Shaw P, Rubens RD, Hayward JL (1983) Sequential bone scanning and chest radiographs in the postoperative management of early breast cancer. Br J Surg 70:517–518

Clyne CAC, Frank JW, Jenkins JD, Smart CJ (1983) The place of ^{99m}Tc-polyphosphonate bone scan in renal carcinoma. Br J Urol 55:174–175

Coleman, RE, Habibollahi R, Rubens RD, Fogelman I (1986) Bone scintigraphy in early breast cancer: The relevance of tumour characteristics in identifying patients for serial scanning. Nucl Med Commun 7:292

Coleman, RE, Rubens, RD (1985) Bone metastases and breast cancer. Cancer Treat Rev 12:251–270

Coleman RE, Rubens RD (1987) The clinical course of bone metastases from breast cancer. Br J Cancer 55:61–66

Coleman RE, Rubens RD, Fogelman I (1988a) Bone scan flare predicts successful systemic therapy for bone metastases. J Nucl Med 29:1345–1349

Coleman RE, Rubens RD, Fogelman I (1988b) A reappraisal of the baseline bone scan in breast cancer. J Nucl Med 29:1045–1049

Coleman RE, Rubens RD, Meier C, Fogelman I (1987) A clinical comparison of two bone scanning agents in breast cancer (Abstract). Nucl Med Commun 8:245–246

Constable AR, Cranage RW (1981) Recognition of the superscan in prostatic bone scintigraphy. Br J Radiol 54:122–125

Corcoran RJ, Thrall JH, Kyle RW (1976) Solitary abnormalities in bone scans of patients with extraosseous malignancies. Radiology 121:663–667

Corrie D, Timmons JH, Bauman JH, Thompson IM (1988) Efficacy of follow-up scans in carcinoma of prostate. Cancer 61:195–202

Daubenton JD, Fisher RM, Karabus CD, Mann MD (1987) The relationship between prognosis and scintigraphic evidence of bone metastases in neuroblastoma. Cancer 59:1586–1589

Davey P, Merrick MV, Duncan W, Padpath AT (1985) Bladder cancer: the value of routine bone scintigraphy. Clin Radiol 36:77–79

Davies CJ, Griffiths PA, Preston BJ, Morris AH, Elston CW, Blamey RW(1977) Staging breast cancer. Role of scanning. Br Med J ii:603–605

DeGroot LJ, Reilly M (1984) Use of isotope bone scans and skeletal survey x-rays in the follow-up of patients with thyroid carcinoma. J Endocrinol Invest 7:175–179

Donato AT, Ammerman EG, Sullesta O (1979) Bone scanning in the evaluation of the patients with lung cancer. Ann Thorac Surg 27:300–304

Drelichman A, Decker A, Al-Sarraf M, Vaitkevicius VK, Muz J (1984) Computerised bone scan. A potentially useful technique to measure response in prostatic carcinoma. Cancer 53:1061–1065

Du Toit JP, Grove DV (1987) Radio-isotope bone scanning for the detection of occult bony metastases in invasive cervical carcinoma. Gynecol Oncol 28:215–219

Edelstyn GA, Gillespie PJ, Grebell FS (1967) The radiological demonstration of osseous metastases: experimental observations. Clin Radiol 18:158–162

El Domeiri AA, Shroff S (1976) Role of preoperative bone scan in carcinoma of the breast. Surg Gynecol Obstet 142:722–724

Fogelman I (1982) Diphosphonate bone scanning agents – current concepts. Eur J Nucl Med 7:506–509

Fogelman I (1987) Tc^{99m} Bone scanning agents. In: Fogelman I (ed) Bone scanning in clinical practice. Springer-Verlag, London, pp 31–40

Fogelman I, Coleman R (1988) The bone scan in breast cancer. In: Freeman L, Weissman H (eds) Nuclear medicine annual. Raven Press, New York, pp 1–38

Fogelman I, McKillop JH, Greig WR, Boyle IT (1977) Absent kidney sign associated with symmetrical and uniformly increased uptake of tracer by the skeleton. Eur J Nucl Med 2:257–260

Fon GT, Wong WS, Gold RH, Kaiser LR (1981) Skeletal metastases of melanoma. AJR 137:103–108

Francis MD, Fogelman I (1987) Tc^{99m} diphosphonate uptake mechanism on bone. In: Fogelman I (ed) Bone scanning in clinical practice Springer Verlag, Berlin Heidelberg New York, pp 7–17

Freeman MH, Tonkin AK (1976) Manifestations of hypertrophic pulmonary osteoarthropathy in patients with carcinoma of the lung. Demonstration by ^{99m}Tc pyrophosphate bone scans. Radiology 120:363–365

Furnival CM, Blumgart LH, Citrin DL, McKillop JH, Fogelman I, Greig WR (1980) Serial scintiscanning in breast cancer: Indications and prognostic value. Clin Oncol 6:25–32.

Galasko CSB (1975) The significance of occult skeletal metastases, detected by scintigraphy, in patients with otherwise early breast cancer. Br J Surg 56:757–764

George MJ (1988) Natural history of localised prostatic cancer managed by conservative therapy alone. Lancet i:494–497

Gerber FH, Goodreau JJ, Kirchner PT, Fonty WJ (1977) Efficacy of preoperative and postoperative bone scanning in the management of breast carcinoma. N Engl J Med 297:300–303

Gilbert HB, Kagan AR (1976) Metastases: incidence, detection and evaluation. In: Weiss L (ed) Fundamental aspects of metastases. Elsevier, Amsterdam pp 385–405

Gillespie PJ, Alexander JL, Edelstyn GA (1975) Changes in ^{87m}Sr concentrations in skeletal metastases in patients responding to cyclical combination chemotherapy for advanced breast cancer. J Nucl Med 16:191–193

Goris ML, Bretille J (1985) Skeletal scintigraphy for the diagnosis of malignant metastatic disease to the bones. Radiother Oncol 3:319–329

Gravenstein S, Peltx MA, Poreis W (1979) How ominous is an abnormal scan in bronchogenic carcinoma? JAMA 241:2523–2524

Gray HW (1987) Soft tissue uptake of bone agents. In: Fogelman I (ed) Bone scanning in clinical practice. Springer-Verlag, Berlin Heidelberg New York, pp 211–235

Greenberg EJ, Chu FCH, Dwyer AJ, Ziminski EM, Dimisch AB Laughlin JS (1972) Effects of radiation therapy on bone lesions as measured by ^{47}Ca and ^{85}Sr local kinetics. J Nucl Med 13:747–751

Harbert JC, Rocha L, Smith FO, Delgado G (1982) The efficacy of radionuclide bone scans in the evaluation of gynecological cancers. Cancer 49:1040–1042

Hatfield DR, DeLand FH, Maruyama Y (1976) Skeletal metastases in pancreatic cancer: a study by isotope bone scanning. Oncology 33:44–47

Hayward JL, Carbone PP, Heuson JC, Kumoaka S, Sgaloff A, Rubens RD (1977) Assessment of response to therapy in advanced breast cancer. Eur J Cancer 13:89–94

Hayward SJ, McIvor J, Burdge AH, Jewkes RF, Williams G (1987) Staging of prostatic cancer with radionuclide bone scintigraphy and lymphography. Br J Radiol 60:79–81

Hetherington JW, Siddall JK, Cooper EH (1988) Contribution of bone scintigraphy, prostatic acid phosphatase and prostatic specific antigen to the monitoring of prostatic cancer. Eur Urol 14:1–5

Hoefnagel CA, Delprat CC, Marcuse HR, de Viilder JJM (1986) Role of thallium-201 total-body scintigraphy in follow-up of thyroid carcinoma. J Nucl Med 27:1854–1857

Hooper RG, Beechler CR, Johnson MC (1978) Radioisotope scanning in the initial staging of bronchogenic carcinoma. Am Rev Resp Dis 118:279–286

Howman-Giles RB, Gilday DL, Ash JM (1979) Radionuclide skeletal survey in neuroblastoma. Radiology 131:497–502

Huben RP, Schellhammer PF (1982) The role of routine follow up bone scans after definitive therapy of localised prostatic cancer. J Urol 128:510–512

Johnson DG, Coleman RE, McCook TA, Dale JK, Wells SA (1984) Bone and liver images in medullary carcinoma of the thyroid. J Nucl Med 25:419–422

Joo KG, Parthasarathy KL, Bakshi SP, Rosner D (1979) Bone scintigrams: Their clinical usefulness in patients with breast carcinoma. Oncology 36:94–98

Kamath CRV, Maruyama Y, De Land FH, van Nagell JR (1982) Value of bone scanning in detecting occult skeletal metastases from adenocarcinoma of the endometrium. Diagn Gynecol Obstet 4:155–158

Kamath CRV, Maruyama Y, De Land FH, van Nagell JR (1983) Role of bone scanning for evaluation of carcinoma of the cervix. Gynecol Oncol 15:171–185

Katz RD, Alderson PO, Rosenhein NB, Bowerman JW, Wagner HN Jr (1979) Utility of bone scanning in detecting occult metastases from cervical carcinoma. Radiology 133:469–472

Kelly RJ, Cason RJ, Ferrie CB (1979) Efficacy of radionuclide scanning in patients with lung cancer. JAMA 242:2855–2857

Khansur T, Haick A, Patel B, Balducci L, Vance R, Thigpen T (1987) Evaluation of bone scan as a screening work-up in primary and loco-regional recurrence of breast cancer. Am J Clin Oncol 10:167–170

Kies MS, Baker AW, Kennedy PS (1978) Radionuclide scans in staging of carcinoma of the lung. Surg Gynecol Obstet 147:175–176

Kim EE, Bledin AG, Gutierrez C, Haynie TP (1983) Comparison of radionuclide images and radiographs for skeletal metastases from renal cell carcinoma. Oncology 40:284–286

Kishi K, Horita T, Matsumoto K, Kakizoe T, Murase T, Fujita J (1981) Carcinoma of bladder: A clinical and pathological analysis of 87 autopsy cases. Urology 125:36–39

Kober B, Hermann HJ, Wetzel E (1979) "Cold lesions" in bone scintigraphy. Fortschr Rotgenstr 131:545–551

Koizumi K, Tonami N, Hisada K (1981) Diffusely increased Tc-99m MDP uptake in both kidneys. Clin Nucl Med 6:362–365

Komaki R, Cox, JD, Eisert RD (1977) Irradiation of bronchial carcinoma. II. Pattern of spread and potential for prophylactic irradiation. Int J Radiat Oncol Biol Phys 2:441–446

Komaki R, Donegan W, Manoli R, Teh EL (1979) Prognostic value of pretreatment bone scans in breast cancer. AJR 132:877–881

Kunkler IH, Merrick MV, Rodger A (1985) Bone scintigraphy in breast cancer: a nine year follow-up. Clin Radiol 36:279–282

Levenson RM, Sauerbrunn BJL, Bates HR, Newman RD, Eddy JL, Ihde DC (1983) Comparative value of bone scintigraphy and radiography in monitoring tumour response in systemically treated prostatic cancer. Radiology 146:513–518

Levenson RM, Saubrunn BJL, Ihde DE et al. (1981) Small cell cancer: radionuclide bone scans for assessment of tumour extent and response. AJR 137:31–35

Lindner A, Dekernion JB (1982) Cost effectiveness of pre cystectomy radioisotopic scans. J Urol 128:1181–1182

Lindholm A, Lundell L, Martenson B, Thulin A (1979) Skeletal scintigraphy in the initial assessment of women with breast cancer. Acta Chir Scand 145:513–518

Lopez-Majano V, Sobti P (1984) Early diagnosis of pulmonary osteoarthropathy in neoplastic disease. J Nucl Med Allied Sci 28:69–76

Lund F, Smith PH, Suciu S (1984) Do bone scans predict prognosis in prostatic cancer? Br J Urol 56:58–63

Marsoni S, Hurson S, Eisenberg M (1985) Chemotherapy of bone metastases. In: Garratini S (ed) Bone resorption, metastasis and diphosphonates. Raven Press, New York, pp 181–194

McGregor B, Tulloh AGS, Quinlan MF, Lovegrove F (1978) The role of bone scanning in the assessment of prostatic carcinoma. Br J Urol 50:178–181

McNeil BJ (1984) Value of bone scanning in malignant disease. Semin Nucl Med 14:277–286

McNeil BJ, Pace PD, Gray EB, Adelstein SJ, Wilson RE (1978) Preoperative and follow-up bone scans in patients with primary carcinoma of the breast. Surg Gynecol Obstet 147:745–748

McNeil BJ, Polak JF (1981) An update on the rationale for the use of bone scans in selected metastatic and primary bone tumours. In: Pauwels EKJ, Schutte HE, Taconis WK (eds) Bone scintigraphy. Leiden University Press, Leiden, pp 187–208

Merrick MV (1987a) The normal bone scan. In: Fogelman I (ed) Bone scanning in clinical practice. Springer-Verlag, Berlin Heidelberg New York, pp 19–20

Merrick MV (1987b) Bone scintigraphy in testicular tumours. Br J Urol 60:167–169

Merrick MV (1989) Bone scintigraphy – an update. Clin Radiol 40:231–232

Merrick MV, Ding CL, Chisholm GD, Elton RD (1985) Prognostic significance of alkaline and acid phosphatase and skeletal scintigraphy in carcinoma of the prostate. Br J Urol 57:715–720

Merrick MV, Merrick JM (1986) Bone scintigraphy in lung cancer: a reappraisal. Br J Radiol 59:1185–1194

Mettler FA, Christie JH, Garcia JF, Baldwin MH, Wicks JD, Barstow SA (1981) Radionuclide liver and bone scanning in the evaluation of patients with endometrial carcinoma. Radiology 141:777–780

Moneypenny IJ, Grieve RJ, Howell A, Morrison JM (1984) The value of serial bone scanning in operable breast cancer. Br J Surg 71:466–468

Muss HB, Richards F, Barnes PL, Willand VV, Cowan R (1979) Radionuclide scanning in patients with advanced malignant melanoma. Clin Nucl Med 4:516–518

Narayam F, Lillian D, Hellstrom W, Hedgcock M, Jajodian PB, Tanagho EA (1988) The benefits of combining early radionuclide renal scintigraphy with routine bone scans in patients with prostatic cancer. J Urol 140:1448–1451

Nomura Y, Kondo H, Yamagata J et al. (1978) Evaluation of liver and bone scanning in patients with early breast cancer, based on results obtained from more advanced patients. Eur J Cancer 14:1129–1136

Nordman E, Marjamaki H, Tannila O (1977) The reliability of Tc^{99m} pyrophosphate scintigraphy in the diagnosis of bony metastases. Ann Clin Res 9:31–34

O'Donoghue EP, Constable AR, Sherwood T, Stevenson JJ, Chisholm GD (1978) Bone scanning and plasma phosphatases in carcinoma of the prostate. Br J Urol 50:172–177

Operchal JA, Bowden RD, Grove RB (1976) Efficacy of radionuclide procedures in the staging of bronchogenic carcinoma. J Nucl Med 17:530 (abstract).

Padmanabhan N, Howell A, Rubens RD (1986) Mechanism of action of adjuvant chemotherapy in early breast cancer. Lancet ii:411–414

Parsarathy KL, Lansberg R, Bakshi SP, Donoghue G, Merrin C (1978) Detection of bone metastases in urological malignancies utilising ^{99m}Tc-labelled phosphate compound. Urology 11:99–102

Paulson DF and the Uro-Oncology Research Group (1979) The impact of current staging procedures in assessing disease extent of prostatic adenocarcinoma. J Urol 121:300–302

Pauwels EKJ, Heslinga JM, Zwaveling A (1982) Value of pre-treatment and follow-up skeletal scintigraphy in operable breast cancer. Clin Oncol 8:25–32

Perez DJ, Powles TJ, Milan J, Gazet JC, Ford HT, McCready VR, Macdonald JS, Coombs RC (1983) Detection of breast carcinoma metastases in bone: Relative merits of x-rays and skeletal scintigraphy. Lancet ii:613–616

Podarsky AER, Stark DD, Hattner RS, Goodling GA, Moss AA (1983). Radionuclide bone scanning in neuroblastoma: skeletal metastases and primary tumour localisation of ^{99m}Tc-MDP. AJR 141:469–472

Pollen JJ, Gerber K, Ashburn WL, Schmidt JD (1981) Nuclear bone imaging in metastatic cancer of the prostate. Cancer 47:1585–1594

Quinn DL, Ostrow LB, Porter DK, Shelton DR, Jackson DE (1986) Staging of non small cell bronchogenic carcinoma. Relationship of clinical evaluation to organ scans. Chest 89:270–275

Ralston S, Fogelman I, Gardner MD, Boyle IT (1982) Hypercalcaemia and metastatic bone disease: is there a causal link? Lancet ii:903–905

Ramsdell JW, Peters RM, Taylor AT, Alazrak NP, Tisi GM (1977) Multiorgan scans for staging of lung cancer: correlation with clinical evaluation. J Thorac Cardiovasc Surg 73:653–659

Rappaport AH, Hoffer PB, Genant HK (1978) Unifocal bone findings by scintigraphy. Clinical significance in patients with known primary cancer. West Med 129:188–192

Reddy PS, Merrick MV (1983) Skeletal scintigraphy in carcinoma of the kidney. Br J Urol 55:171–173

Rosen PR, Murphy KG (1984) Bone scintigraphy in the initial staging of patients with renal cell carcinoma. J Nucl Med 25:289–291

Rosenthall L, Stern J, Arzoumanian A (1982) A clinical comparison of MDP and DMAD. Clin Nucl Med 7:403–406

Rossleigh MA, Lovegrove FTA, Reynolds PM et al. (1984) The assessment of response to therapy of bone metastases in breast cancer. Aust NZ J Med 14:19–22

Roth JA, Eilber FR, Bennett LR, Morton DL (1975) Radionuclide photoscanning. Usefulness in preoperative evaluation of melanoma. Arch Surg 110:1211–1212

Shafer RB, Reinke DB (1977) Contribution of the bone scan, serum acid and alkaline phosphatase and radiographic bone survey to the management of newly diagnosed carcinoma of the prostate. Clin Nucl Med 2:200–203

Shearer RJ, Constable AR, Girling M, Hendry WF, Fergusson JD (1974) Radiographic bone scintigraphy with the gamma camera in the investigation of prostatic cancer. Br Med J ii:362–365

Shih WJ, Purcell M, Domstad PA (1986) Evolving scintigraphic pattern of skeletal metastases from prostatic carcinoma. J Nucl Med 27:1786–1788

Sklaroff RB, Sklaroff DM (1976) Bone metastases from breast cancer at the time of radical mastectomy. Cancer 38:107–111

Smith FW, Gilday DL, Ash JM, Reid RH (1980) Primary neuroblastoma uptake of 99m-technetium methylene diphosphonate. Radiology 137:501–504

Smith ML, Martin W, McKillop JH, Fogelman I (1984) Improved lesion detection with dimethyl-amino-diphosphonate: A report of two cases. Eur J Nucl Med 9:519–520

Soloway MS, Hardeman SW, Hickey D, Raymond J, Todd BN, Soloway S, Moinuddin M (1988) Stratification of patients with metastatic prostatic cancer based on extent of disease on initial bone scan. Cancer 61:195–202

Spencer GR, Khan M, Bird C, Seymour R, Brown TR, Collins CD (1981) Is bone scanning of value in patients with breast cancer? Acta Chir Scand 147:247–248

Sundkvist CMG, Ahlgren L, Lilja B, Mattson S, Abrahamson PA, Wadstrom LB (1988) Repeated quantitative bone scintigraphy in patients with prostatic carcinoma treated with orchiectomy. Eur J Nucl Med 14:203–206

Sven NR, Karstens JH, Gloeckner W, Steinstrasser A, Schwarz A, Ammon J, Buell U (1989) Radioimmunoimaging for diagnosis of bone marrow involvement in breast cancer and malignant lymphoma. Lancet i:299–301

Terry DW, Isitman AI, Holmes RA (1975) Radionuclide bone images in hypertrophic pulmonary osteoarthropathy. AJR 124:571–576

Thomas JH, Panoussopoulus D, Liesmann GE, Jewell WR, Preston DF (1979) Scintiscans in the evaluation of patients with malignant melanoma. Surg Gynecol Obstet 149:574–576

Thomsen HS, Rasmussen D, Munck O, Lund JO, Gerhard-Nielsen V, Terkildsen T, Dombernowsky P, Andersen KW (1987). Bone metastases in primary operable breast cancer. The role of a yearly scintigraphy. Eur J Cancer Clin Oncol 23:779–781

Turner P, Haggith JW (1981) Preoperative radionuclide scanning in bronchogenic carcinoma. Br J Dis Chest 75:291–294

Vest SA (1954) Prostatic malignancy. Clin Symp 6:93–103

Vider M, Maruyama Y, Narvaez R (1977) Significance of the vertebral venous (Batson's) plexus in metastatic spread in colorectal cancer. Cancer 40:67–71

Wahner HW, Kyle RA, Beabout JW (1980) Scintigraphic evaluation of the skeleton in multiple myeloma. Mayo Clin Proc 55:739–746

Waxman AD, Siensen JK, Levine AM (1981) Radiographic and radionuclide imaging in multiple myeloma: the role of gallium scintigraphy. J Nucl Med 22:232–236

Wickerham L, Fisher B, Cronin W, members of the NSABP Committee for treatment failure. (1984)

The efficacy of bone scanning in the follow-up of patients with operable breast cancer. Breast Cancer Res Treat 4:303–307

Wilkinson MJS, Howell A, Harris M, Adam NM, Lupton E, Johnson RJ, Sellwood RA (1985) Retroperitoneal tumour infiltration detected by bone scanning in patients with infiltrating lobular carcinoma of the breast. Br J Surg 72:626–628

Wolfe JA, Rowe LD, Lowry LD (1979) Value of radionuclide scanning in the staging of head and neck carcinoma. Ann Otol Rhinol Laryngol 88:832–836

Wolfenden JM, Pitt MJ, Durie BGW, Moon TE (1980) Comparison of bone scintigraphy and radiology in multiple myeloma. Radiology 134:723–728

Yeates MG, Tan PKS, Broadfoot E, Green D, Morris JG (1972) Bone scanning with technetium polyphosphate. Preliminary results. Australas Radiol 16:393–400

4 Radiology

Sheila Rankin

Skeletal Survey

The skeleton is a common site for metastases from many primary tumours. The apparent distribution and frequency of metastases are influenced by the method of investigation used to identify them.

The initial radiological investigation for the diagonsis of bone metastases is a skeletal survey which, based on the usual distribution of metastases, normally includes a lateral skull and cervical spine, antero-posterior (AP) and lateral thoracic and lumbar spine, an AP pelvis and a chest radiograph at low KVp to visualise the ribs optimally. Extremity radiographs are not normally performed unless there is a clinical indication. The alternative investigation is an isotope bone scan which is described in detail in Chap. 3. Of skeletal metastases in men, 60% arise from the prostate and in women 70% come from the breast. In children the commonest primaries giving rise to skeletal deposits are neuroblastoma and Ewing's sarcoma.

Distribution and Routes of Spread

The axial skeleton is predominantly affected. This is rich in red marrow with a large capillary network and sluggish blood flow which may be suitable for the growth of tumour. The lumbar spine is most commonly affected, followed by the thoracic and cervical spine. This may be due to Batson's plexus and the large bone mass in the spine, although in part the effect may be spurious, due to sampling techniques, as the spine is the most accessible part at post mortem. The other common sites in order of decreasing frequency are pelvis, ribs, sternum, femur, humeral shaft and skull. Many of these sites contain red marrow and most metastases are in the medulla with secondary involvement of the cortex. The mandible is rarely affected although it is typically involved in myeloma. The patella and the extremities distal to the elbow and knee are unusual sites for metastases, probably because the route of access is arterial only and there is no red bone marrow.

Metastases may be cortical only. The cortex is supplied by two distinct but anastomosing vascular systems. One arises from the nutrient artery and the other from the endosteal and periosteal vascular supply. Cortical metastases may develop from tumour emboli caught in this vascular network. The diaphysis of long bones is the site for 77% of cortical metastases, perhaps because cortical metastases are dependent on the cortical dimensions and the blood flow, which is maximal in the mid-shaft. Cortical metastases, which are nearly always lytic, were initially thought to be specific for bronchogenic cancer, but Coerkamp and Kroom (1988) found the primary to be renal in 31%, lung in 23% and the remaining primaries included hepatoma, thyroid, breast, melanoma and gastro-intestinal malignancy (Fig. 4.1).

There are four routes that may result in skeletal metastatic disease.

1. *Direct Invasion*. Soft tissue tumours may involve adjacent bone by direct extension into the underlying bone structures e.g., a Pancoast tumour (Fig. 4.2) involving the underlying ribs or a nasopharyngeal tumour extending through the base of the skull, although this would probably not be called true metastatic disease. Primary tumours may also metastasise and the metastases may involve adjacent bony structures e.g., lung cancer spreading into the mediastinum and then extending into the adjacent thoracic vertebrae. Invasion of bone by an adjacent tumour mass means there is a prominent soft tissue component with osseous destruction and stimulation of periosteal reaction. The outer cortex is

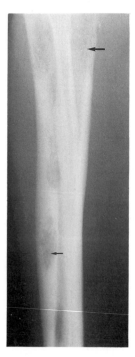

Fig. 4.1. Lytic metastases in the anterior cortex of the tibia (*small arrow*) from bronchogenic carcinoma. Larger deposit involving the medulla (*large arrow*).

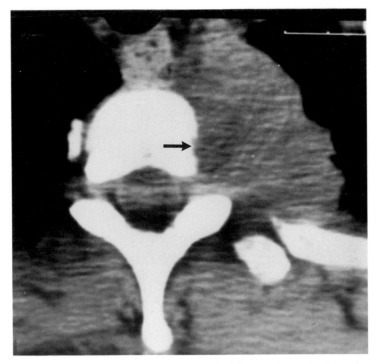

Fig. 4.2. Pancoast tumour eroding the underlying vertebral body (*arrow*).

involved initially with later involvement of the entire cortex and medulla. There is cortical erosion with a fluffy periosteal reaction and "moth-eaten" or permeative bone destruction associated with a soft tissue mass; this is well shown on computed tomography (CT) or plain radiographs. This allows differentiation from an intraosseous tumour which will affect the inner margin of the cortex and then the periosteum, with a secondary, usually smaller, soft tissue mass.

2. *Lymphatic Spread.* This is a relatively unimportant mode of spread. Deposits may occur in regionally draining lymph nodes which can secondarily affect adjacent bony structures. An important example is the vertebral destruction seen in pelvic malignancy, especially in carcinoma of the cervix. The presence of lumbar spine metastases with absent pulmonary metastases supports the theory of local spread via the lymphatic and venous plexus into the lumbar spine, rather than haematogenous dissemination.

Radiographically there is a paraspinal soft tissue mass with scalloped erosion of the underlying vertebral bodies. This occurs more frequently on the left than the right, supposedly related to the lymph nodes being closer to the spine on the left (Fig. 4.3). These changes are not specific for cervical cancer as they may be seen in lymphoma and myeloma.

3. *Haematogenous Spread.* This may be via the arterial or venous route. Venous involvement is commoner than arterial invasion. The venous route involves Batson's plexus of veins which surrounds the vertebrae. This is an intercommunicating system of thin-walled vessels with extensive communication

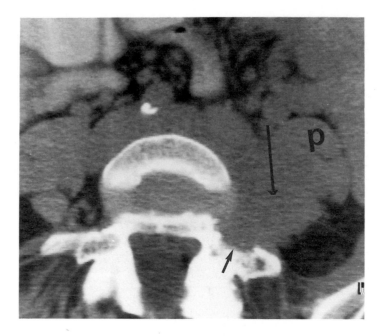

Fig. 4.3. Carcinoma of the cervix with lymph node deposits (*long arrow*) invading the transverse process of L4 (*arrow*). P, the psoas muscle.

with the veins of the spinal cord as well as the portal, caval, azygous, intercostal, pulmonary and renal venous systems. The plexus also communicates with veins from the breast, head and neck and the major vasa-vasorum of the extremities. The variety of the direction of flow means tumours from many sites may go anywhere in the course of the vessels.

4. *Intraspinal Spread.* The cerebrospinal fluid (CSF) is an additional pathway for the dissemination of secondaries from intracranial neoplasms. These seed down the spine as subarachnoid seedlings. One of the commonest tumours to do this is medulloblastoma in children, which gives rise to osteoblastic lesions in the vertebral bodies.

Radiographic Appearances

Radiographs are relatively insensitive in the diagnosis of skeletal metastases, particularly if medullary rather than cortical. More than 50% of the bone mineral content has to be lost before a metastasis is identifiable on a radiograph. Earlier recognition occurs if there is cortical involvement, but metastatic disease predominantly involves cancellous bone with cortical destruction a late manifestation. The alteration in bone density and architecture gives rise to three radiographic patterns: lytic, sclerotic and mixed.

Lytic metastases are the most common arising from breast, lung, thyroid, renal, adrenal and gastro-intestinal malignancies, but also occur in uterine cancer, Wilms' tumours, hepatomas and phaeochromocytomas (Fig. 4.4). The decrease in density is due either to bone destruction by the malignant cells or osteoclast stimulation with bone resorption. There is thinning or loss of trabecula and the margins are usually ill-defined, representing regions of partially destroyed trabeculae between the central destruction and the radiologically normal bone. The width of the margin reflects the aggressiveness of the lesion, with a narrow zone of transition in the less aggressive and, in the more aggressive, a poorly defined margin with a wide zone of transition. If the metastasis is in the medulla there is endosteal scalloping, with sub-periosteal scalloping or a focal cortical defect if the lesion is in the periosteum. The appearance of lesions may change during the course of the disease under the influence of local and systemic factors. Expansile metastases usually arise from kidney, thyroid or hepatoma and occasionally from the prostate.

Sclerotic metastases are usually from cancers of the prostate, lung, bladder and gastro-intestinal tract, but also from medulloblastoma, neuroblastoma and the breast. The sclerosis is due to stimulation of osteoblasts by the tumour cells or a host response with an attempt at healing with thickening and coarsening of the trabeculae (Aoki at al. 1986). The metastases are nodular, rounded, discrete and fairly well circumscribed (Fig. 4.5) or mottled irregular zones of increased bone density with ill-defined margins. There may be areas of normal appearing

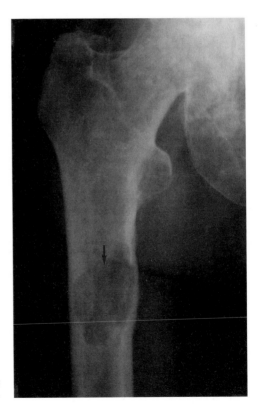

Fig. 4.4. Lytic metastasis (*arrow*) in the proximal femur from carcinoma of the breast.

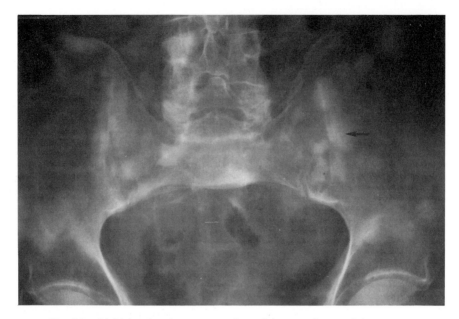

Fig. 4.5. Multiple sclerotic metastases (*arrow*) from carcinoma of the prostate.

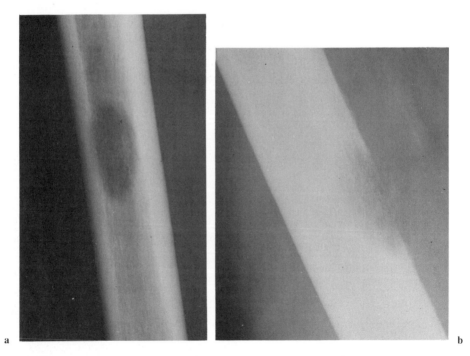

a   b

Fig. 4.6. **a** Lytic metastasis which appears to lie in the medulla on the AP film. **b** The importance of the lateral film which shows that it is actually in the cortex.

bone in an area of diffuse deposits. Periosteal reaction may be minimal or absent; however, if there is periosteal or endosteal deposition of bone deformity may occur similar to Paget's disease.

Metastases in the long bones are usually in the medulla of the diaphysis or metaphysis and are rarely cortical or subperiosteal. If they occur in the periosteum they are usually lytic and destructive with concave scalloping of the cortex. They may be ill-defined or sharply marginated depending on the growth rate. To separate cortical from medullary deposits two views at right angles may be required (Fig. 4.6). Pathological fractures may be the presenting feature in metastatic disease, as the metastases cause osseous weakening (Fig. 4.7). Tubular bones and the proximal portion of the femur are frequent sites of fracture. It is usually easy to separate benign from pathological fractures as the latter are through areas of rarefied bone with trabecular destruction and endosteal scalloping. In the spine there is compression or collapse of tumour-containing vertebrae with or without spinal cord compression. The danger of imminent fracture is poorly recognised on radiographs. It is likely to occur if more than 50% of the cortical surface is involved. CT may be a more accurate way of assessing the extent of cortical involvement and predicting fracture.

Soft tissue reaction is generally not a prominent feature with metastases, except in the ribs where there may be a large extrapleural mass. Soft tissue calcification may occur with or without local adjacent bony involvement,

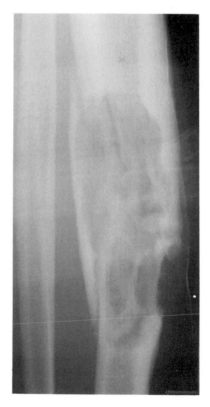

Fig. 4.7. Pathological fracture through a lytic metastasis from a soft tissue angiosarcoma.

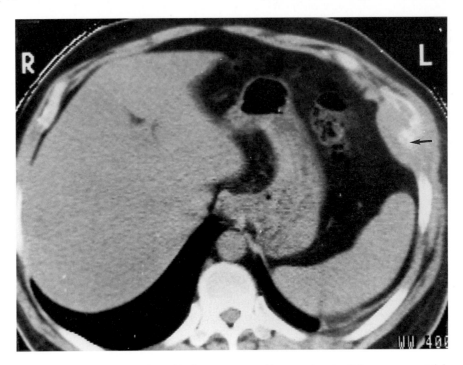

Fig. 4.8. Carcinoma of the colon with rib metastases, with a prominent soft tissue mass containing amorphous calcification (*arrow*).

especially in colonic, gastric, breast, lung and transitional cell cancer. The extent of the soft tissue abnormality and the ossification are better visualised on CT (Fig. 4.8).

Most metastases are multiple and, if the appearances are classical in a patient with known malignancy, the diagnosis is not usually in doubt. However 10% of bone metastases are solitary especially from lung, thyroid and kidney and if there is any doubt biopsy of the lesion should be undertaken.

Computed Tomography(CT)

CT scans have excellent soft tissue and contrast resolution and are superb for defining the soft tissue masses associated with bone metastases and also in demonstrating extradural deposits and nerve root compression. Associated lymphadenopathy is well visualised, although the presence of enlarged lymph nodes does not always indicate metastatic involvement as CT cannot differentiate between reactive hyperplasia in nodes and malignant lymphadenopathy. Bony destruction and sclerotic deposits are well shown. The CT signs in the spine indicative of metastases include:

1. Cortical bone discontinuity
2. Focal medullary trabecular loss
3. Focal medullary sclerosis unassociated with discogenic disease or other pathology
4. Soft tissue mass with bone destruction

CT is more sensitive than radiography in diagnosing spinal metastases. However, as the entire spine connot readily be scanned, CT is normally reserved for assessment of patients with positive isotope scans, but with negative radiographs, in an attempt to clarify the pathology (Fig. 4.9). Of patients with breast cancer with positive isotope scans and normal radiographs 50% had obvious bony metastases on CT, 25% had a benign cause for the increased uptake and in 25% no abnormality was demonstrated as a cause for the positive scan (Muindi et al. 1983) and none of these patients subsequently developed metastases. Similar results were obtained by Redmond et al. (1984).

CT should also be used in cases where the isotope scan is negative or suggests only degenerative disease especially if there are persisting clinical signs such as

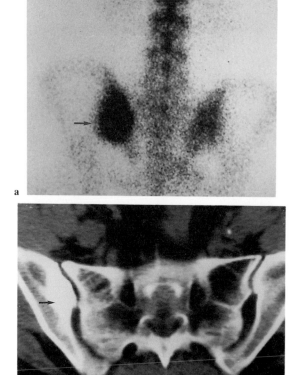

Fig. 4.9. a Area of increased tracer uptake in the right sacro-iliac joint in a patient with known breast cancer. Normal radiograph. Bone scan reversed to correspond with the CT scan. **b** CT scan shows sclerotic metastasis in the iliac wing (*arrow*).

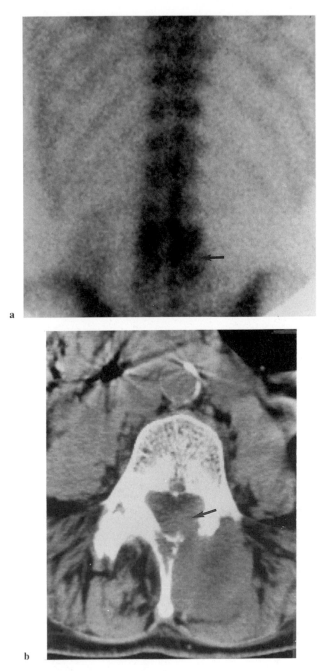

Fig. 4.10. **a** Bone scan reported as probable degenerative disease (*arrow*). Patient had severe back pain which was out of proportion to the degenerative changes on the radiographs. **b** CT scan shows destruction of the lamina of L4 with an associated soft tissue mass and extradural extension (*arrow*). Biopsy confirmed adenocarcinoma of unknown primary.

bone pain or neurological deficit to suggest focal deposits (Fig. 4.10). Isotope scans may be negative with very aggressive tumours; although an area of reduced uptake may be seen, this is more difficult to identify than an area of increased activity. It may be helpful to undertake CT, even if the radiographs are positive as the extent of the soft tissue mass and nerve compression is better seen (Fig. 4.11).

There have been no large clinical trials comparing the use of magnetic

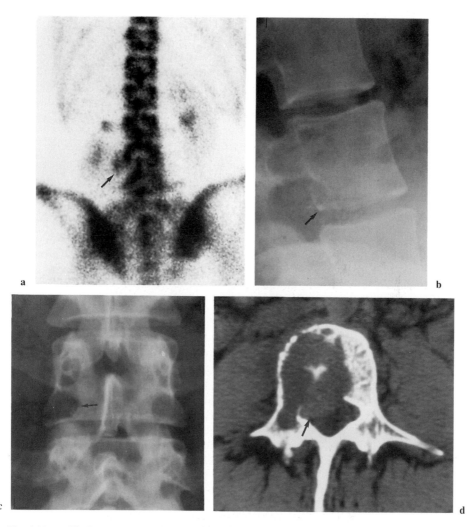

Fig. 4.11. **a** The bone scan was reported as showing increased uptake in the right transverse process of L4 (*arrow*) in a patient with known breast cancer and severe sciatica on the right. Bone scan reversed to correspond with the radiographs. **b** The lateral spinal radiograph shows a lytic metastasis in L4 with cortical irregularity (*arrow*) especially when compared with the vertebral body above. **c** The AP view shows subtle alteration in the bone density on the right (*arrow*). **d** The CT scan confirmed the metastasis but showed it was much more extensive than suspected and demonstrated the extradural component with compression of the nerve root and theca (*arrow*).

resonance imaging (MRI), CT and isotope scans, although undoubtedly MRI is very sensitive to changes in the medulla and there have already been case reports of positive MRI and CT scans with negative bone scans (Mehta et al. 1989), and MRI will no doubt be used more frequently in the future.

Radiological Appearances at Specific Sites

Skull. Osteolytic metastases vary in size and may be single or multiple. The edges are ill-defined and irregular, often with sclerotic margins. The metastases may involve the inner table, the outer table or the diploic space either alone or in combination. The differential diagnosis of a solitary lytic metastasis includes an epidermoid, haemangioma, eosinophilic granuloma or fibrous dysplasia. The osteosclerotic metastases are usually from carcinoma of the prostate and any part of the cranium may be involved; however, the base of the skull is a well-recognised site of involvement. The differential diagnosis includes Paget's disease, fibrous dysplasia and meningioma.

Spine. This is a frequent site of involvement, particularly of the lumbar and thoracic vertebrae. Large deposits may be present with relatively few symptoms. The patient may develop an enlarging mass with a pathological fracture and vertebral instability, leading to spinal cord compression which occurs in about 5% of cases. Of patients with epidural spinal metastases, 85% will have vertebral bone involvement, but extradural or intradural deposits may occur distant from the site of bony disease and therefore the plain films cannot be relied on to localise the level. Myelography or MRI will be required adequately to localise the level of cord compromised prior to surgery or radiotherapy. CT without intrathecal contrast can identify extradural deposits in the lower lumbar or upper cervical spine but for the remainder of the spine, and for intrathecal deposits, intrathecal contrast will required. A myelogram is usually performed initally via the lumbar route as the whole spine can be examined. If there is a complete block, a localised CT at the level of the block may obviate the need for the cervical puncture for, even if there appears to be no contrast going past the block on the conventional films, it will often be visualised on CT with its superior contrast resolution. CT may show the full extent of the block and any associated paraspinal soft tissue mass (Fig. 4.12), otherwise introduction of contrast via a cervical puncture may be required to outline the extent of the block. Myelography is an invasive procedure which may make the symptoms of the spinal cord compression worse and MRI will, in the future, be the investigation of choice.

Vertebral collapse due to metastatic breast, lung or prostate cancer may be difficult to differentiate from other non-neoplastic causes. Metastases are the most frequent cause if the upper thoracic spine is involved, particulary if there is an associated soft tissue mass with destruction and angulation, or irregular deformity of the end plates. The degree of collapse is greater with metastases and complete plattening (vertebra plana) may occur. If there is anterior wedging of the vertebral bodies and the involvement is non-uniform then osteoporosis should be considered. Unfortunately these appearances may co-exist with metastatic disease and biopsy may be required for differentiation.

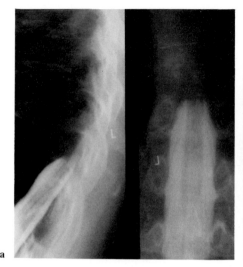
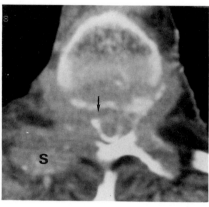

a   b

Fig. 4.12. **a** Myelogram showing complete block at the level of a collapsed thoracic vertebra in a patient with breast cancer and bony deposits. **b** CT scan performed after the myelogram demonstrates the extradural (*arrow*), bony and soft tissue deposits(s).

Sclerosis of vertebral bodies occurs in prostatic cancer, lymphoma, chordoma and rarely myeloma. The differential diagnosis includes Paget's disease and vertebral haemangioma. The pedicles may be involved in either sclerotic or lytic metastases. This helps to differentiate metastases from myeloma as the pedicles are rarely involved in this condition.

Radiological Appearance of Specific Metastases

Breast. The metastases are osteolytic or mixed and rarely blastic, although the morphology changes in response to therapy. Pathological fractures are common.

Lung. Both direct extension into adjacent ribs and distant metastases are common. The deposits may be sclerotic, lytic or mixed.

Prostate. Usually sclerotic. Occasionally sunburst periosteal reaction, where there is spiculated new bone formation will be observed (Bloom et al. 1987).

Renal. Direct extension into the renal lymphatics and the para-aortic nodes with involvement of the mediastinal nodes and there may also be direct invasion of the renal veins and thus the vascular system. Bony metastases are common in the spine, ribs and femora and tend to be osteolytic and expansile.

Thyroid. Metastases are single or multiple. They tend to be expansile and lytic and to involve the axial skeleton. The method of spread is haematogeneous. Medullary thyroid cancer metastases are often osteosclerotic.

Uterine and Cervical. These metastases invade the venous system and the regional lymphatics and there may be erosion of the underlying bones. The metastases tend to be osteolytic rather than osteosclerotic or mixed.

Comparison of Skeletal Survey and Isotope Bone Scans

Radiographs are not as sensitive as bone scanning in the detection of bone metastases. In a series of patients with breast cancer, isotope scans were positive in 84% and radiographs positive in 50%, with the additional lesions seen on the scans taking up to 18 months to become apparent on the radiographs (Galasko 1972).

These findings were confirmed, using radiographs or bone scans as the standard, with sensitivity 82% and specificity 79% for bone scans and sensitivity 72% with specificity 97% for radiographs (Hortobagyi et al. 1984). There was agreement in the initial detection in 51%–73% depending on the anatomical area involved, with radiographs better for the pelvis and ribs rather than the spine. In a much larger series of patients with breast cancer, using radiographs as the standard, isotope scans were positive in 96% with sensitivity 96%, in 14% of patients with positive bone scans and negative radiographs there were positive bone marrow aspirates (Kamby et al. 1987). Thus x-rays under-estimate the

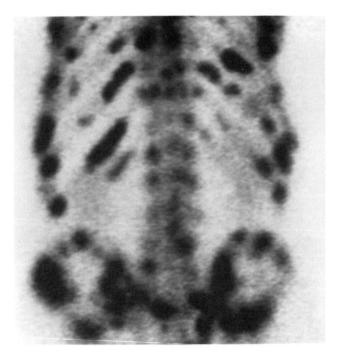

Fig. 4.13. Classical positive bone scan with multiple areas of increased uptake in a patient with prostatic cancer.

extent of disease, having a low sensitivity mainly because the cells grow in the marrow without involving the cortex.

Therefore the initial survey should be an isotope bone scan with radiographs of the abnormal areas, although many centres would perform a base-line skeletal survey. If there are clinical symptoms or a raised alkaline phosphatase, radiographs may be performed at the outset. The classical appearance of metastases on isotope scans is of multiple areas of increased uptake (Fig. 4.13). If a solitary focal abnormal area is identified it is very important to assess it fully as 34% of patients with known malignancy and solitary lesions on bone scans had a benign cause for the isotope abnormality (Corcoran et al. 1976). The probability of metastatic disease depended, to a certain extent, on the site of the lesion. In the axial skeleton 80% were metastases, but in the ribs only 17% were metastatic. When the results were correlated with the x-ray films, of the 58 who had metastases only 21 had abnormal radiographs. Similar results were obtained by Collins et al. (1979) and Mink (1987) who used both CT and isotope scans to guide the bone biopsy of questionable lesions.

Response to Treatment

The response of bony metastases to treatment has been well documented by Libshitz and Hortobagyi (1981), in a series of patients with breast cancer. The response on radiographs followed an orderly evolution and response was often identified within 3 months of commencing therapy. Lytic metastases, which are the easiest to evaluate and that are responding, develop a sclerotic rim. This may also be seen around lesions that were not previously detected and as healing progresses the area fills in centripetally until it is uniformly blastic, which may take several months or a year. The trabecular pattern may remain abnormal, but if healing continues the blastic area will regress with a return to normal of the density and trabecular appearance (Fig. 4.14). If there is progression of disease the lesions will increase in size or new areas of destruction may develop

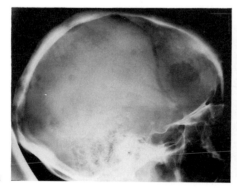
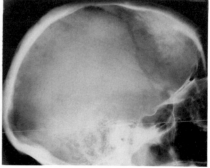

a   b

Fig. 4.14. **a** Multiple lytic metastases from breast cancer. **b** 5 months after treatment the bone texture has virtually returned to normal.

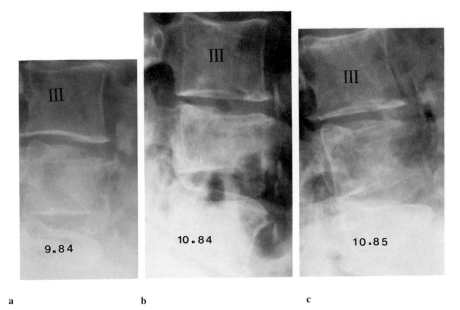

a   b   c

Fig. 4.15. a Lytic deposit in the vertebral body of L4 from carcinoma of the breast (September 1984). **b** After 6 weeks of treatment, there has been some healing with sclerosis and reformation of the anterior cortex (October 1984). **c** 1 year later the patient has relapsed with further bony destruction in previously involved areas (October 1985).

(Fig. 4.15). If there has been an initial response, then progression may be more difficult to identify. In these cases the size of the metastasis is identified by the sclerotic rim and if this area increases, then progression has occurred even if the sclerotic response is still identified. Progression may also be identified by loss of the sclerotic response in an area of previous disease. It is important to note the extent of response as it may be difficult to separate recrudescence of disease from generalised fading of a blastic lesion indicating healing.

Mixed lesions can be thought of as lytic metastases which have demonstrated a response and individual lesions can be evaluated in the same way. The appearance of a new mixed lesion during early follow-up may be confusing, as it may indicate healing in a previously undetected lesion, rather than progression. It is important to note the size of the area involved as response occurs at the periphery of the lesion, so an increase in size indicates progression, as does loss of an area of blastic response. Sclerotic lesions which respond fade to the normal trabecular pattern and density. Either an increasing area of blastic response or development of destruction in the sclerotic area indicates progression of disease. However, early focal destruction is difficult to differentiate from diffuse fading. Response to treatment may be difficult to evaluate due to the natural variability of metastases and if there is no base-line study it is impossible to distinguish between lytic metastases responding to treatment and the development of new mixed lesions.

There is some dispute over which modality should be used to monitor response. Hortobagyi et al. (1984) found agreement between the clinical response and the radiological evaluation in 79% of patients at 3 months and 85% at 6 months. The correlation for bone scans and clinical response was 36% at 3 months and 57% at 6 months. Although the bone scans were more sensitive they were less specific, thus a decrease in the activity on the scan may indicate improvement, or progression due to a decrease in osteoblastic activity in response to a growing metastasis, and an increase in activity could be due to progression or the "flare" response which indicates healing (see Chap. 3). These authors concluded that scans were insufficient for assessing response and that radiographs should continue to be used. Similarly in a small series of breast cancer patients treated with aminoglutethamide or adrenalectomy the clinical and radiological status concurred in 16 of 17 sites (Barry et al. 1981).

However, only 10% of patients with breast cancer who responded were correctly identified radiologically (Citrin et al. 1981). This low figure may partly be due to the small number of patients with lytic deposits in this series and the difficulty in assessing mixed and sclerotic lesions. In the patients who progressed on bone scans, radiography correctly identified 63%, and these authors suggested that isotope scans should be used to monitor response, with radiographs used as a supplementary investigation for lytic metastases and to confirm progression identified on the scans. Radiographs were also better for assessing pathological fractures.

Both serial scanning and radiographs were poor in showing objective response with a concordance with clinical findings in 12% for scans and 8% for radiographs (Bitran et al. 1980). Serial radiographs may be unreliable in assessing the significance of the flare response, distinguishing between healing flare and progressive disease in only 10% (Rossleigh et al. 1984). These authors found clinical response with an improvement in bone pain was very helpful in distinguishing between the healing flare response and progression.

The importance of clinical pain relief was stressed by Coombes et al. (1983) as changes on the radiographs occurred late or not at all. Isotope scans showed either progression or regression at an earlier stage, but pain relief was a good guide to response. These authors suggested that bone scans, particularly if there was a greater than 50% reduction in activity, and relief of bone pain were the most useful parameters of response to therapy.

Bellamy et al. (1987) compared CT and skeletal surveys in the assessment of lytic metastases and found CT helpful in assessing the response of lytic metastases to treatment. Using regions of interest and electronic callipers small changes in the attenuation of lesions can be assessed, but it is important to ensure that exactly the same region has been used each time and that the scanner is calibrated against an external standard if quantitative measurements are to be made. The signs of healing on CT include a decrease in associated soft tissue mass, remodelling of cortical bone and medullary architecture and an increase in the CT number (Hounsfield units) within the lesion. In many cases the changes are obvious and electronic measurements are not required (Fig. 4.16). CT concurred with the clinical impression in 67%, and in 86% where there was healing. The skeletal survey was concurrent in only 35% although this increased to 50% if localised views were performed. Bellamy et al. suggested that follow-up skeletal surveys to monitor clinical response were not justified and that a limited CT scan was a more sensitive and accurate method of monitoring response to therapy.

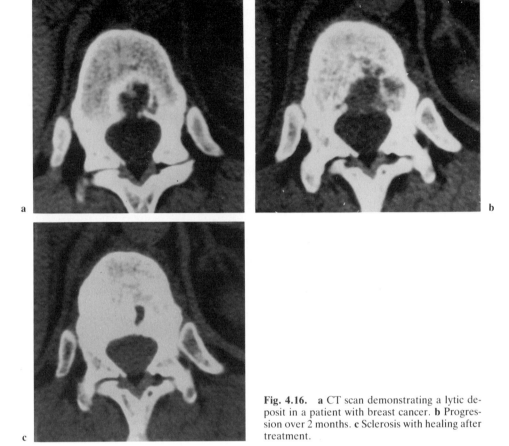

Fig. 4.16. **a** CT scan demonstrating a lytic deposit in a patient with breast cancer. **b** Progression over 2 months. **c** Sclerosis with healing after treatment.

Summary

Isotope bone scans are the investigation of choice for the initial assessment of bony metastases. Many units will also perform a skeletal survey at the same time to act as a base-line for later follow-up and also to confirm that there are not extensive aggressive lytic metastases that may be missed by the scan. If a skeletal survey is not performed, radiographs of abnormal areas in the bone scan should be undertaken to confirm lesions and for monitoring response. Monitoring response can also be by isotope scans, with localised radiographs of abnormal new areas and to confirm progression. Radiographs should be undertaken for localised bone pain and the assessment of suspected pathological fractures and may be used to follow lytic bone lesions.

More specific imaging may be required for particular clinical problems. MRI scans will become the preferred investigation for suspected spinal cord compression, and may be used increasingly for diagnosis and follow-up of metastatic disease. In the presence of specific neurological deficit or localised bone pain, particularly if the bone scan and radiographs are negative, other imaging modalities such as CT or MR should be undertaken to assess the full extent of the disease. With increasing availability, CT will be used more frequently to monitor response.

References

Aoki J, Yamamoto I, Hino M, Shigeno C, Kitamura N, Sone T et al. (1986) Sclerotic bone metastasis. Radiologic-pathologic correlation. Radiology 159:127–132

Barry WF, Wells SA, Cox E, Haagensen DE Jr(1981) Clinical and radiographic correlation in breast cancer patients with osseous metastases. Skeletal Radiol 6:27–32

Bellamy EA, Nicholas D, Ward M, Coombes RC, Powles TJ, Husband JE (1987) Comparison of computed tomography and conventional radiology in the assessment of treatment response of lytic bony metastases in patients with carcinoma of the breast. Clin Radiol 38:351–355

Bitran JD, Bekerman C, Desser RK (1980) The predictive value of serial bone scans in assessing response to chemotherapy in advanced breast cancer. Cancer 45:1562–1568

Bloom RA, Libson E, Husband JE, Stoker DJ (1987) The periosteal sunburst reaction to bone metastases. A literature review and report of 20 additional cases. Skeletal Radiol 16:629–634

Citrin DL, Hougen C, Zweibel W, Schlise S, Pruitt B, Ershler W et al. (1981) The use of serial bone scans in assessing response to bone metastases to systemic treatment. Cancer 47:680–685

Coerkamp EG, Kroon HM (1988) Cortical bone metastases. Radiology 169:525–528

Collins JD, Bassett L, Main GD, Kagan C (1979) Percutaneous biopsy following positive bone scans. Radiology 132:439–442

Coombes RC, Dady P, Parsons C, McCready VR, Ford HT, Gazet J-C et al. (1983) Assessment of response of bone metastases to systemic treatment in patients with breast cancer. Cancer 52:610–614

Corcoran RJ, Thrall JH, Kyle RW, Kaminski RJ, Johnson MC (1976) Solitary abnormalities in bone scans of patients with extraosseous malignancies. Radiology 121:663–667

Galasko CSB (1972) Skeletal metastases and mammary cancer. Ann R Coll Surg Engl 50:3–28

Hortobagyi GN, Libshitz HI, Seabold JE (1984) Osseous metastases of breast cancer. Clinical, biochemical, radiographic and scintigraphic evaluation of response to therapy. Cancer 53:577–582

Kamby C, Vejorg I, Daugaard S, Guldhammer B, Dirksen H, Rossing N et al. (1987) Clinical and radiologic characteristics of bone metastases in breast cancer. Cancer 60:2524–2531

Libshitz HI, Hortobagyi GN (1981) Radiographic evaluation of therapeutic response in bony metastases of breast cancer. Skeletal Radiol 7:159–165

Mehta RC, Wilson MA, Perlman SB (1989) False-negative bone scan in extensive metastatic disease. CT and MR findings. J Comput Assist Tomogr 13:717–719

Mink J (1987) Percutaneous bone biopsy in the patient with known or suspected osseous metastases. Radiology 161:191–194

Muindi J, Coombes RC, Golding S, Powles TJ, Kahn O, Husband JE (1983) The role of computed tomography in the detection of bone metastases in breast cancer patients. Br J Radiol 56:233–236

Redmond J 3rd, Spring DB, Munderloh SH, George CB, Mansour RP, Volk SA (1984) Spinal computed tomography scanning in the evaluation of metastatic disease. Cancer 54:253–258

Rossleigh MA, Lovegrove FT, Reynolds PM, Byrne MJ, Whitney BP (1984) The assesment of response to therapy of bone metastases in breast cancer. Aust NZJ Med 14:19–22

5   Magnetic Resonance Imaging

M.A. Richards

Introduction

Although the phenomenon of nuclear magnetic resonance was first reported in the 1940s (Bloch et al. 1946; Purcell et al. 1946), its potential for clinical imaging was not recognised for a further quarter of a century (Lauterbur 1973). At about the same time, Damadian (1971) observed that cancerous tissues examined in vitro have different magnetic resonance characteristics from those of normal tissues. It is only in the past few years, however, that magnetic resonance imagers capable of giving good quality images of the whole body have been developed. Assessment of the usefulness of this new technology is, therefore, still at a relatively early stage (Franken et al. 1986; Kent and Larson 1988), particularly when compared with other imaging techniques such as plain radiography and radionuclide bone scanning.

Principles of Magnetic Resonance Imaging

Mobile hydrogen nuclei (protons) in body tissues tend to align themselves in the direction of a strong external magnetic field. They can be deflected from this alignment by an appropriate radiofrequency pulse. When the radiofrequency pulse is stopped the protons return to their original alignment inducing a radiofrequency signal in a receiver coil. During the period of re-alignment the protons lose energy to the surrounding macromolecular environment (the lattice). This process occurs exponentially with a time constant called the spin-lattice relaxation time (T1). Each proton precesses around the direction of the external magnetic field, in the same way as a spinning top precesses around the direction of the earth's gravitational field. Because of local interactions between neighbouring protons, some protons will precess slightly faster than others and phase coherence is lost. The time constant for this process is called the spin-spin relaxation time (T2).

By applying suitable gradients to the external magnetic field, nuclei in selected slices of the body can be excited. Within the selected slice, protons in different anatomical locations will be subject to small differences in magnetic field strength. The complex signal emitted from all the affected nuclei can be reconstructed by a computer to give a grey-scale image of the body. The intensity of the signal from a particular tissue depends on the number of protons present and on the T1 and T2 characteristics of the tissue. The relative contribution of these different factors to the final image can be altered by changing the intervals between the components of the excitatory spin-echo radiofrequency pulse. Details of the physical principles of magnetic resonance imaging (MRI) are fully explained elsewhere (Partain et al. 1983; Kean and Smith 1986). The most commonly used radiofrequency pulses are those which emphasise either the T1 component of the signal (T1-weighted images) or the T2 component (T2-weighted) (Fig. 5.1a,b). On T1-weighted images, tissues with long T1 appear hypointense (dark) and those with short T1 appear hyperintense

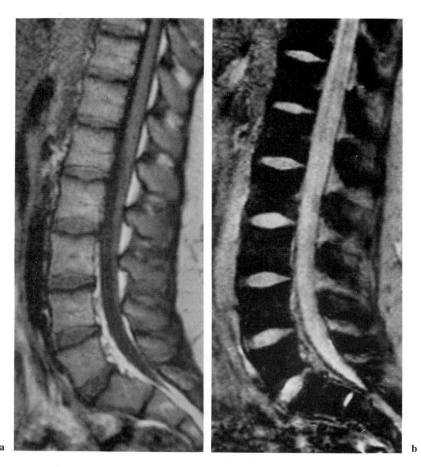

a   b

Fig. 5.1. **a** T1-weighted image of normal lumbar spine. **b** STIR image of normal lumbar spine illustrating differences in intensity between vertebral bone marrow, intervertebral discs and cerebrospinal fluid.

(bright). However, on T2-weighted images tissues with long T2 values appear bright.

Technical Considerations

General

Magnetic resonance imaging has several potential advantages when compared with x-ray CT. First, the multiplanar capacity of MRI enables sagittal and coronal slices to be imaged in addition to the transverse images available using CT. Second, contrast between soft tissues is generally greater using MRI than with CT. Third, no ionising radiation is required. Against these advantages must be set the higher cost of MRI and the longer imaging time generally required. In addition, a small proportion of patients cannot tolerate MRI because of claustrophobia.

The safety profile of MRI is good and is considered similar to that for non-contrast CT and better than that for contrast-enhanced CT, invasive CT or myelography (Kent and Larson 1988). However, patients with cardiac pacemakers, intracranial aneurysm clips and metal workers, who may have small ferromagnetic fragments in or around the eye (Kelly et al. 1986), should not be evaluated by MRI. Perhaps the greatest danger to patients undergoing MRI is from loose ferromagnetic objects carried into the MR unit. It is, therefore, essential that strict procedures for checking staff and visitors are maintained.

Bone and Bone Marrow

The solid constituents of cortical bone give no signal on MRI and therefore appear black on images. Fat and erythropoietic bone marrow, however, give strong signals. Thus MRI of bone and bone marrow differs markedly from plain x-ray and CT, in which the bright signal is almost entirely due to the solid bone matrix.

Detection of bone metastases by MRI depends on differences in MR parameters between tumour tissue and normal bone marrow. Metastatic tumour is, therefore, visualised directly, in contrast with the indirect changes observed by x-ray or radionuclide bone scanning. On x-ray films the presence of metastases is inferred from destruction of the bone matrix (lytic deposits) or new bone formation (sclerotic deposits). It has been estimated that between 30% (Ardan 1951) and 70% (Edelstyn et al. 1967) of the bone matrix must be lost before a lytic deposit is observable on plain x-ray. Metastatic "hot spots" on radionuclide bone scanning result from localised areas of increased osteoblastic activity rather than from the metastatic tumour per se.

As with CT, imaging of the whole skeleton is not feasible with MRI because of time constraints. Imaging of the spine in the sagittal plane is, however, relatively simple and the pelvis and upper femora can be imaged in the coronal plane. Other parts of the skeleton can, of course, be imaged if clinical findings or abnormalities detected by other imaging techniques make this important.

The duration of an MRI examination depends both on the number of areas scanned and on the number of different pulse sequences used. Although it is feasible to image the whole spine in a single examination, better anatomical detail can be achieved using surface coils placed under the patient's back with the patient lying supine to image the cervical, thoracic and lumbosacral regions separately. For many purposes, T1-weighted pulse sequences alone are sufficient and, in general, such examinations can be completed within an hour. In certain circumstances additional information may be gained by using T2-weighted or other sequences such as Inversion Recovery (IR), Short Tau Inversion Recovery (STIR) and Fast Field Echo (FFE).

MRI of Normal Bone Marrow

The MR appearances of normal bone marrow have been studied both in healthy volunteers (Richards et al. 1988a) and in patients not suspected of having any bone marrow abnormality (Dooms et al. 1985; Jenkins et al. 1986; Daffner et al. 1986). In most cases the patients were being investigated for suspected lumbar disc abnormalities.

Normal bone marrow has a moderately high signal intensity on T1-weighted images due to the short T1 of fat and the somewhat longer T1 of erythropoietic marrow. In the series of 100 control patients studied by Daffner et al. (1986), none had abnormal signal from their marrow areas, either in terms of focal or diffuse changes in signal intensity.

In normal adults the vertebrae and pelvis are the major areas of active erythropoietic bone marrow (Kricun 1985). In contrast the femoral heads contain fatty (yellow) marrow. In keeping with this, the T1 of femoral heads is shorter than that for vertebral bone marrow (Richards et al. 1988a). On T1-weighted images, the femoral heads give a somewhat brighter signal than that from vertebrae.

Some authors have shown that T1 signals from vertebral marrow decrease with age (Dooms et al. 1985; Richards et al. 1988a). Jenkins et al. (1986), however, detected no such effect. The decrease in marrow T1 with age within the adult population is not generally appreciated on visual inspection of T1-weighted images and is, therefore, only of importance in studies which attempt to quantify T1 values.

MRI of Pathological Bone Marrow

Infiltration of bone marrow by metastatic cancer or by haematological malignancies results in prolongation of T1 and a consequent reduction of signal intensity on T1-weighted images. The abnormal signal may either be diffuse or focal. Changes in T2 with neoplasia are less consistent, although in many cases metastases give high signal intensity on T2-weighted images.

These changes are not specific for malignancy as many pathological processes result in similar T1 changes. It is therefore not generally possible to differentiate between malignant infiltration and, for example, either osteomyelitis or eosinophilic granuloma on the basis of changes in T1-weighted signal intensity (Paushter and Modic 1984; Han et al. 1983; Sugimura et al. 1987).

Comparison of Malignant and Osteoporotic Vertebral Collapse

MRI may be useful in elucidating the cause of a vertebral compression fracture. Yuh and colleagues (1989) studied 109 vertebral compression fractures in 64 patients. The final diagnosis was made by follow-up CT and MR examinations combined with clinical history. Twenty-five of the fractures were due to malignancy and 23 were the result of known trauma. The remaining 61 fractures occurred in patients with no known malignancy and with no history of trauma and were presumed to be osteoporotic in origin. The appearances of the marrow on sagittal T1-weighted images were classified into three categories: complete replacement, incomplete replacement and complete preservation of normal marrow. In 47 of the 61 (77%) cases of presumed osteoporotic collapse, normal marrow appearances were completely preserved. The other 14 non-traumatic benign fractures had incomplete changes in the marrow. In contrast, 22 of the 25 malignant fractures showed complete marrow replacement. Two of the other 3 cases had incomplete marrow replacement and one had normal marrow on T1-weighted images but diffusely abnormal signal on a T2-weighted scan. Traumatic fractures showed very variable marrow appearances. Thus Yuh and colleagues (1989) concluded that, in the large majority of cases (94%), analysis of signal intensity in combination with the pattern of abnormality on T1-weighted images allowed differentiation between metastatic and osteoporotic vertebral collapse.

MRI may also help in the diagnosis of a benign cause for back pain in patients with known malignancy. Goldberg and coworkers (1988) described 2 patients with carcinoma of the breast in whom thoracic disc protrusion could be identified as the cause of the patient's symptoms, even though one had coexisting bone metastases. Hypointensity of the vertebral body on T1-weighted images may be observed in association with a prolapsed disc, but the area of hypointensity is confined to a zone around the intervening disc, helping to exclude malignancy as the cause.

Patterns of Vertebral Metastases

The anatomical localisation of vertebral metastases has been studied in depth by Asdourian and his colleagues (1990) in 25 patients with breast cancer. T1- and T2-weighted sagittal images were made in each case using surface coils. A total of 579 vertebrae were examined. Each vertebra was divided into three regions: the vertebral body, the pedicles and the posterior elements (spinous process, lamina, facets and transverse processes). Vertebrae which were not adequately visualised in all three regions or which showed involvement of all three regions were excluded from the analysis. Forty-four vertebrae (2 cervical, 28 thoracic and 14 lumbar) were suitable for this part of the study. In 27 vertebrae only the body was abnormal. A further 15 vertebrae showed involvement of the body and at least one pedicle. Involvement of the pedicle and posterior elements without involvement of the vertebral body was observed in only 2 cases. Thus the authors established that the vertebral body was the area of the vertebra most frequently involved with metastatic disease. This contrasts with radiographic findings in which an absent pedicle is often the first sign of vertebral metastasis (Jacobson et al. 1958). Findings similar to those reported by Asdourian et al. have also been observed on CT scanning of spinal metastases (Braunstein and Kuhns 1983).

In the second part of their study, Asdourian et al. (1990) examined the distribution of metastatic deposits within vertebral bodies. Seventy-six vertebral bodies (13 cervical, 46 thoracic and 17 lumbar) fulfilled the authors' criteria of adequate visualisation of the vertebral body combined with incomplete metastatic involvement. The posterior half of the body was involved more frequently than the anterior half in both the cervical ($p<0.05$) and thoracic ($p<0.01$) regions (Fig. 5.2) Posterior involvement was also more frequently observed than anterior involvement in the lumbar spine, but the difference was not statistically significant. No significant differences in metastatic involvement were observed between the superior and inferior halves of the vertebral bodies, nor between the right and left sides.

These MRI findings are consistent with the hypothesis that metastatic spread of breast and prostatic cancer to vertebrae occurs via the valveless vertebral venous system (Batson 1942; Coman and deLong 1951). The posterior half of the vertebral body lies closest to the vertebral venous plexus and might, therefore, be expected to be the first site of establishment of a metastatic seedling.

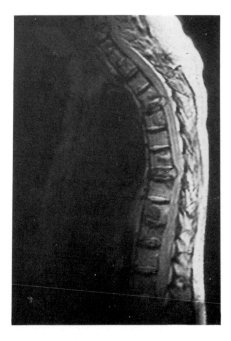

Fig. 5.2. T1-weighted image of thoracic spine showing partial involvement of vertebrae by metastatic cancer. (Note also spinal cord compression.)

Sensitivity of MRI

Primary Bone Marrow Disorders

Leukaemia. Most of the early MRI studies of bone marrow focussed on the detection of abnormalities in patients with primary haematological disorders rather than on the detection of metastases from solid tumours. Abnormalities of bone marrow on MRI have been reported in children (Cohen et al. 1984) and adults (Richards et al. 1988b) with acute leukaemia, and in adults with chronic myeloid leukaemia (Olson et al. 1986; McKinstry et al. 1986). In haematological malignancies resulting in diffuse infiltration of marrow by neoplastic cells, quantification of vertebral T1 in patients and in control populations may increase the accuracy of MRI (Moore et al. 1985; Thomsen et al. 1986; Richards et al. 1988b).

Lymphoma. MRI appearances of bone marrow in patients with lymphoma have been compared with the results of bone marrow aspirate and biopsy specimens (Shields et al. 1987; Richards et al. 1988c; Dohner et al. 1989). In general, a high level of concordance has been found between the two techniques. Some false-negative MRI examinations have, however, been reported in patients with low grade non-Hodgkin's lymphomas (Dohner et al. 1989; Richards et al. 1988c). A false-negative T1-weighted scan in a patient with lymphoma was also observed by Shields et al. (1987), but in this case the abnormality was detected using the STIR technique. All three studies noted cases in which MRI was positive in the presence of normal bone marrow histology. Clinical evidence of subsequent response to chemotherapy or progression of disease suggests that in these cases the MRI findings were truly positive with false-negative biopsy findings. It is well known that marrow involvement in both Hodgkin's disease and non-Hodgkin's lymphoma can be patchy and that single bone-marrow biopsies are subject to sampling errors (Brunning et al. 1975). With MRI it is possible to image a large volume of marrow, and thus it may be possible to use MRI to detect likely sites of bone marrow involvement as a guide for subsequent biopsy.

Myeloma. Daffner and colleagues (1986) studied 30 patients with multiple myeloma by MRI using a T1-weighted pulse sequence. All patients were studied by plain radiographs and radionuclide bone scan as well as by MRI. Fifteen were studied by CT. Normal appearances of marrow on MRI were established by imaging 80 control patients with suspected lumbar disc disease and 20 patients with suspected avascular necrosis of the hip.

  MRI detected abnormalities in all 30 patients, and these were confirmed by needle aspiration of bone marrow. Radionuclide bone scan, as might be expected in myeloma, was only positive in 6 of the 30 cases. Abnormalities seen on plain x-ray were abnormal in each of these 6 cases and in a further 14 patients. Radiographs were, however, normal in the remaining 10 cases. Four of the 15 patients who underwent CT scanning had studies that were indistinguishable from osteoporosis. Thus MRI may well prove to be the most sensitive imaging technique in patients with myeloma. Avrahami et al. (1989) included 4 patients with myeloma in their series of 40 patients with known malignancy but normal radionuclide bone scan examined by MRI for possible spinal metastases. In each case the MRI examination was abnormal. In 3 of the 4 cases a mosaic pattern due to multiple small foci with strong or weak signal intensity was noted both on T1- and T2-weighted images. This pattern was not observed amongst 17 patients with abnormal spinal MRI from breast, kidney or prostatic cancer.

Bone Metastases from "Solid Tumours"

The sensitivity of MRI in the detection of bone metastases from solid tumours has been demonstrated both in individual case reports (Mehta et al. 1989; Khurana et al. 1989) and in several larger studies (Frank et al. 1989; Daffner et al. 1986; Sarpel et al. 1987; Avrahami et al. 1989). The criteria for undertaking MRI studies have, however, varied widely and as yet there have been very few prospective studies confined to particular cancer types.

Daffner et al. (1986) examined 50 patients with known primary tumours, all of whom were suspected of having skeletal metastases. In all cases radionuclide bone scan was abnormal. Plain radiographs showed evidence of metastases in 33 of the cases. MRI was abnormal in these 33 cases and in a further 7 patients. The remaining 10 patients had changes on plain radiographs indicative of arthritis (7) or old fractures (3) to account for the abnormality on radionuclide bone scan. In each of these 10 patients the bone marrow appeared normal on MRI. The authors, therefore, concluded that there were no false-positive and no false-negative MRI examinations in that study.

Avrahami et al. (1989) studied 36 patients with known breast, kidney or prostatic cancer and back pain by MRI using T1-weighted plus T2-weighted images and a spinal coil. CT and radionuclide bone scanning were undertaken in all cases and were normal. Seventeen of the 36 patients had abnormalities on at least one of the pulse sequences used. All of these patients subsequently underwent needle biopsy of the abnormal vertebra. Nine patients had reduced signal intensity on T1-weighted images. T2-weighted images in these patients showed a variety of patterns and added little. Conversely, 5 cases with obvious increased signal intensity on T2-weighted images had normal T1-weighted images. Lesions with similar primary pathology had different MRI patterns. The authors concluded that MRI is the most sensitive procedure for the demonstration of bone-marrow metastases in the spine and that both T1- and T2-weighted sequences are required to maximise the sensitivity of the technique (Fig. 5.3a, b).

A higher level of sensitivity of MRI compared with radionuclide bone scan has also been reported by Frank et al. (1989) in 106 patients with either primary or metastatic bone tumours. Histological confirmation was established by biopsy. In 32 cases both MRI and radionuclide bone scan were positive and in 41 cases both examinations were negative. 30 patients had positive MRI, but negative bone scan, while only 3 patients had positive bone scan but negative MRI. Two of the last 3 patients were found to have benign lesions on bone biopsy. Overall, MRI was significantly more sensitive than bone scan (p<0.001).

Two recent studies from the Royal Marsden Hospital have examined the use of MRI in specific types of cancer, namely neuroblastoma (Oliff et al. 1989) and

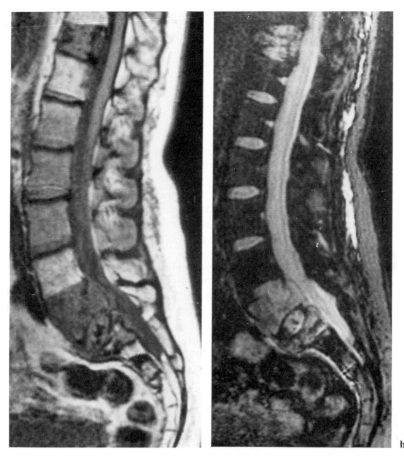

Fig. 5.3. **a** T1-weighted image of spine with metastases in T11 and L5 appearing darker than normal marrow. **b** STIR image of spine from the same patient with metastases appearing brighter than normal marrow.

breast cancer (Jones et al. 1990). Thirty MRI examinations were undertaken in 20 children with neuroblastoma and results were compared with those from metaiodobenzylguanidine (mIBG) scanning and from bone-marrow aspirates. In general, MRI and mIBG were of equivalent sensitivity and both were more sensitive than bone-marrow aspiration. However, (MRI) frequently demonstrated more extensive disease, particularly in the femora.

Eighty-four patients with breast cancer were examined by MRI in another study from the same hospital (Jones et al. 1990). All patients either presented with "high risk" early breast cancer (defined by primary tumour size larger than 5 cm or positive axillary nodes) or had soft tissue recurrence of breast cancer. Patients with "definite" metastases on bone scan were excluded. In the presence of a normal bone scan and negative skeletal survey, 7% of patients were found to have positive MRI. In patients with equivocal bone scans, 50% had positive MRI.

Spinal Cord Compression

One of the major advantages of MR imaging of the spine is its potential for detecting spinal cord compression. On sagittal images both the vertebrae and the spinal cord can be clearly imaged without the need for intrathecal contrast injection (Fig. 5.4). In patients with a complete block of the subarachnoid space, MRI can delineate the upper limit of the block without the need for a high cervical injection of contrast, which is required for full myelographic examination. Furthermore, acute deterioration of neurological function is a well-recognised complication of myelography (Hollis et al. 1986) which should be avoided by using MRI. Early diagnosis of spinal cord compression or compression of the subarachnoid space by tumour could potentially be of major therapeutic significance. It has been estimated that only 7% of patients who are paraplegic at the time of diagnosis of extradural metastasis become ambulatory after treatment, while 60% of ambulatory patients remain so (Bruckman and Bloomer 1978).

What is the current evidence regarding the relative sensitivity of MRI and myelography (with or without CT) for the diagnosis of spinal cord compression? In the majority of published series in which at least 20 patients have been studied by both techniques, MRI is considered to be at least as informative as myelography (Godersky et al. 1987; Williams et al. 1989; Carmody et al. 1989) although at least one study favours myelography (Hagenau et al. 1987).

The largest single reported study is that by Carmody et al. (1989) in which 70 patients underwent both MRI and myelography. Sixty-four of the patients had a

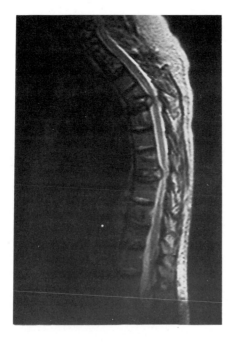

Fig. 5.4. T2-weighted image of thoracic spine showing spinal cord compression at two separate levels; note associated bone metastases. (Same patient as in Fig. 5.2.)

known primary tumour and all satisfied at least one of the following criteria: myelopathy, radioculopathy, back pain or radiological evidence of spinal metastases. Receiver operating characteristic (ROC) analysis (Metz 1978) was used to compare the accuracy of the two procedures, viewed by a panel of neurologists. Extradural masses were observed in 46 patients, 25 of whom had cord compression. No significant difference was observed between the two modalities for the diagnosis of cord compression. Extradural masses without cord compression were generally better visualised on MRI, though the difference in sensitivity of the two techniques was not statistically significant. As expected, MRI was much more sensitive in the detection of bone metastasis. Subarachnoid spread of tumour was, however, much more clearly shown by myelography. The insensitivity of MRI in the diagnosis of meningeal carcinomatosis has been observed by others (Krol et al. 1988; Godersky et al. 1987; Williams et al. 1989). This problem may be overcome either by the use of T2-weighted sequences (Carmody et al. 1989) or by using gadolinium-DTPA enhanced T1-weighted sequences (Sze 1988). In summary, it seems reasonable to use non-invasive MRI as the first procedure for patients with suspected cord compression, reserving myelography with or without CT for patients in whom MRI is not feasible or does not satisfactorily explain neurological findings. If MRI is to be used in cases of suspected spinal cord compression, the entire cord should be imaged, as approximately 10% of patients will have multiple levels of cord impingement (Bonner and Lichter 1990; Bernat et al. 1983).

Monitoring Response to Treatment

As bone metastases are visualised directly by MRI, in contrast with the indirect signs provided by plain radiography and radionuclide scanning, it might be expected that MRI would be useful for monitoring response to treatment. Surprisingly little work has been published in this area, especially on MRI of metastases from solid tumours.

Serial MRI examinations have been performed in patients receiving treatment for leukaemia (McKinstry et al. 1986; Richards et al. 1988b) and lymphoma (Richards et al. 1987). In patients with leukaemia a paradoxical increase in bone marrow T1 may be observed within the first few days of treatment, followed by a fall in T1 to within the normal range (Fig.5.5). The explanation for this is not known, but such changes could result from necrosis of neoplastic cells. In all cases, the early rise in bone marrow T1 was accompanied by a marked decrease in leukaemic cells in the peripheral blood, suggesting that the treatment was effective (Richards et al. 1988b). Further studies are clearly warranted, but these early changes could potentially be a useful method for detecting a response to treatment.

Following chemotherapy, persistent T1 prolongation or persistent hypointense marrow signal on T1-weighted images almost certainly reflects the presence of active disease. The sensitivity of MRI for the detection of small volumes of residual disease following treatment needs further investigation. Following radiotherapy, vertebrae usually give an intense white signal on T1-weighted images, reflecting fatty change and loss of erythropoietic marrow

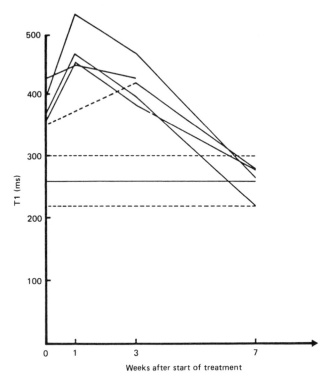

Fig. 5.5. Changes in bone marrow T1 in patients with acute leukaemia before and after the start of chemotherapy: there is an early rise in T1 value followed by a fall to below pre-treatment levels.

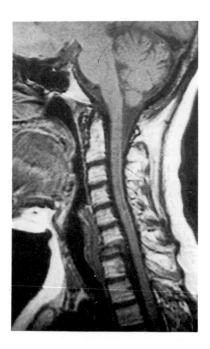

Fig. 5.6. Intense signal from irradiated vertebrae seen on T1-weighted image.

(Ramsey and Zacharias 1985) (Fig. 5.6). These changes in intensity of marrow signal may persist for at least 10 years. Long-term reduction in bone marrow T1 has also been observed following successful chemotherapy for leukaemia, but in general the effects are less marked than those observed with radiotherapy.

Serial MRI examinations have been undertaken in 10 patients receiving primary chemotherapy for osteosarcoma (Hogeboom et al. 1989). Changes in MR parameters were compared with CT findings and with histological appearances from bone biopsies taken after chemotherapy. The authors concluded that an increase in T2 following treatment was an indicator of tumour necrosis and that MRI may be superior to CT for monitoring response. Clearly, similar studies need to be conducted prospectively in patients undergoing treatment for bone metastases where assessment of response is difficult using conventional methods.

Conclusions

It is still too early to define the role of MRI in clinical management of patients with bone metastases. However, current evidence suggests that MRI is a highly sensitive method for detecting tumour in bone marrow, and in many cases is more sensitive than radionuclide bone scanning. Its use is, however, limited by the cost of MRI, the relatively small number of MR scanners available and the inability of MRI to evaluate the whole skeleton.

In cases of suspected spinal cord compression, MRI is an acceptable non-invasive alternative to myelography. The future challenge will be to identify which patients should undergo MRI before neurological complications develop, in the hope that such patients will be able to receive effective prophylactic treatment.

There is considerable potential for MRI as a method for monitoring response to treatment. Further studies in this area are required.

References

Ardan GM (1951) Bone destruction not demonstrable by radiotherapy. Br J Radiol 24:107–109

Asdourian PL, Weidenbaum M, DeWald RL, Hammerberg KW, Ramsey RG (1990) The pattern of vertebral involvement in metastatic vertebral breast cancer. Clin Orthop 250:164–70

Avrahami E, Tadmor R, Dally O, Hadar H (1989) Early MR demonstration of spinal metastases in patients with normal radiographs and CT and radionuclide bone scans. J Comput Assist Tomogr 13:598–602

Batson OV (1942) The role of the vertebral veins in metastatic processes. Ann Intern Med 16:38–45

Bernat JL, Greenberg ER, Barrett J (1983) Suspected epidural compression of the spinal cord and cauda equina by metastatic carcinoma: Clinical diagnosis and survival. Cancer 51:1953–1957

Bloch F, Hansen WW, Packard M (1946) Nuclear induction. Phys Rev 69:127

Bonner JA, Lichter AS (1990) A caution about the use of MRI to diagnose spinal cord compression. N Engl J Med 322:556–557

Braunstein EM, Kuhns LR (1983) Computed tomographic demonstration of spinal metastases. Spine 8:912–915

Bruckman JE, Bloomer WD (1978) Management of spinal cord compression. Semin Oncol 5:135–140

Brunning RD, Bloomfield DC, McKenna RW, Peterson L (1975) Bilateral trephine bone marrow biopsies in lymphoma and other neoplastic diseases. Ann Intern Med 82:365–366

Carmody RF, Yang PJ, Seeley GW, Seegar JF, Unger EC, Johnson JE (1989) Spinal cord compression due to metastatic disease: diagnosis with MR imaging versus myelography. Radiology 173:225–229

Cohen MD, Klatte EC, Baehnes R et al. (1984) Magnetic resonance imaging of bone marrow disease in children. Radiology 151:715–718

Coman DR, deLong RP (1951) The role of the vertebral venous system in the metastasis of cancer to the spinal column. Cancer 5:610–618

Daffner RH, Lupetin AR, Dash N, Deeb ZL, Sefczek RJ, Schapiro RL (1986) MRI in the detection of malignant infiltration of bone marrow. AJR 146:353–358

Damadian R (1971) Tumour detection by nuclear magnetic resonance. Science 171:1151–1153

Dohner H, Guckel F, Knauf W, Semmler W, van Kaick G, Ho AD, Hunstein W (1989) Magnetic resonance imaging of bone marrow in lymphoproliferative disorders: correlation with bone marrow biopsy. Br J Haematol 73:12–17

Dooms GC, Fisher MR, Hricak H et al. (1985) Bone marrow imaging: Magnetic resonance studies related to age and sex. Radiology 155:429–432

Edelstyn GA, Gillespie PJ, Grebbel FS (1967) The radiological demonstration of osseous metastases: experimental observations. Clin Radiol 18:158–162

Frank J, Ling A, Patronas N, Carrasquillo J, Horvath K, Dwyer A (1989) Comparison of magnetic resonance imaging and radionuclide bone scan in the evaluation of primary and metastatic disease in the bone. Proc ASCO 8:7 (abstr 25)

Franken EA, Berbaum KS, Dunn V, Smith WL, Erhardt JC, Leiritz GS, Breckenridge RE (1986) Impact of MR imaging on clinical diagnosis and management: a prospective study. Radiology 161:377–380

Godersky JC, Smoker WR, Knutzon R (1987) Use of magnetic resonance imaging in the evaluation of metastatic spinal disease. Neurosurgery 21:676–680

Goldberg AL, Rothfus WE, Deeb ZL, Khoury MB, Daffner RH (1988) Thoracic disc herniation versus spinal metastases: optimizing diagnosis with magnetic resonance imaging. Skeletal Radiol 17:423–426

Hagenau C, Grosh W, Currie M, Wiley RG (1987) Comparison of spinal magnetic resonance imaging and myelography in cancer patients. J Clin Oncol 5:1663–1669

Han JS, Kaufman B, El Yousef SJ et al. (1983) NMR imaging of the spine. AJR 141:1137–1145

Hogeboom WR, Hoekstra HJ, Mooyaart EL, Oosterhuis JW, Postma A, Veth RPH, Schraffordt Koops H (1989) Magnetic resonance imaging (MRI) in evaluating in vivo response to neoadjuvant chemotherapy for osteosarcomas of the extremities. Eur J Surg Oncol 15:424–430

Hollis PH, Malis LI, Zappula RA (1986) Neurological deterioration after lumbar puncture below complete spinal subarachnoid block. J Neurosurg 64:253–256

Jacobson HG, Poppel MH, Shapiro JH, Grossberger S (1958) The vertebral pedicle sign: a roentgen finding to differentiate metastatic carcinoma from multiple myeloma. AJR 80:817–821

Jenkins JPR, Stelling M, Hillier VF, Hickey DS, Isherwood I (1986) Magnetic resonance imaging of vertebral bodies: a T1 and T2 study. Proc Soc Mag Res Med: Works in Progress 197–198

Jones AL, Williams MP, Powles TJ, Oliff JFC, Hardy J, Cherryman GR, Husband JE (1990) Magnetic resonance imaging in the detection of skeletal metastases in patients with breast cancer. Br J Cancer 62:296–298

Kean DM, Smith MA (1986) Magnetic resonance imaging: principles and applications. Heinemann, London

Kelly WM, Paglen PG, Pearson JA, San Diego AG, Soloman MA (1986) Ferromagnetism of intraocular foreign body causes unilateral blindness after MR study. AJNR 1986 7:243–245

Kent DL, Larson EB (1988) Magnetic resonance imaging of the brain and spine: Is clinical efficacy established after the first decade. Ann Intern Med 108:402–424

Khurana JS, Rosenthal DI, Rosenberg AE, Mankin HJ (1989) Skeletal metastases in liposarcoma detectable only by magnetic resonance imaging. Clin orthop 243:204–207

Kricun ME (1985) Red-yellow marrow conversion: its effects on the location of some solitary bone lesions. Skeletal Radiol 14:10–19

Krol G, Sze G, Malkin M, Walker R (1988) MR of cranial and spinal meningeal carcinomatosis: comparison with CT and myelography. AJNR 9:709–714

Lauterbur PC (1973) Image formation by induced local interactions: examples employing nuclear magnetic resonance. Nature 242:190–191

McKinstry CS, Jones L, Steiner RE, Bydder GM (1986) NMR imaging of the bone marrow in leukaemia treated by bone marrow transplantation. Proc Soc Mag Res Med 2:577–578

Mehta RC, Wilson MA, Perlman SB (1989) The false-negative bone scan in extensive metastatic disease: CT and MR findings. J Comput Assist Tomogr 13:717–719

Metz CE (1978) Basic principles of ROC analysis. Semin Nucl Med 8:283–298

Moore S, Gooding C, Ehman R, Brasch R (1985) Intensity measurement of the marrow in patients with acute lymphocyte leukaemia. Proc Soc Mag Res Med 2:1183

Oliff JFC, Moyes JSE, Pinkerton CR, Williams MP, Cherryman GR, Meller ST, Husband JE (1989) Magnetic Resonance (MR) imaging of the marrow in patients with neuroblastoma: a comparison between MRI, MIBG and marrow aspirates. 75th scientific assembly and annual meeting of the Radiological Society of North America, Chicago, Nov 1989

Olson DO, Shields AF, Scheurich CJ, Porter BA, Moss AA (1986) Magnetic resonance imaging of the bone marrow in patients with leukaemia, aplastic anaemia and lymphoma. Invest Radiol 21:540–546

Partain CL, James AE, Rollo FD, Price RR (1983) Nuclear magnetic resonance imaging. WB Saunders, Philadelphia

Paushter DM, Modic MT (1984) Magnetic resonance imaging of the spine. Appl Radiol 13:61–68

Purcell EM, Torrey HC, Pound RV (1946) Resonance absorption by nuclear magnetic moments in a solid. Phys Rev 69:37–38

Ramsey RG, Zacharias CE (1985) MR imaging of the spine after radiation therapy: easily recognisable effects. AJR 144:1131–1135

Richards MA (1987) Magnetic resonance imaging in lymphoma – the role of spin lattice relaxation time measurement. Cancer Surv 6:315–341

Richards MA, Webb JAW, Jewell SE, Gregory WM, Reznek RH (1988a) In vivo measurement of spin lattice relaxation time (T1) of bone marrow in healthy volunteers: the effect of age and sex. Br J Radiol 61:30–33

Richards MA, Webb JAW, Malik S, Jewell SE, Amess JAL, Lister TA (1988b) Low field strength magnetic resonance imaging of bone marrow in acute leukaemia. Haematol Oncol 6:285–290

Richards MA, Webb JAW, Jewell SE, Amess JAL, Wrigley PFM, Lister TA (1988c) Low field strength magnetic resonance imaging of bone marrow in patients with malignant lymphoma. Br J Cancer 57:412–415

Sarpel S, Sarpel G, Yu E, Hyder S, Kaufman B, Hindo W, Ezdinli E (1987) Early diagnosis of spinal-epidural metastasis by magnetic resonance imaging. Cancer 59:1112–1116

Shields AF, Porter BA, Churchley S, Olson DO, Appelbaum FR, Thomas ED (1987) The detection of bone marrow involvement by lymphoma using magnetic resonance imaging. J Clin Oncol 5:225–230

Sugimura K, Yamasaki K, Kitagaki H, Tanaka Y, Kono M (1987) Bone marrow disease of the spine: differentiation with T1 and T2 relaxation times in MR imaging. Radiology 165:541–544

Sze G (1988) Gadolinium-DTPA in spinal disease. Radiol Clin North Am 26:1009–1024

Thomsen C, Grundtvig P, Karle H, Henriksen O, Christofferson P (1986) In vivo estimation of relaxation processes by magnetic resonance in the bone marrow in patients with acute leukaemia. Proc Soc Mag Res Med 2:277–278

Williams MP, Cherryman GR, Husband JE (1989) Magnetic resonance imaging in suspected metastatic spinal cord compression. Clin Radiol 40:286–290

Yuh WT, Zachar CK, Barloon TJ, Sato Y, Sickels WJ, Hawes DR (1989) Vertebral compression fractures: distinction between benign and malignant causes with MR imaging. Radiology 172:215–218

6 Assessment of Response to Treatment

R.E. Coleman

There are many treatments available for bone metastases and radiotherapy, endocrine manipulation and chemotherapy may all produce significant clinical improvement. Control of the tumour by systemic therapy reduces osteoclast activity allowing bone healing, mediated by osteoblasts, to occur. However, as assessment of response for most tumours is based on changes seen on serial plain radiographs, the precise effect of therapy is difficult to measure objectively. In 1977, on behalf of the Union Internationale Contre le Cancer (UICC), Hayward et al. defined criteria for objective assessment of response in advanced breast cancer (Table 6.1). These criteria have since been applied to assessment of response in other tumour types and although they are internationally accepted and have standardised the reporting of clinical trials, response in bone remains an imprecise entity.

New methods of assessing response are needed, both to improve patient management and to evaluate specific treatments. A number of alternatives have been suggested and radionuclide bone scanning (Rossleigh et al. 1984), biochemical parameters of bone metabolism (Hortabagyi et al. 1984; Coleman et al. 1988a), tumour markers such as carcino-embryonic antigen (Palazzo et al. 1986) and measurement of symptomatic response (Coombes et al. 1983) have all been proposed as useful alternatives or adjuncts to assessment based on plain radiographs. None are ideal, each having advantages and disadvantages as outlined below.

Imaging of Bone Metastases

Plain Radiology

Metastatic bone destruction results from the invasion of malignant cells from the bone marrow cavity. These cells secrete paracrine factors which stimulate

Table 6.1.   The UICC criteria for assessment of response in bone metastases

Complete response (CR)	Complete disappearance of all lesions on x-ray for at least 4 weeks
Partial response (PR)	Partial decrease in size of lytic lesions, recalcification of lytic lesions, *or* decreased density in blastic lesions. No new lesions appearing
No change (NC)	No change in number or size of lesions, for at least 8 weeks
Progressive disease (PD)	Increase in the size of existing lesions or appearance of new lesions

osteoclasts to resorb bone and disturb the normal coupling between osteoblast and osteoclast function (Mundy 1987). When bone resorption predominates, areas of lysis will be visible on plain radiographs and, conversely, areas of sclerosis indicate increased osteoblast activity (Galasko and Bennett 1976).

It is generally accepted that sclerosis of lytic metastases with no radiological evidence of new lesions constitutes tumour regression (Fig. 6.1). However, some patients will have a mixture of sclerotic and lytic lesions before starting therapy, making interpretation of serial radiographs difficult. In prostate cancer, sclerotic metastases are usual and radiological assessment of response usually impossible (Aabo 1987). Even when radiological evidence of response to successful therapy is obtained, it is often not evident for 6 months and may be delayed for more than a year (Scher and Yagoda 1987). Complete response in non-osseous sites occurs in 10%–20% of patients but a complete response in bone with return of the normal trabecular pattern, or resolution of sclerotic metastases, as shown in Fig. 6.2, are rare.

In breast cancer, clinical trials using the UICC criteria of response have usually reported lower response rates in bone than the overall response achieved with a treatment. In a review of clinical studies of endocrine therapy for advanced breast cancer, the overall response rate was 31% (640/2093), com-

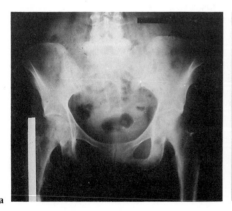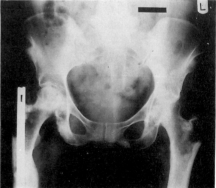

a   b

Fig. 6.1a,b. Plain radiographs **a** before and **b** 6 months after treatment with tamoxifen and prednisolone. Areas of lysis have been replaced by sclerotic new bone.

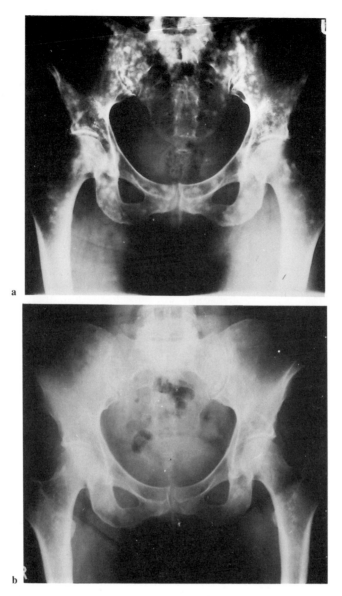

Fig. 6.2a,b. Plain radiographs **a** before and **b** 18 months after treatment of multiple sclerotic metastases by ovarian irradiation and prednisolone.

pared with 26% (206/796) in bone (p<0.02) (Coleman and Rubens 1985). Similarly, response rates in bone to chemotherapy appear to be less (Chlebowski and Block 1981). Although this could be a true phenomenon, indicating metastases in bone are biologically different from those in other sites and relatively refractory to treatment, it seems likely that the difference is more apparent than real, reflecting the insensitivity of assessment methods.

Radionuclide Imaging

The radionuclide bone scan is now well established as the most sensitive method for detecting pathological change in the skeleton. The sensitivity is high, dependant only on the presence of an osteoblastic response at the site of disease, but the specificity of the technique is low and complementary investigations are necessary to confirm metastatic involvement of the skeleton.

The use of bone scanning in assessment of response to therapy has always been contentious and certainly when lytic metastases predominate is often unreliable. A reduction in the intensity and number of lesions on the bone scan (hot spots) was previously considered to represent response, and progressive disease assumed if an increase in intensity or number of hot spots were seen. However, this interpretation is too simplistic. Following successful therapy for metastatic disease the increased production of immature new bone, and hence the cause of the hot spot, eventually ceases and isotope uptake gradually falls. However, healing causes an initial increase in uptake, akin to callus formation, and scans performed during this phase may be incorrectly interpreted as progression of disease (Rossleigh et al. 1984). Conversely, a reduction in isotope uptake is occasionally seen in rapidly progressive disease when the overwhelming destruction allows little chance for new bone formation; appearances which this time are easily mistaken for improvement (Goris and Bretille 1985). These different patterns of response are illustrated in Fig 6.3.

In the ICRF Clinical Oncology Unit at Guy's Hospital, we recently studied the value of performing serial bone scans during systemic therapy for bone metastases from advanced breast cancer (Coleman et al. 1988b). Pre-treatment

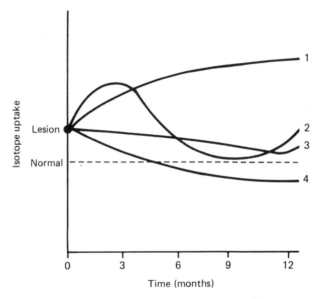

Fig. 6.3. Schematic demonstration of different observed patterns of ^{99m}Tc-labelled diphosphonate uptake following treatment of bone metastases. (1) progression of disease, (2) flare response to successful therapy and subsequent relapse, (3) "typical" response to successful therapy and subsequent relapse, (4) rapidly progressing lytic disease.

bone scans showed multiple sites of abnormal tracer uptake in all 53 patients. During the next 6 months 16 patients showed unequivocal radiographic evidence of response. At 3 months after starting treatment a repeat bone scan was performed. In 12 responding patients (75%) this bone scan showed increased activity in base-line lesions and the appearance of new lesions suggesting, erroneously, progressive disease. There was no change in the bone-scan appearances in 2 responders and improvement, with reduced activity in base-line lesions and no new areas of tracer uptake, in only 1 responding patient (Table 6.2).

After treatment for 6 months, the bone scan showed "improvement" in 14/16 responding patients when compared with the scan performed after just 3 months treatment and was unchanged in the other 2 patients. "Improvement" was most marked in the 12 patients whose 3-month scans had shown a "deterioration" from base-line. Even after 6 months the bone-scan appearances still often looked worse than the base-line scan, although new lesions appearing after 6 months reflected either progressive disease or a fracture site.

The deterioration followed by subsequent improvement in the bone-scan appearances following successful therapy corresponds to a transient increase in osteoblast activity during the early phase of healing and has been termed the flare response. An example of this flare response is shown in Fig. 6.4. In 10 of 14 patients with progressive disease the bone-scan appearances at 3 months had deteriorated with increased activity and/or new lesions – appearances which were indistinguishable from those seen in responding patients. A further confounding feature in 1 patient was a reduction in uptake at sites of rapidly progressive lytic disease.

New lytic lesions on plain radiographs indicate progression, but new scan lesions may appear in healing lesions which are initially either too small to be detectable or fail to promote a discernible osteoblastic response. New lesions on the 3-month scan were seen in 12 of 16 (75%) responders, 2 of 13 (15%) with stable disease and 9 of 14 (64%) with progressive disease.

Table 6.2. Changes in the bone scan appearances 3 months after a change in systemic therapy

Bone scan appearances		UICC Response category[a]		
		PR	NC	PD
Number of lesions	Increased	12	2	9
	Unchanged	4	11	5
	Reduced	0	0	0
Activity of lesions	Increased	12	2	10
	Unchanged	2	5	3
	Reduced	1	4	1
	Mixed change[b]	1	1	0
	Other[c]	0	1	0
Increase in activity and number of lesions		12	2	9
No change in activity or number of lesions		2	5	2
Scan not repeated		0	1	9

[a] PR, partial response; NC, no change; PD, progressive disease.
[b] Activity increased in some lesions and reduced in others.
[c] Diffuse increased activity (super scan) became more focal.

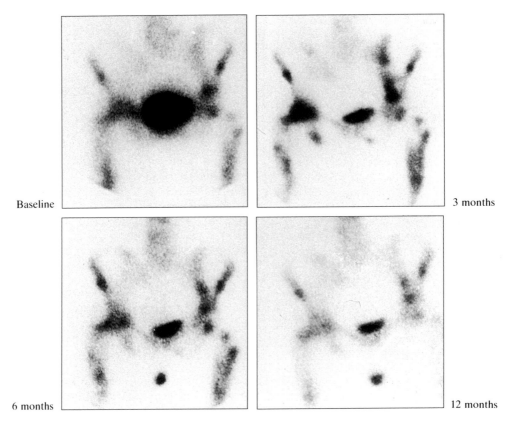

Baseline   3 months

6 months   12 months

Fig. 6.4. Serial bone scans of a patient responding to endocrine therapy with tamoxifen and prednisolone, to illustrate the flare response. The base-line, 3-, 6-, and 12-month bone scans are shown. Increased activity in base-line lesions and new scan lesions are seen at 3 months followed by improvement at 6 and 12 months. The corresponding radiographs of the pelvis before and 6 months after starting treatment are shown in Fig 6.1 and confirm response with sclerosis of lytic disease.

Bone scans in advanced disease should be interpreted with caution within 6 months of a change in therapy and are most useful for restaging on relapse to identify sites for radiological assessment and sites at risk of pathological fracture.

Quantitative bone scanning has been investigated by Parbhoo (1983). In metabolic bone disease, when the pathological process is diffuse, clearance of tracer with time is useful, but for metastatic disease, where the involvement is focal, "regions of interest" (ROI) scans are more appropriate. The counts from an abnormal area are compared with an adjacent normal area of similar size and the relative counts expressed as a ratio; e.g., second lumbar vertebra: fourth lumbar vertebra. This technique has confirmed the flare response with an increase in the number of counts from the region of interest during the early months of a response (Parbhoo 1983). Although this technique gives more accurate assessment of individual lesions, visual interpretation is probably as reliable for evaluating widespread metastatic disease (Condon et al. 1981).

Computed Tomography

Computed tomography (CT) offers three-dimensional information and high quality images. The density discrimination is far superior to that found with conventional x-ray examination, providing excellent bone to soft tissue resolution. Bone destruction can be identified early and extra-osseus, soft tissue and intra-osseous medullary spread assessed. When the marrow cavity is replaced by tumour, higher attenuation of the x-ray beam is observed in comparison to unaffected marrow (Mazess and Vetter 1985). CT has been quite widely used to identify or confirm the presence of a bone lesion (Rafii et al. 1986), but only occasionally evaluated as a parameter of response in metastatic disease (Crone-Munzebrock 1987, Bellamy et al 1987).

Metastatic involvement of the skeleton results in gross structural changes and usually involves both cortical and trabecular bone. Detection of minor changes in mineralisation are technically difficult, but this is probably not relevant in the context of metastatic disease as only a major change in the size of a lesion or its mineralisation are likely to be acceptable as response criteria. Indeed quantitative assessment of bone mineralisation has been used to monitor healing of bone metastases following radiotherapy (Crone-Munzebrock 1987) and systemic therapy (Bellamy et al. 1987; Coleman and Rubens 1985).

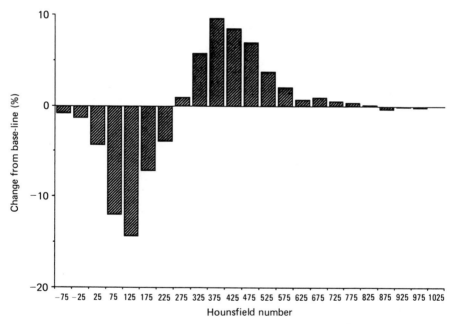

Fig. 6.5. Diagrammatic representation of the change in Hounsfield spectrum within a vertebral body following radiotherapy. A spectrum obtained before irradiation is taken as base-line. The change in the percentage distribution of pixels for each 50-Hounsfield band width of the spectrum obtained 6 weeks after radiotherapy is shown as a histogram. The spectrum has shifted to the right as lytic disease is replaced by denser sclerotic bone. There is a fall in the proportion of pixels of Hounsfield value −50 to +200 and a corresponding increase in the proportion between +250 and 600.

Metastatic lesions are selected (target lesions) which are considered to be representative of the metastatic process and suitable for serial examination. To enable accurate repositioning of the patient, only target lesions in the spine, limb girdles or proximal ends of the humerus or femur are used. Three-millimetre-thick transverse sections with a standard window width and level appropriate for bone are optimum. The ROI can be defined and the spectrum of Hounsfield values within it calculated by the computer. Changes in the spectrum with time can be determined, a shift in the spectrum to the right (more positive) indicating

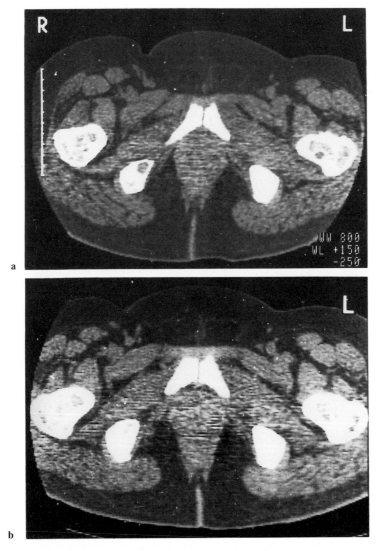

Fig. 6.6a,b.   CT appearances of diffuse sclerotic metastatic disease in the pelvis. Islands of lysis in **a** are seen, which have undergone sclerosis following treatment, in **b**.

replacement of lytic bone with low Hounsfield values by new sclerotic bone with a relatively high Hounsfield number (Fig. 6.5).

Sclerotic bone disease is considered non-assessable by UICC criteria. Fading of sclerotic metastases on plain radiographs is seen occasionally (Fig. 6.2), but it is more typical to see either no change in the appearances, new areas of sclerosis or increase in their size; changes which are usually uninterpretable. Clearly in these patients new bone formation predominates, but, within sclerotic metastases, areas of osteolysis are usually present as well. CT is able to identify these areas of lysis. Fig. 6.6 shows serial CT sections through the pelvis of a patient with diffuse sclerotic disease on plain radiographs. This patient subjectively responded to treatment and the follow-up CT scan shows sclerosis of the lytic component. Conversely, CT scans of the left femoral head in another patient show new areas of lysis as well as increased sclerosis; the latter appearance was seen on the plain films and interpreted as responding disease (Fig. 6.7).

Magnetic Resonance Imaging

Magnetic resonance imaging (MRI) is not yet widely available in Europe, but shows promise in evaluating bone metastases. It is impractical to image more than a limited part of the skeleton with CT, but with magnetic resonance imaging sagittal sections allow large sections of the skeleton to be assessed. Cortical bone does not produce a signal on MRI, but the modality is highly sensitive for detecting medullary bone disease. Bone metastases produce a reduced signal on T1-weighted sequences, reflecting replacement of marrow fat (Daffner et al. 1986). Early diagnosis of bone metastases is possible and preliminary reports suggest MRI is superior to CT for lesion detection (Frank et al. 1989).

MRI is also an excellent technique for visualising the spinal cord. The multiplanar capabilities of MRI are very useful for accurately defining the extent and position of lesions and changes seen following treatment. MRI offers several advantages over myelography, including identification of additional bone lesions and sites of compression, assessment of paravertebral extension, lack of discomfort for the patient and no exacerbation of compression by contrast media (Smoker et al. 1987).

The use of MRI for monitoring response to treatment is at present anecdotal. Because of limited machine availability, MRI is unlikely to be suitable for routine use, but, as in primary bone tumours, may have a role for detailed evaluation of a specific lesion, for example prior to surgery.

Biochemical Monitoring

There is no specific marker to monitor the progress of metastatic disease in the skeleton. However, metastatic involvement of bone disturbs bone cell function and perturbs a variety of biochemical parameters. Major changes in bone-cell activity are seen within the first few weeks of starting effective therapy, reflecting the changes in rates of bone formation and resorption that occur (Coleman et al. 1988a).

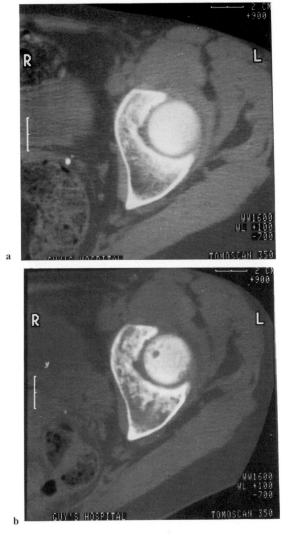

Fig. 6.7a. CT appearances of mixed lytic and sclerotic disease in the proximal femur. **b** Some increased sclerosis is seen on treatment, but new areas of lysis have appeared, particularly in the femoral head.

In a search for more sensitive response criteria, a prospective study of alternative assessment criteria was performed at Guy's Hospital in 70 women with advanced breast cancer and radiographically confirmed progressing bone metastases (Coleman et al. 1988a). Correlation with the UICC response was made and parameters which predicted radiological response identified. No attempt was made to select patients on a particular treatment with half receiving an endocrine treatment and the others chemotherapy. Assessment of the UICC response on plain radiographs was possible in 53 patients. Sixteen (30%) patients achieved a UICC partial response (PR) in bone, 14 showed no change

(NC) and 23 had progressive disease (PD). No patient had a complete response. The median duration of response was 12 months (range 5–33+ months).

Osteoblast activity was monitored by serial measurements of alkaline phosphatase bone isoenzyme (ALP-BI) using a heat-inactivation technique (Moss and Whitby 1975) and osteocalcin (BGP) by radio-immunoassay. Serum calcium, tartrate-resistant acid phosphatase (TRP) (Efstradiatis and Moss 1985), and molar ratios of urinary calcium and hydroxyproline to creatinine (Grant et al. 1984) were measured to assess osteoclast activity. Symptomatic response was assessed by a questionnaire completed by the patient. Severity of pain and mobility were rated by the patient and combined with a scoring of analgesic consumption and the WHO performance status to produce an overall symptom score (Coleman et al. 1988c).

Markers of Bone Formation

Osteoblasts are rich in alkaline phosphatase and the serum concentration is a reflection of their activity. Measurement of total alkaline phosphatase is routine, but to exclude the contribution from the liver, bone isoenzyme estimation is required. Raised levels reflect new bone formation and correlate with hydroxyproline excretion and bone scan activity (Stepan et al. 1978). The highest values are found with osteoblastic metastases or in response to healing (Parbhoo 1985). In prostate cancer, alkaline phosphatase is a sensitive marker of response with raised levels falling to normal a few months after androgen ablation (Urwin et al. 1985).

Osteocalcin (Bone GLA protein, BGP) is also synthesised in osteoblasts. This small protein contains three residues of the vitamin K-dependent amino acid α-carboxyglutamic acid and is unique to bone and tooth dentine. Osteocalcin binds strongly to hydroxyapatite, but a small fraction of newly synthesised protein appears in the circulation from which it is rapidly cleared by the kidney. Measurement of serum levels is possible by radio immunoassay (Price and Nishimoto 1980). Levels reflect new bone formation and correlate with alkaline phosphatase activity and the bone mineralisation rate (Brown et al. 1984).

Raised levels are found in Paget's disease, hyperparathyroidism and osteoporosis (Gundberg et al. 1984). In metastatic disease raised levels are usual, the highest values occurring in patients with a large sclerotic component to their disease and low values, sometimes subnormal, in patients with rapidly advancing lytic destruction or hypercalcaemia (Coleman et al. 1988d).

During treatment in the Guy's Hospital study a transient rise in ALP-BI, maximal at 1 month, and BGP, maximal at 2 months, was seen in responding patients, followed by a gradual fall over subsequent months as the osteoblastic reaction induced by successful therapy subsided. After 1 month 15/16 (94%) responding patients showed a >10% rise in ALP-BI and BGP (Fig. 6.8) compared with 7/22 (31%) with progressive disease (p<0.001). The flare in ALP-BI subsided more quickly than BGP, suggesting these two markers may reflect different aspects of osteoblast function (Fig. 6.9 a,b).

Patients with radiologically stable disease showed a less consistent pattern, although some showed biochemical changes which were similar to those seen in responding patients. The fact that the survival prospects of patients with no change is similar to that of responding patients (Coleman and Rubens 1985)

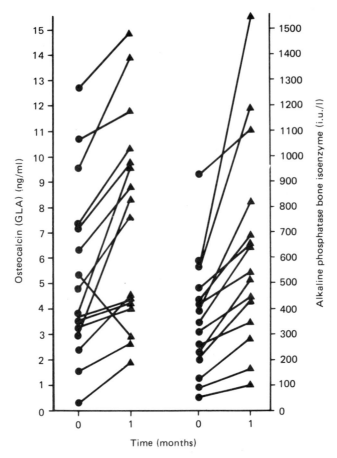

Fig. 6.8. Osteocalcin (GLA) and alkaline phosphatase bone isoenzyme (ALP-BI) before and 1 month after successful systemic therapy (n=16).

suggests a tumour response probably does occur. Nevertheless, it seems, on the evidence of both plain radiography and biochemical monitoring, that the usual end-result of a tumour response, that is remineralisation, does not occur to a significant degree in these patients. In patients with progressive disease, an increase in parameters of osteoblast activity was seen in some patients, presumably reflecting an increase in the sclerotic component of the disease.

A transient rise in alkaline phosphatase during the first month of treatment has been noted before (Hortabagyi et al. 1984), but in that study was not seen in all responders, possibly because isoenzyme measurements were not performed. In another study (Coombes et al. 1983), changes in ALP were unhelpful, but here repeat measurements were not made until 2–4 months, a time when osteoblast activity is falling again.

Similar findings are found in multiple myeloma, a disease characterised usually by impaired osteoblast activity (Valentin-Opran et al. 1982). Here response to therapy results in an increase in BGP from subnormal to normal as coupling is restored (Bataille et al. 1987).

Markers of Bone Resorption

Resorption of bone releases hydroxyproline, a major amino-acid constituent of collagen, from the matrix and the mineral components calcium and phosphate into the circulation. Much of the hydroxyproline is oxidised by the liver, but approximately 15% appears in the urine. Measurements are made on either a 24-h urine collection or the second voided early morning sample after an overnight fast (Mundy 1979).

Serum calcium measurements are routinely performed, but changes within the normal range give little guide to disease activity. Hypercalcaemia usually indicates progressive skeletal disease, but occasionally develops shortly after starting tamoxifen without evidence of progressive disease (Villalon et al. 1979). In the Guy's study, serum calcium did not change significantly and changes within the normal range could not be used to predict response. However, hypercalcaemia developed in 6 patients and this invariably indicated progressive disease.

Hypocalcaemia may occur when osteoblastic metastases predominate. 23/143 (16%) of patients in one series (Raskin et al. 1973) and 10/28 (36%) of another had hypocalcaemia (Smallridge et al. 1981).

Urinary calcium excretion is a more sensitive indicator of alterations in calcium homeostasis. The molar ratio of calcium to creatinine in an early morning urine sample after an overnight fast is a convenient reproducible method of quantifying calcium excretion (Peacock et al. 1969) and has been reported as a marker of response (Campbell et al. 1983). The Guy's study confirmed this with a fall in urinary calcium excretion with a nadir at 1 month occurring in responding patients. At 1 month 15 (94%) responders had a >10% reduction in calcium excretion compared with 10/21 (48%) with progressive disease (p<0.01). No patient with responding or static disease for more than 6 months had a rise in calcium excretion at 1 month (Fig. 6.9c).

Increased hydroxyproline excretion may reflect either increased bone resorption or formation and measuring urinary excretion cannot distinguish between the two. Hydroxyproline excretion has a circadian rhythm with a peak in the early morning and is strongly influenced by diet, age and soft-tissue destruction. Not surprisingly, its value as a marker of malignant disease in bone has been controversial. Hydroxyproline excretion has been proposed as a marker for diagnosis of bone metastases, documenting progression and monitoring therapy (Dequecker et al. 1983). However, others have been unable to confirm this (Coombes et al. 1983) and in the Guy's study serial measurements correlated poorly with response. Despite a reduction in calcium excretion and evidence of bone healing, levels of hydroxyproline remained high in many responding patients. A rise was seen in 73% of non-responders, but levels fell in only 50% of responders.

Acid phosphatases are produced by several cell types and the tartrate-labile isoenzyme is used as a marker of disease activity in prostate cancer. The tartrate-resistant isoenzyme is mainly derived from osteoclasts and is a marker of the rate of osteoclastic bone resorption (Efstradiatis and Moss 1985). Levels rise with progressive metastatic bone disease and a fall correlates with response to endocrine therapy (Zweig and Ihde 1985). In the Guy's study, although levels did not often fall as a result of effective therapy, a rise was more common in progressive disease (p<0.02) and an increase in tartrate-resistant acid

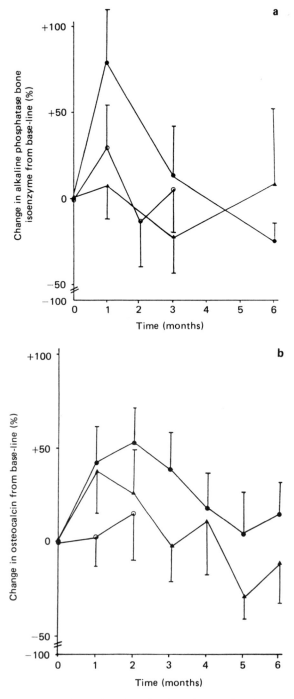

Fig. 6.9a–d. Mean percentage change from base-line in **a** alkaline phosphatase bone isoenzyme, **b** osteocalcin, **c** urinary calcium excretion and **d** symptom score for the three UICC response groups. *Closed circles*, partial responders; *triangles*, no change patients; *open circles*, progressive disease. Error bars are SEM.

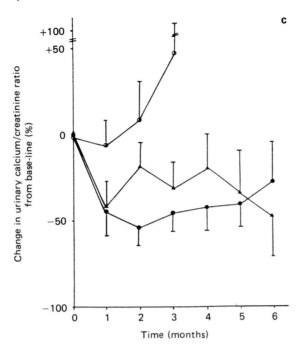

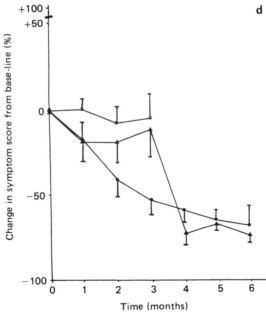

phosphatase after 3 months occurred in 13/17 patients with progressive disease compared with 2 of 9 responders (p<0.05).

Subjective Assessment

The relief of symptoms is the principal aim of palliative therapy and rationally should be the most important manifestation of response to treatment. However, the use of pain relief as a marker of response in clinical trials has not found universal acceptance because measurement is difficult and confounded by analgesic usage. Nevertheless, the use of a linear analogue scale or pain score plus a record of analgesic consumption and mobility (performance status) enables an approximate measurement of pain and provides useful corroboration of objective response (Coombes et al. 1983).

The pain questionnaire used in the Guy's study (Table 6.3) was completed by the patient and provided a semi-quantitative assessment of pain, mobility and analgesic use. From these data a symptom score was easily computed. Symptomatic response to treatment occurred quite slowly. After 1 month, only 8 responders (50%) reported symptomatic benefit, but by 3 months symptomatic improvement had occurred in all responding patients (Fig. 6.9d). Patients progressing had, at best, only a slight and transient relief of symptoms, usually

Table 6.3. Key to the derivation of a symptomatic assessment from a patient-completed questionnaire

Parameter	Description	Score
Pain	None	0
	Mild	1
	Moderate	2
	Severe	3
	Very severe	4
	Intolerable	5
Analgesic use	None	0
	Simple analgesic or NSAID[a]	1
	Simple analgesic + NSAID	2
	Moderate analgesic (eg Dihydrocodeine)	3
	Opiates (<40 mg morphine daily)	4
	Opiates (>40 mg morphine daily)	5
Mobility	Normal	0
	Vigorous exercise/activity impaired	1
	Climbing stairs/walking/bending impaired	2
	Difficulty with dressing/washing	3
	Difficulty with all activities	4
	Totally dependant and bedbound	5
Performance status	Normal	0
	Light work possible	1
	Up and about > 50% of the day	2
	Confined to bed >50% of the day	3
	Completely bed-bound	4
Symptom score expressed as a percentage of maximum total		19 (100%)

[a] NSAID, non-steroidal anti-inflammatory drug

attributable to local radiotherapy. Steady worsening of symptoms invariably indicated progressive disease, although an abrupt and transient flare in pain is well-recognised shortly after starting hormone treatment and often heralds a response.

Tumour Markers

The use of beta human chorionic gonadotrophin (β-HCG) and alphafetoprotein (AFP) in monitoring response in testicular cancer and, to a lesser extent CA-125 in ovarian cancer, has had a major beneficial effect on the management of these diseases. However, there is no comparable tumour marker for breast cancer although some cases of breast cancer do produce tumour antigens which can be detected by radio-immunoassay. The most widely studied is carcinoembryonic antigen (CEA), a β-1-glycoprotein normally found in foetal gut. Among patients with metastatic breast cancer 50%–80% produce CEA (Loprinzi et al. 1986). Raised CEA levels may be useful in predicting response (Palazzo et al. 1986) and monitoring treatment, a fall in CEA correlating with response (Mughal et al. 1983). However, Loprinzi et al. (1986) found serial CEA levels to be of minimal clinical value and reported an initial rise in CEA during the first 3 months of successful treatment, changes indistinguishable from progressive disease.

The antigen CA 15-3 may be a more sensitive marker than CEA (Colomer et al. 1989). Levels of the antigen are elevated more commonly, particularly when the disease has metastasised and serial values appear to correlate with objective response (Kerin et al. 1989). Although it is clear that CA 15-3 is not a useful marker for screening for breast cancer, a detailed prospective evaluation of CA 15-3 in advanced breast cancer when the majority of patients will have elevated levels does seem justified.

In prostate cancer, the tumour product prostatic acid phosphatase (PAP) has been used as a marker of disease activity for many years (Rubinstein et al. 1988). About one half of patients with disseminated disease will have PAP concentrations more than twice the upper limit of the normal range (Buamah et al. 1988). More recently, prostate-specific antigen (PSA) has been studied and is a more reliable marker. All patients with metastatic carcinoma had PSA levels more than twice the upper limit of the reference range (Buamah et al. 1988). Levels of PSA correlate with tumour volume and extent of disease (Stamey et al. 1989a); serial measurements are useful in monitoring response to therapy with anti-androgens. An initial and often dramatic decrease in PSA levels was seen in 72% of patients during the first 6 months of therapy (Stamey et al. 1989b).

Response to treatment in multiple myeloma has been defined as either a 50% (Chronic Leukaemia-Myeloma Task Force 1973) or 75% (Alexanian et al. 1973) decrease in serum myeloma protein level or urinary myeloma protein excretion. Bone healing is unusual in myeloma, even when a fall in myeloma protein has occurred and, therefore, is not included in response assessment. Recently, intensive treatment incorporating high-dose chemotherapy and autologous bone-marrow transplantation has increased the response rate and new criteria for complete remission in myeloma have been proposed. These are based on

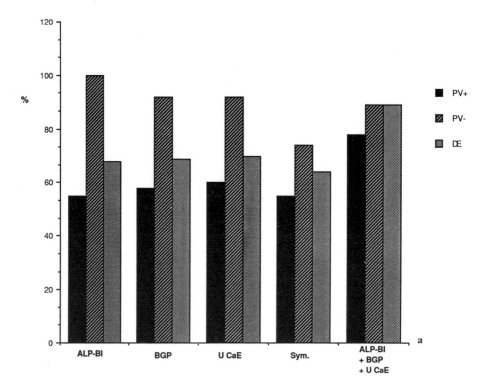

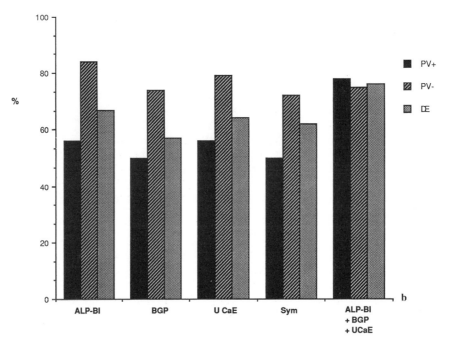

complete disappearance of the myeloma protein from blood and urine and clearing of the bone marrow of excess plasma cells (Gore et al. 1989).

Suggestions for Future Study

Although the plain radiograph and the UICC criteria of response remain the "gold standard" for assessing the effects of treatment it is clear that reliable alternatives are necessary. The development of reliable tumour markers would perhaps provide the most direct method and attempts to identify new markers are under way in many laboratories. The modern imaging modalities will undoubtedly be refined and their role more clearly defined. However, state of the art imaging is likely to remain expensive, time consuming and confined to specialist centres. Monitoring of bone metabolism shows the most promise and appears the most likely method to replace the plain radiograph. The tests are relatively straightforward and could be readily made available to most centres.

The Guy's study demonstrated that biochemical monitoring of bone cell function could predict eventual radiological response. Successful therapy resulted in a flare in osteoblast activity and reduction in the rate of bone resorption, changes which were significantly different from those seen with progressive disease.

The positive and negative predictive values (PV+ and PV−) and diagnostic efficiency (DE) (Galen and Gambino 1975) of changes in ALP-BI, BGP, urinary calcium excretion and symptom score after 1 month's treatment were calculated. A 10% change from base-line (increase for ALP-BI and BGP, decrease for urinary calcium excretion and symptom score) was selected as the cut-off. The negative predictive value of single biochemical parameters was high, but the more clinically useful positive predicting value and diagnostic efficiency relatively low. Combining parameters, however, improved the discrimination and a combination of a >10% rise in ALP-BI and BGP with a >10% fall in calcium excretion was the most useful (Fig. 6.10). The diagnostic efficiency for discriminating between response and progression was 89%. When patients with radiologically stable disease were included, the diagnostic efficiency fell slightly to 76% for discriminating between progression after more than six months from progression within the first 6 months of treatment (Fig. 6.10).

In conclusion, biochemical monitoring appears to be a good alternative to plain radiography as it provides an indication of response long before radiological changes can be expected. Independant prospective studies to try to confirm and refine this alternative approach are now indicated.

←──

Fig. 6.10a,b. The positive (PV+) and negative (PV−) predictive values and diagnostic efficiency (DE) of alternative parameters of response. **a** The ability to discriminate between responders (n=16) and progressive disease (n=22). **b** The discrimination between time to progression (TTP) of more than 6 months (n=22) compared with TTP of less than 6 months (n=31). ALP-BI, alkaline phosphatase bone isoenzyme; BGP, osteocalcin; UCaE, urinary calcium: creatinine ratio; Sym, Symptom score.

References

Aabo K (1987) Prostate cancer: evaluation of response to treatment, response criteria, and the need for standardization of the reporting of results. Eur J Cancer Clin Oncol 23:231–237

Alexanian R, Gehan E, Bonnet J et al. (1973) Combination chemotherapy for multiple myeloma. Semin Haematol 10:135–147

Bataille R, Delmas P, Sany J (1987) Serum bone gla-protein in multiple myeloma. Cancer 59:329–334

Bellamy EA, Nicholas D, Ward M, Coombes RC, Powles TJ (1987) Comparison of computed tomography and conventional radiology in the assessment of treatment response of lytic bony metastases in patients with carcinoma of the breast. Clin Radiol 38:351–355

Brown JP, Delmas PD, Malaval L, Edouard C, Chapuy MC, Meunier PJ (1984) Serum bone GLA protein: a specific marker for bone formation in postmenopausal osteoporosis. Lancet i:1091–1093

Buamah PK, Johnson P, Skillen AW (1988) Comparative study of the clinical usefulness of prostate specific antigen and prostatic acid phosphatase in prostatic disease. Br J Urol 62:581–583

Campbell FC, Blamey RW, Woolfson AMJ et al. (1983) Calcium excretion CaE in metastatic breast cancer. Br J Surg 70:202–204

Chlebowski RT, Block JB (1981) Chemotherapy of bone metastasis (1). In: Weiss L, Gilbert HA (eds) Bone metastases. GK Hall, Boston, pp 312–324

Chronic Leukaemia-Myeloma Task Force (1973) Proposed guidelines for protocol studies. II. Plasma cell myeloma. Cancer Treat Rep 4:145–158

Coleman RE, Rubens RD (1985) Breast cancer and bone metastases. Cancer Treat Rev 12:251–270.

Coleman RE, Mashiter G, Fogelman I et al. (1988a) Osteocalcin: a marker of metastatic bone disease. Eur J Cancer Clin Oncol 24:1211–1217

Coleman RE, Rubens RD, Fogelman I (1988b) The bone scan flare following systemic therapy for bone metastases. J Nucl Med 29:1354–1359

Coleman RE, Whitaker KD, Moss DW, Mashiter G, Fogelman I, Rubens RD (1988c) Biochemical monitoring predicts response in bone metastases to treatment. Br J Cancer 58:205–210

Coleman RE, Woll PJ, Miles M, Scrivener W, Rubens RD (1988d) Treatment of bone metastases from breast cancer with (3-amino-1-hydroxypropylidene)-1, 1-bisphosphonate (APD), Br J Cancer 58:621–625

Colomer R, Ruibal A, Salvador L (1989) Circulating tumour marker levels in advanced breast carcinoma correlate with the extent of metastatic disease. Cancer 64:1674–1681

Condon BR, Buchanan R, Garvie NW et al. (1981). Assessment of progression of secondary bone lesions following cancer of the breast or prostate using serial radionuclide imaging. Br J Radiol 54:18–23

Coombes RC, Dady P, Parsons C et al. (1983) Assessment of response of bone metastases to systemic treatment in patients with breast cancer. Cancer 52:610–614

Crone-Munzebrock RP (1987) Quantification of recalcification of irradiated vertebral body osteolyses by dual-energy computed tomography. Eur J Radiol 7:1–5

Daffner RH, Lupetin RH, Dash N et al. (1986) MRI in the detection of malignant infiltration of the bone marrow. AJR 149:457–469

Dequecker J, Mbuyi-Muamba JM, Holvoet G (1983) Hydroxyproline and bone metastasis. In: Stoll BA, Parbhoo S (eds) Bone metastasis: monitoring and treatment. Raven Press, New York, pp 181–199

Efstradiatis T, Moss DW (1985) Tartrate resistant acid phosphatase of human lung: Apparent identity with osteoclastic acid phosphatase. Enzyme 33:34–40

Frank J, Ling A, Patronas N et al. (1989) Comparison of magnetic resonance imaging and radionuclide bone scan in the evaluation of primary and metastatic disease to bone. Proc ASCO 8:7

Galasko CSB, Bennett A (1976) Mechanism of bone destruction in the development of skeletal metastases. Nature 263:507–508

Galen RS, Gambino SR (1975) How to determine the predictive value and efficiency of a test when reading a scientific paper. In: Galen RS, Gambino SR (eds) Beyond normality: the predictive value and efficiency of medical diagnosis. John Wiley & Sons, New York, pp 30–51

Gore ME, Selby PJ, Viner C, Clark PI et al. (1989) Intensive treatment of multiple myeloma and criteria for complete remission. Lancet ii:879–881

Goris ML, Bretille J (1985) Skeletal scintigraphy for the diagnosis of malignant metastatic disease to the bones. Radiother Oncol 3:319–329

Grant CS, Hoare SA, Millis RR, Hayward JL, Wang DY (1984) Urinary hydroxyproline and prognosis in human breast cancer. Br J Surg 71:105–108

Gundberg CM, Lian JB, Gallop PM, Steinberg JJ (1984) Urinary gamma-carboxyglutamic acid and serum osteocalcin as bone markers: studies in osteoporosis and Paget's disease. J Clin Endocrinol Metab 57:1221–1225

Hayward JL, Carbone PP, Heuson JC, Kumaoka S, Segaloff A, Rubens RD (1977) Assessment of response to therapy in advanced breast cancer. Eur J Cancer Clin Oncol 13:89–94

Hortabagyi GN, Libshitz HI, Seabold JE (1984) Osseous metastases of breast cancer. Clinical, biochemical, radiographic and scintigraphic evaluation of response to therapy. Cancer 55:577–582

Kerin MJ, McAnena OJ, O'Malley VP, Grimes H, Given HF. (1989) CA 15–3: its relationship to clinical stage and progression to metastatic disease in breast cancer. Br J Surg 76:838–839

Loprinzi CL, Tormey DC, Rasmussen P et al. (1986) Prospective evaluation of carcinoembryonic antigen levels and alternating chemotherapeutic regimens in metastatic breast cancer. J Clin Oncol 4:46–56

Mazess A, Vetter J (1985) The influence of marrow on measurement of trabecular bone using computed tomography. Bone 6:349–351

Moss DW, Whitby LG (1975) A simplified heat-inactivation method for investigating alkaline phosphatase isoenzymes in serum. Clin Chim Acta 61:63–71

Mughal AW, Hortobagyi GN, Fritsche HA, et al. (1983) Serial plasma carcinoembryonic antigen level measurements during treatment of metastatic breast cancer. JAMA 249:1881–1886

Mundy A (1979) Urinary hydroxyproline excretion in carcinoma of the prostate: a comparison of 4 different modes of assessment and its role as a marker. Br J Urol 51:570–574

Mundy GR (1987) The hypercalcaemia of malignancy. Kidney Int 31:142–155

Palazzo S, Liguori V, Molinari B (1986) Is the carcino-embryonic antigen test a valid predictor of response to medical therapy in disseminated breast cancer? Tumori 72:515–518

Parbhoo SP (1983) Serial scintiscans in monitoring patients with bone metastases In: Stoll BA, Parbhoo SP (eds) Bone metastasis: monitoring and treatment. Raven Press, New York, pp 201–239

Parbhoo SP (1985) Usefulness of current techniques in detecting and monitoring bone metastases from breast cancer. J R Soc Med 78:(Suppl 9) 7–10

Peacock M, Robertson WD, Nordin BEC (1969) Relation between serum and urinary calcium with particular reference to parathyroid activities. Lancet i:384–386

Price PA, Nishimoto SK (1980) Radioimmunoassay for the vitamin K-dependant protein and its discovery in plasma. Proc Natl Acad Sci USA 77:2234–2238

Rafii M, Firooznia H, Golimbu C, Beranbaum E (1986) CT of skeletal metastasis. Semin Ultrasound, CT MR 7:371–379

Raskin P, McClain C, Medager T (1973) Hypocalcaemia associated with metastatic bone disease. Arch Intern Med 132:539–543

Rossleigh MA, Lovegrove FTA, Reynolds PM, Byrne MJ, Whitney BP (1984) The assessment of response to therapy of bone metastases in breast cancer. Aust NZ J Med 14:19–22

Rubinstein M, Guinan PD, McKiel CF, Dubin A (1988) Review of acid phosphatase in the diagnosis and prognosis of prostatic cancers. Clin Physiol Biochem 6:241–252

Scher HI Yagoda A (1987) Bone metastases: pathogenesis, treatment, and rationale for use of bone resorption inhibitors. A J Med 82:(suppl 2A) 6–28

Smallridge RC, Wray HL, Schaaf F (1981) Hypocalcaemia with osteoblastic metastases in a patient with prostate carcinoma, A cause of secondary hyperparathyroidism. A J Med 71:184–188

Smoker WRG, Godersky JC, Knutzon RK, Keyes WD, Norman D, Bergman W (1987) The role of MR imaging in evaluating metastatic spinal disease. A J N R 6:901–908

Stamey TA, Kabalin JN, McNeal JE et al. (1989a) Prostate specific antigen in the diagnosis and treatment of adenocarcinoma of the prostate. II. Radical prostatectomy treated patients. J Urol 141:1076–1083

Stamey TA, Kabalin JN, Ferrari M, Yang N (1989b) Prostate specific antigen in the diagnosis and treatment of adenocarcinoma of the prostate. IV. Anti-androgen treated patients. J Urol 141:1088–1090

Stepan J, Pacovsky V, Horn V et al. (1978) Relationship of the activity of the bone isoenzyme of serum alkaline phosphatase to urinary hydroxyproline excretion in metabolic and neoplastic bone diseases. Eur J Clin Invest 8:373–377

Urwin GH, Percival RC, Yates AJP et al. (1985) Biochemical markers and skeletal metabolism in carcinoma of the prostate. Br J Urol 57:711–714

Valentin-Opran A, Charhon SA, Meunier PJ, Edouard CM, Aelot ME (1982) Quantitative histology of myeloma-induced bone changes. Br J Haematol 52:601–610

Villalon AH, Tattersall MH, Fox RM, Woods RL (1979) Hypercalcaemia after tamoxifen for breast
    cancer: a sign of tumour response. Br Med J ii:1329–1330
Zweig M, Ihde D (1985) Assessment of serum and enzymatic prostatic acid phosphatase activity in
    prostate cancer. JAMA 245:1501–1504

7   The Systemic Treatment of Bone Metastases

D.J. Dodwell and A. Howell

Introduction

Skeletal involvement is one of the most distressing and common complications of many solid cancers, particularly breast, lung, prostate, thyroid and kidney. The high incidence of many of these cancers and the frequency of bone involvement means that those treating patients with metastatic bone disease face a large scale clinical problem.

Different types of cancer have preferred patterns of blood-borne metastases. It is still unclear whether haematogenous dissemination is dependent on the vascular supply of host organs or whether particular biological environments are favoured by clumps of tumour cells – the "seed and soil" hypothesis – although a combination of these factors may operate.

The reported incidence of bone involvement in different malignancies is dependent on the method of determination. Post mortem studies indicate that as many as 85% of women dying from breast cancer have bone metastases and corresponding figures for patients with prostate and lung cancer are 85% and 60% (Stoll 1983). The more meticulous the pathological and histological examination the higher the reported incidence and it is likely that because of sampling problems the true incidence of skeletal disease in patients with advanced forms of these common malignancies is even higher.

Tofe et al. (1975) reported a series of 1355 patients who had been submitted to isotope scintigraphy for various reasons. The incidence of "positive" scans ranged from 43% to 67% and the proportion positive was apparently independent of tumour type. Clearly such patients had symptoms or signs suggestive of bone involvement and are therefore highly selected. However the sensitivity of isotope scintigraphy is dependent on an osteoblastic response and this is only likely to be seen once a metastasis is of the order of 2–3 mm in size. It is also obvious in the clinic that many patients are asymptomatic despite widespread skeletal involvement and the prevalence of bony involvement within populations of cancer patients is likely to be underestimated.

There is also increasing evidence that bone involvement is by no means a late complication of malignancy. The incidence of bone marrow involvement in small cell lung cancer at the time of presentation has been reported to be from 20% to 50% (Trillet et al. 1989) depending on the methods used to detect tumour cells. Mansi et al. (1987) used a cytokeratin antibody to show that malignant cells could be detected in bone marrow smears in 25% of women undergoing surgery for primary breast cancer if multiple aspirates were taken at the time of surgery. The presence of malignant cells within the marrow also predicted early recurrence. Sharp et al. (1989) have shown that when marrow is harvested from women with "early" breast cancer and filtered prior to cryopreservation, breast cancer cells can be grown from the material collected on the filter in 50% of cases. This is of concern for those using autologous marrow rescue after high-dose chemoradiotherapy for patients with small cell lung cancer and breast cancer, even if there is no radiographic evidence of bone involvement.

The morbidity from skeletal metastases is considerable. Bone metastases are the commonest cause of cancer pain (Twycross 1982) and in addition cause immobility, pathological fracture, bone marrow failure, cord compression and hypercalcaemia. Patients with bone metastases, particularly those from breast cancer, tend to survive longer than those with other organ sites such as liver or lung (Coleman and Rubens 1987) and, therefore, may have prolonged periods of morbidity.

The current management of patients with skeletal metastases is directed towards symptom palliation; other than in certain rare exceptions, cure is an unrealistic aim. Treatment may encompass the specialties of radiotherapy, oncology, surgery and palliative care, but the contribution from each will depend heavily on tumour type, stage of disease and local resources.

Available treatments for bony metastases may be local or systemic. Although the purpose of this chapter is to discuss the systemic treatment of skeletal metastases, it may be useful to mention local therapy in order to place the medical treatment in context and to serve as a reminder that the successful management of patients with bone metastases is highly dependent on a multidisciplinary approach.

External beam radiotherapy is the treatment of choice for localised metastatic bone pain and is successful in relieving the pain arising from bony metastases in approximately 85% of cases; however, relief may not be evident for 2 weeks. There is no clear evidence of a dose-response effect in terms of the degree of pain relief, and the mode of action of radiotherapy may involve factors other than tumour shrinkage. A single dose appears to be as effective as fractionated treatment and is clearly more convenient. The role of radiotherapy in asymptomatic lesions is, however, uncertain and it is unlikely that the risk of pathological fracture is reduced by radiotherapy.

The incidence of pathological fracture in weight-bearing bones where there is lytic destruction is high and related to the extent of cortical involvement (Fidler 1981). This has led to the recommendation that lesions involving the cortex are surgically stabilised prior to irradiation, and prosthetic surgery has also been shown to provide good pain relief from large lytic lesions (Galasko 1986). However, this may be difficult surgery and major procedures may not be feasible in patients who are often a poor anaesthetic risk.

Systemic Therapy

The clinical effects of bone metastases are produced by tumour cell proliferation and interactions between tumour cells and host cells. The cellular interactions are mediated by a variety of growth factors and cytokines and are described in detail in Chap. 2. Systemic therapy for bone metastases may be directed against the tumour cell in order to reduce cell proliferation and the production of mediators or may be directed against blocking the effect of mediators on host cells. Chemotherapy, endocrine therapy and bone-seeking isotopes have direct anti-tumour effects whereas agents such as the bisphosphonates and calcitonin are effective by preventing host cells (primarily osteoclasts) from reacting to tumour products. Thus systemic therapies may have direct or indirect actions.

Direct Anti-tumour Therapy

The systemic treatment for bone metastases from various malignancies tends to parallel available treatments for other metastatic manifestations and can only be discussed according to tumour type. In this regard we will discuss the medical treatment of bone metastases from breast and prostate cancer predominantly as these tumours have effective, available systemic treatments and represent the majority of patients with bone metastases. These treatments are endocrine therapy and chemotherapy. We will attempt to summarise information for the treatment of tumours which are less common or produce skeletal metastases uncommonly.

Breast Cancer

Introduction

Approximately one quarter of women with primary breast cancer have identifiable tumour cells within the bone marrow at the time of mastectomy (Mansi et al. 1987). The skeleton is the commonest site of distant recurrence after surgery for breast cancer and at least 70% of patients with advanced breast cancer develop clinically identifiable bone metastases at some time during the course of their disease (Coleman and Rubens 1987; McNeil 1984).

It has also been shown that patients with skeletal metastases only have a more protracted clinical course compared to other metastatic sites, with a median survival from relapse of 24–52 months (Coleman and Rubens 1987; Sherry et al. 1986; Leone et al. 1988). The development of extra-skeletal disease in lung or liver is associated with a much poorer prognosis. The prolonged survival of patients with metastases only in bone may be related to the tendency for receptor-positive well-differentiated tumours to spread to this site (Coleman and Rubens 1987).

Endocrine Therapy

The results of endocrine treatment of osseous metastases in breast cancer are derived from both uncontrolled phase II and comparative studies of differing forms of endocrine therapy, designed to evaluate response and survival in patients with all advanced manifestations of the disease.

It is usually possible to derive data concerning response in bone from these studies, but they rarely give response duration in bone or survival in patients with bone metastases only. Thus, in most cases, only the response rates to differing forms of endocrine therapy can be compared between studies. Uncontrolled studies of additive endocrine therapy in post-menopausal women with advanced breast cancer which adequately provide bone response data are listed in Table 7.1.

In order that these forms of endocrine therapy may be adequately compared, only published studies which report response classified according to UICC criteria are included. Tamoxifen has become the treatment of choice in post-menopausal women with advanced breast cancer and, as can be seen, skeletal response rates differ considerably. In the study of Brule (1978), only 4 of 75 patients with evaluable skeletal disease responded to tamoxifen whereas 7 of 18 patients responded in the study of Lerner et al. (1976). More recently Rubens et al. (1988) reported a higher overall response rate, response duration and survival when prednisolone was added to ovarian ablation or tamoxifen in the treatment of pre- and post-menopausal women with advanced breast cancer. The response rate in bone was also higher in the prednisolone-treated arms.

There is little available information in terms of bone response to aminoglutethimide when used as first-line therapy after relapse and consequently this agent has been evaluated predominantly as second-line therapy. In this situation bone response rates vary from 0% (Kaye et al. 1982) to 50% (Smith et al. 1978). There appears to be little evidence of a dose response effect to aminoglutethimide (Bonneterre et al. 1985; Harris et al. 1989).

Response rates to progestogens where these are used as second-line therapy also appear to vary widely. Blackledge et al. (1986) reported no responses in 13 patients with evaluable bone disease treated with megestrol acetate whereas Hortobagyi et al. (1985) saw 9 responses in 18 evaluable patients.

When randomised studies are considered (Table 7.2) conflicting results are seen. Smith et al. (1981) and Lipton et al. (1982) reported higher response rates to aminoglutethimide in bone compared to tamoxifen. However, the differences were not significant within their individual studies because of relatively small numbers but became significant when the results of the studies were combined. Van Veelen et al. (1986) compared tamoxifen and medroxyprogesterone acetate (MPA) as first-line therapy and reported a slightly higher overall response rate and also a higher response rate in bone (40% compared to 23%) using MPA. In contrast, Mouridsen et al. (1979) found that the overall and bone response rates to tamoxifen were reduced (albeit not significantly) when MPA was given in addition. In the randomised studies of second-line additive endocrine therapy summarised in Table 7.2, aminoglutethimide appears to have a slight but consistent advantage over other forms of additive endocrine therapy and, in view of this, is widely held to be superior for this particular metastatic site (Harmsen and Porsius 1988). However, the greater toxicity of aminoglutethimide is likely to outweigh any possible advantage that it may have in the treatment of bone

Table 7.1. Uncontrolled studies of additive endocrine therapy in the treatment of bone metastases from breast cancer

Author	Year	Drug	Number of evaluable patients	Response rate classified by UICC criteria		Response duration for patients with bone dominant disease
				All sites	Bone only	
Brule	1978	Tamoxifen (f)	177	29/177 (16%)	4/75 (5%)	NR
Ribeiro	1977	Tamoxifen (f)	141	36/141 (25%)	1/24 (4%)	NR
Lerner et al.	1976	Tamoxifen (f)	74	35/74 (47%)	7/18 (39%)	NR
Valavaara et al.	1988	Toremifene (f)	46	25/46 (54%)	1/6 (13%)	NR
Kaye et al.	1982	Aminoglutethimide (s)	52	10/52 (19%)	0/30	NR
Murray and Pitt	1981	Aminoglutethimide (s)	53	24/53 (45%)	20/36 (56%)	NR
Ceci et al.	1985	Aminoglutethimide (m)	53	22/53 (43%)	5/16 (31%)	NR
Smith et al.	1978	Aminoglutethimide (m)	40	15/40 (37%)	19/36 (50%)	NR
Hoffken et al.	1986	Aminoglutethimide (s)	38	5/38 (13%)	5/38 (13%)	13 mths
Harris et al.	1989	Aminoglutethimide (m)	101	25/101 (25%)	4/41 (9%)	NR
Hortobagyi et al.	1985	Medroxyprogesterone (m)	39	17/39 (44%)	9/18 (50%)	NR
Alexieva-Figuschi	1980	Megestrol (m)	160	48/160 (30%)	1/31 (3%)	NR
Gregory et al.	1985	Megestrol (m)	110	29/110 (26%)	16/51 (31%)	NR
Blackledge et al.	1986	Megestrol (m)	37	9/37 (25%)	0/13	NR
Minton et al.	1981	Prednisolone (s)	91	13/91 (14%)	4/40 (10%)	NR

f, used as first-line therapy.
s, used as second line therapy.
m, used both first and second-line within the study.
NR, not reported.

Table 7.2.   Randomised trials of additive endocrine therapy in breast cancer

Author	Drugs	Number of patients evaluable	Response Rate (UICC criteria)	
			All sites	Bone
First-line therapy				
Alonso-Munoz et al.	Tamoxifen	34	18/34 (53%)	2/4 (50%)
(1988)	Aminoglutethimide	31	15/31 (48%)	3/4 (75%)
	Tam + aminoglut.	29	11/29 (38%)	2/2 (100%)
Van Veelen et al.	Tamoxifen	68	24/68 (35%)	7/31 (23%)
(1986)	Medroxyprogesterone	61	27/61 (44%)	11/23 (48%)
Mouridsen et al.	Tamoxifen	46	20/46 (45%)	9/20 (45%)
(1979)	Tam + medroxyprog.	55	14/55 (26%)	4/18 (22%)
Rubens et al. (1988)	Tamoxifen	77	24/77 (31%)	6/41 (15%)
	Tamoxifen + prednisolone	85	39/85 (46%)	12/41 (29%)
	Ovarian ablation	15	4/15 (27%)	0/8 (0%)
	Ovarian ablation + pred.	16	10/16 (63%)	4/6 (67%)
Second-line therapy				
Canney et al. (1988)	Aminoglutethimide	106	29/106 (27%)	6/24 (25%)
	Medroxyprogesterone[a]	102	35/102 (31%)	6/35 (17%)
Lundgren et al.	Medroxyprogesterone	74	23/74 (31%)	6/39 (15%)
(1989)	Aminoglutethimide	76	26/76 (33%)	8/27 (30%)
Smith et al.[b] (1981)	Tamoxifen	60	18/60 (30%)	5/29 (17%)
	Aminoglutethimide	57	17/57 (18%)	11/31 (35%)
Lipton et al. (1982)	Tamoxifen	39	15/39 (38%)	4/27 (15%)
	Aminoglutethimide	36	13/36 (36%)	9/27 (33%)

[a] At high dose.
[b] Includes some previously untreated patients.

metastases from breast cancer and tamoxifen, because of its efficacy and lack of toxicity, should remain standard first-line therapy in most cases. (The problem of tamoxifen-resistant disease will, however, arise in the near future because of the large numbers of patients given this drug as adjuvant treatment.)

Comparing response rates alone gives some indication of the possible magnitude of a palliative effect with treatment, but response duration, survival and quality of life are equally, if not more, important. Unfortunately most published studies do not provide this information for bone metastases.

In the majority of cases response rates in bone are less than the overall response rate: the possible reasons for this are discussed below.

Chemotherapy

Chemotherapy is normally reserved for endocrine-resistant disease in the treatment of metastatic breast cancer in all but a few exceptions such as inflammatory cancer or rapidly progressive or life-threatening visceral disease. Bone-response data are derived from studies reporting the results of treatment of patients with all metastatic sites. A series of recent chemotherapy studies giving UICC-classifiable bone-response data are shown in Table 7.3.

Table 7.3. Chemotherapy studies in advanced breast cancer

Author	Drug/s	Response rates classified according to UICC criteria	
		Overall	Bone
Non-randomised studies			
Mattsson et al.[a] (1982)	Mitomycin C + 5-fluorouracil	29/50 (58%)	5/9 (56%)
De Lena et al.[a] (1988)	CMF	26/60 (43%)	5/15 (33%)
Carmo-Pereira et al.[b] (1988)	Mitoxantrone + prednisolone	13/37 (35%)	3/15 (20%)
Di Costanzo et al.[c] (1986)	Mitomycin C + vindesine	5/31 (16%)	1/15 (7%)
Randomised studies			
Henderson et al.[c] (1989)	Doxorubicin vs. mitoxantrone	47/160 (29%) 34/165 (21%)	4/28 (14%) 2/33 (6%)
Parvinen and Numminen[a] (1985)	Doxorubicin + cyclophosphamide vs. Vincristine, cyclophosphamide, methotrexate, 5-fluorouracil + prednisolone	15/47 (32%) 19/55 (35%)	2/9 (22%) 0/4 (0%)
Muss et al.[a] (1982)	Vincristine, doxorubicin + cyclophosphamide vs. Low-dose cyclophosphamide, methotrexate + 5-fluorouracil	20/45 (44%) 7/44 (16%)	10/26 (38%) 0/15 (0%)
Randomised studies of combined hormone and chemotherapy			
Brunner et al.[d] (1977)	"Chemotherapy" vs. "Hormone and chemotherapy"	56/108 (52%) 64/105 (61%)	9/29 (31%) 16/38 (42%)
Perry et al.[b] (1987)	Cyclophosphamide, doxorubicin + 5-fluorouracil vs. + Tamoxifen	105/190 (55%) 118/185 (64%)	22/38 (58%) 17/33 (52%)

[a] Studies involving both groups of patients
[b] First-line.
[c] Second-line.
[d] A variety of hormone and cytotoxic treatments in both pre- (42) and post-menopausal (171) women were analysed. All patients were chemotherapy naive but 75 post-menopausal patients had received prior hormone therapy.

Whitehouse (1985) has also reviewed several chemotherapy studies in advanced breast cancer and found that response rates in bone varied from between 0% and 30%. The data indicate that there is no convincing evidence for the superiority of any single drug or regimen. In general, response rates in bone are lower than overall response rates and response rates at other sites. The rapid relief of bone pain which may occur in hormone-responsive disease is also less common after chemotherapy (Whitehouse 1985).

Evaluation of Response

The reported response rates to endocrine and cytotoxic therapy for bone metastases from breast cancer are usually lower than response rates at other metastatic sites (Stoll 1985; Smith and Macaulay 1985; Whitehouse 1985). The criteria of the UICC (Hayward et al. 1977) stipulate that radiological evidence of recalcification of lytic disease is required for classification as a response. The low response rates in bone may be artefactual. Reasons for the apparent lack of response to systemic treatment and the difficulties inherent in studies of systemic therapy are:

1. The numbers of evaluable patients in reported studies becomes low as patients with sclerotic metastases are excluded because they are non-evaluable, as are patients with single skeletal lesions which have been previously irradiated
2. Changes of systemic treatment are often influenced by extra-skeletal disease as this is more readily evaluable
3. Radiological recalcification requires not only tumour regression but also a healing response and as such may not be evident for 4–6 months after the start of therapy
4. As the median response duration to most forms of systemic treatment in extra-skeletal disease is between 7 and 18 months, this may not be a sufficient time for healing and therefore sclerosis to occur
5. Changes in treatment are often influenced by subjective criteria such as pain or skeletal events such as pathological fracture, vertebral collapse or spinal cord compression which do not necessarily signify progressive disease
6. It is likely that large lytic lesions in bone are avascular and are unlikely to heal even after complete tumour regression

The low response rate may be genuinely lower than at other sites, but the high prevalence of receptor-positive disease within the skeleton makes it unlikely with respect to endocrine therapy. If the more subjective criteria of pain relief are used, then the response rates in bone to endocrine therapy are as high as, if not higher than, those at visceral or locoregional sites (Stoll 1985). A further problem in the analysis of response rates is the inadequate reporting of the response rate within bone in many older published trials.

Because of the problems in the assessment of response in bone the "no change" category of response has recently been adopted. We have shown that those patients achieving "no change" after systemic treatment for breast cancer for at least 6 months had a similar proportion of receptor-positive tumours, similar disease-free intervals and a similarity in the range of pathological grades compared to those patients achieving a partial remission. Survival was also identical to those patients achieving partial remission (Howell et al. 1988).

The adoption of these criteria has, however, been criticised (Scher and Yagoda 1987) because of the possibility of observer bias and the recognition that the radiological progression of skeletal disease is often slow. Nevertheless, Coleman et al. (1987) and Harris et al. (1989) have also shown that patients with bone metastases responding or achieving "no change" to systemic treatment have a similar survival. The "no change" category is valid and useful as long as there is clear evidence of progressive disease prior to entry to the study and may give a truer indication of response in bone.

Prostate Cancer

Introduction

Bone is the major site of metastatic disease in prostate cancer and, in general terms, the treatment of metastatic prostate cancer is the treatment of skeletal disease. The appearances on plain radiography are predominantly osteoblastic and, because of this radiological response, are notoriously difficult to evaluate. Serial scintigraphy may be more helpful in this regard but fortunately the availability of relatively specific tumour markers (acid phosphatase and prostate-specific antigen) means that systemic treatments can be objectively evaluated.

Endocrine Therapy

At least 80% of prostate tumours exhibit some degree of hormone responsiveness (Solowat 1984). The most commonly used form of endocrine therapy in advanced prostate cancer remains surgical castration and patients responding to this procedure have a reduction in bone pain and an increased survival compared to non-responders. The advent of many new forms of endocrine treatment such as luteinising hormone releasing hormone (LHRH) agonists (Mauriac et al. 1988), flutamide (Sogani et al. 1984) and combined endocrine therapy (Belanger et al. 1988) do not show an improvement over surgical orchidectomy but may be preferable to some patients. Oestrogen therapy, with its feminising effects and its cardiovascular risks in an elderly male population (Lyss 1987), should probably no longer form part of modern oncological practice. Other forms of endocrine manipulation have, however, been evaluated in a number of phase II and phase III trials.

A recent three-arm EORTC phase III trial (Pavone-Macaluso et al. 1986) demonstrated that diethylstilboestrol and cyproterone acetate were of equal efficacy in the treatment of advanced prostatic cancer, but medroxyprogesterone acetate was less effective with a shorter survival and time to progression. Cardiovascular side effects were more frequent in the oestrogen-treated group.

Other treatment modalities that are currently being investigated include ketoconazole which, apart from its well-known anti-fungal action, causes castrate levels of testosterone, if given at high doses, within 1–2 days after initiation of treatment (Bamberger and Lowe 1988). Johnson et al. (1988) treated 22 patients with progressive metastatic prostate cancer, despite androgen deprivation therapy, with ketoconazole. Pain relief which lasted 1–8 months was apparent in 13 of 16 patients in whom pain was a prominent feature.

Elomaa et al. (1988) used aminoglutethimide and hydrocortisone in 20 patients with hormone-resistant advanced prostate cancer and painful bone metastases. Pain relief was seen in 75% of patients but improvements in bone-scan appearances were only seen in 4 patients (22%), whereas a reduction in acid phosphatase level was seen in 50% (8 of 16 patients). Levels of testosterone and dihydrotestosterone have also been shown to be reduced during aminoglutethimide therapy (Worgul et al. 1983).

In 1982 Labrie et al. introduced a new concept in the hormonal treatment of metastatic prostate cancer based on complete androgen blockade. Neri et al. (1989) treated 47 previously untreated patients with advanced prostate cancer. They were given an LHRH agonist (Buserelin) plus a pure anti-androgen (flut-amide). Circulating testosterone was reduced to castrate levels and the overall response rate (including stable disease) was 90% with a median duration of 12 months. Newer forms of endocrine therapy are, however, not known to be more effective than surgical castration and phase III trials, to compare newer agents to this standard form of treatment, are in progress. (For a comprehensive review of current trials and results of newer forms of endocrine therapy in prostate (and breast) cancer see Jackson et al. 1989.)

Chemotherapy

The more contentious issue concerning the treatment of metastatic prostate cancer is the use of cytotoxic chemotherapy. Relief of pain from bone metastases has been reported in 11% (Eagen et al. 1978) to 54% (Scott et al. 1987) of patients. There is, as yet, no good evidence that combination treatment is better than single agent therapy (Muss et al. 1981). P.H.Smith et al. (1986) reported a randomised phase III study of the urological group of the EORTC where estramustine (a drug with both weak oestrogenic and cytotoxic activity) was compared to diethylstilboestrol in advanced prostate cancer. Local tumour response was higher in the diethylstilboestrol-treated group but for bone metastases there was no difference in efficacy between treatments. Cardiovascu-lar toxicity was higher in the oestrogen-treated group. Similar results were reported by Johansson et al. (1987).

Androgen priming has recently been tested as a method to enhance the tumour chemosensitivity in men with stage III prostate cancer refractory to orchidectomy. Manni et al. (1986) reported a higher response rate but not response duration or survival in androgen-primed patients compared to a control group. However, Muss et al. (1985) reported that androgen priming was an unsatisfactory method of improving responses to chemotherapy in a group of 23 hormone-resistant patients with advanced prostate cancer and bone metastases.

Patients with advanced prostate cancer tend to be elderly and often of poor performance status; as such their tolerance of toxic chemotherapeutic regimens is often poor. There is no evidence that cytotoxic drugs prolong survival in such patients and they are generally used with palliative intent. It is important that physicians treating these patients address the issues of pain control, mobility and quality of life in addition to tumour response.

Other Tumours

Johnson et al. (1976) reported an autopsy series of testicular germ cell tumours (GCT) where 47% of bony metastases was seen among patients with seminoma.

Skeletal involvement at presentation is uncommon in patients with germ cell tumours but has been reported to be an adverse prognostic feature (Bosl et al. 1986; Williams et al. 1987). In contrast, Hitchins et al. (1988) reported a low incidence (7/251; 3%) of bone metastases in patients presenting with testicular and extragonadal GCT. The incidence was 9% (4 of 46) at relapse. At a median follow-up of 4 years, survival amongst patients presenting with bone disease was similar to the survival in the whole group and better than those presenting with liver or central nervous system metastases.

Bone involvement at diagnosis in Hodgkin's disease and non-Hodgkin's lymphoma (NHL) has also been reported, although uncommonly. Localised bone involvement appears not to be an adverse prognostic feature in Hodgkin's disease but widespread bone involvement commonly occurring in NHL carries an adverse prognosis. However, because of the paucity of published studies describing bone involvement in both of these chemosensitive tumours few conclusions can be drawn. Prolonged survival of patients presenting with bone involvement in lymphomas and germ cell tumours is not uncommon and it is clear, therefore, that bone does not represent a "sanctuary site" for these tumours.

Bone involvement in solid tumours which are primarily chemoresistant has also been reported. Fon et al. (1981) has reported a poor prognosis (median survival 4.7 months) in patients with melanoma who had bone involvement. There is a high incidence of bone involvement in patients with lung cancer. Frytak et al. (1988) have reported that 30% of patients with lung cancer will develop bone metastases at some time and metastases at this site are associated with a poor prognosis. There are, however, no published data concerning the response of bone metastases to systemic therapy for patients with these two forms of malignancy.

Inhibitors of Tumour Effects on Host Cells

Introduction

Bone turnover is normally a tightly regulated physiological process and, in normal health, bone resorption and bone formation are closely coupled. Physiological bone resorption, for example during growth, development and bone remodelling after fracture, is dependent on osteoclast activity. The absence of effective osteoclasts results in a generalised increase in skeletal mass as seen in osteopetrosis. This condition provides evidence for the haemopoeitic origin of osteoclast progenitors as it may be cured by bone marrow transplantation (Marks and Popoff 1988). Pathological bone resorption, an integral part of the effect of skeletal metastases, is also osteoclast-mediated (Marks and Popoff 1988) and tumours frequently metastasising to bone have been shown to release diffusable substances capable of stimulating osteoclastic bone resorption. It was originally thought that this osteoclast-activating-factor (OAF) was a single entity, but it soon became clear that a number of cytokines including interleukin-1, transforming growth factor alpha (TGFα), parathyroid hormone-related peptide and the tumour necrosis factors were capable of stimulating osteoclast activity (Marks and Popoff 1988). Although osteoclast-mediated mechanisms may predominate in many situations, the relative role and importance of direct bone destruction by tumours, independent of osteoclasts, remains to be established (Galasko 1976) and there is no evidence that osteoclast stimulation is an obligate requirement for the development of skeletal metastases. Inhibition of osteoclastic overactivity represents a possible therapeutic target in the systemic treatment of bone metastases. The most widely used agents of this class are the bisphosphonates although other "resorption inhibitors" will be discussed. Most agents in this class have been used successfully for the treatment of tumour-induced hypercalcaemia (a syndrome almost always characterised by excessive osteoclastic activity). Uncontrolled and controlled studies of these agents in the treatment of metastatic bone disease are listed in Tables 7.4 and 7.5.

Mithramycin

Mithramycin is a cytotoxic antibiotic with powerful effects on osteoclast activity which has been used for the treatment of malignant hypercalcaemia and Paget's disease for many years. The first report of the effect of mithramycin in the treatment of bone metastases was from Davies et al. (1979), who treated 15 patients with widespread painful skeletal metastases from breast cancer with mithramycin. All patients were refractory to other systemic therapy and were given intravenous mithramycin at doses usually used for treating Paget's disease. Relief of pain was reported in 10 patients, and was marked and of rapid in onset in 7. There was an improvement in mobility in 4 patients but no anti-tumour effect was seen, in that there was no healing of established bone lesions. In fact further lesions developed during treatment. To our knowledge there have been no controlled trials of mithramycin in the treatment of bone metastases. Mithramycin has unpredictable marrow and hepatic toxicity and has been largely superseded by the bisphosphonates.

Calcitonin

The effects of calcitonin have been assessed in both phase II (Table 7.4) and a small number of phase III (Table 7.5) trials in patients with painful osteolytic metastases. Roth and Kolaric (1986) studied the analgesic effect of salmon calcitonin in a double-blind, randomised, controlled trial in 40 female patients with painful bone metastases. Twenty patients were given subcutaneous calcitonin for 28 days and the control group of 20 patients received physiological saline. Systemic treatment other than calcitonin or placebo was left uncontrolled but was not changed during the 3-month run up to the trial. Treatment with calcitonin resulted in a significant reduction in analgesic consumption and level of pain compared with placebo. There was, however, no improvement in patients' functional capacity. No effect was seen on serum calcium levels, radiology or bone scintigraphy and calcitonin had no apparent anti-tumour effect in bone.

Gennari et al. (1989) in a further placebo-controlled study demonstrated a decreased pain intensity and a reduction in bone turnover as assessed by reduced

Table 7.4. Uncontrolled trials of "resorption inhibitors" in metastatic bone disease

Author	Drug	Number of patients	Findings
Breast			
Davies et al. (1979)	Mithramycin (iv)	15	Reduced pain in 10 patients, improved mobility in 4 patients, no anti-tumour effect
Siris et al. (1983)	Clodronate (oral)	10	Improvement in pain symptoms in some patients
Jung et al. (1983)	Clodronate (oral)	10	Reduced pain in some patients
Morton et al. (1988)	Pamidronate (iv)	16	Improvement in pain, sclerosis of lytic mets in 4 patients, falling tumour markers in 3 patients
Coleman et al. (1988)	Pamidronate (iv)	28	Improvement in pain, sclerosis of lytic mets in 4 patients
Dodwell et al. (1990)	Pamidronate (oral)	16	No analgesic effect, no tumour responses in bone seen
Prostate			
Carey and Lippert (1988)	Etidronate (oral)	12	Improvement in pain in 10 patients, reduced narcotic use
Clarke (1990) (unpublished)	Pamidronate (iv)	26	Reduction of pain in 10 of 18 patients, stabilisation of deteriorating bone scans and reversal of rising acid phosphatase in some patients
Scher et al. (1987)	Gallium nitrate (iv)	23	7 patients had a reduction in bone pain, 2 short partial remissions

Table 7.5. Controlled trials of "resorption inhibitors" in metastatic bone disease

Author	Drug	Number of patients	"Skeletal morbidity"	Anti-tumour effect	Survival
Breast					
Roth and Kolaric (1986)	Calcitonin	40	Reduced pain	None	Not reported
van Holten-Verzantvoort et al. (1987)	Pamidronate (oral)	131	Significantly reduced	Fewer patients with progression on x-ray	No different
Elomaa et al. (1985)	Clodronate (oral)	34	Reduced	Formation of new osteolytic foci inhibited	Significantly improved due to hypercalcaemia in controls
Blomqvist et al. (1988)	Calcitonin	49	No improvement in pain	None seen	No different
Gennari et al.[a] (1989)	Calcitonin	60	Reduced pain	Delay in time to progression. CEA level "stabilised"	Not reported
Prostate					
Smith (1989)	Etidronate[b]	57	No improvement in pain seen	None	No different
Myeloma					
Merlini et al. (1990)	Clodronate (iv)	60	Reduced fractures	Reduced formation of new osteolytic foci	Survival 45 vs. 30 months (p = NS)

[a] Breast, lung and gastric cancer studied but beneficial effects only seen in breast cancer patients.
[b] Intravenous and oral.

alkaline phosphatase and urinary hydroxyproline measurements in patients treated with calcitonin. A fall in the mean plasma prostaglandin E-2 level was seen in the calcitonin-treated group. The authors also report little change in the mean values of carcinoembryonic antigen in patients receiving calcitonin, whereas those randomised to receive placebo injections had an increase in this tumour marker. No UICC-classifiable responses were reported in either group of patients, but at 6 months there was progression of skeletal disease in 14 of 16 patients in the placebo group and 5 of 15 patients in the treatment group, suggesting that concurrent administration of calcitonin delayed disease progression. However, this apparent anti-tumour effect was seen only in patients with bone metastases from breast cancer and did not appear to influence the course of skeletal disease from gastric and lung cancer. Calcitonin may cause nausea and abdominal pain and is expensive. Its usage in the treatment of hypercalcaemia and bone metastases has declined since the advent of the bisphosphonates. (For a review of the role of calcitonin in the management of bone pain see Gennari and Agnusdei 1988.)

Bisphosphonates

Bisphosphonates (diphosphonates) are structural analogues of pyrophosphate, which is the natural regulator of bone mineral precipitation and dissolution. The bisphosphonates are characterised by the presence of a P-C-P bond as compared with the P-O-P bond of pyrophosphate (Fig. 7.1). This biochemical substitution of a carbon atom for oxygen renders bisphosphonates resistant to pyrophosphatase activity. These compounds have profound effects on skeletal pathophysiology and can cause both inhibition of bone mineralisation and bone resorption. The currently available bisphosphonates are etidronate (Didronel, Norwich Eaton), which is licensed for use in the UK for the treatment of malignant hypercalcaemia and Paget's disease of bone. This agent has the undesirable effect of significantly inhibiting bone mineralisation (Fleisch 1988). Clodronate (Boerhinger) has only minimal inhibition of bone mineralisation, but at the time of writing is not licensed for use in the UK. Pamidronate (Aredia, Ciba Geigy) is the most effective bisphosphonate for the treatment of malignant hypercalcaemia (Ralston et al. 1989a) and is licensed for the treatment of hypercalcaemia in the UK. It has the advantage of minimal inhibition of bone mineralisation. The structure of the available bisphosphonates in relation to pyrophosphate is given in Fig. 7.1.

Although the effects of bisphosphonates on skeletal homeostasis are well known their mechanism of action is incompletely understood. Bisphosphonates bind to bone mineral with strong affinity and thereby alter the surface charge on hydroxyapatite, exerting a marked physico-chemical effect on hydroxyapatite crystal physiology. The ionic make-up of the hydration layer surrounding developing crystals is changed with displacement of orthophosphate and attraction of calcium. The calcium-x-phosphate product is grossly altered and further crystal development is consequently inhibited. Whilst this form of chemical interaction may account for the effect of bisphosphonates on bone mineralisation and even impair the ability of osteoclasts to "recognise" bone mineral binding sites, direct cellular mechanisms are required to explain the effect of bisphosphonates on osteoclastic bone resorption. Ultrastructural

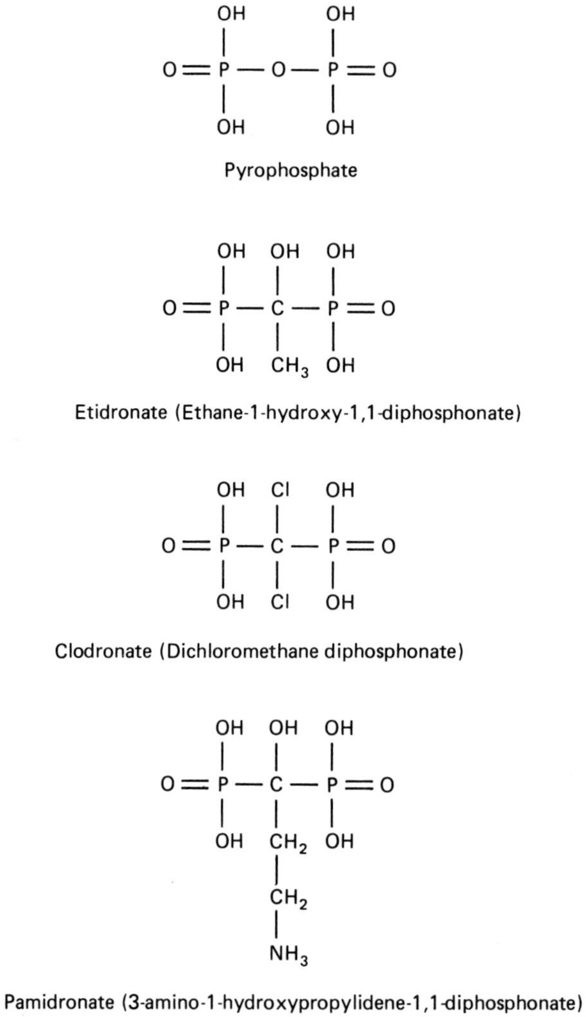

```
       OH        OH
       |         |
O = P — O — P = O
       |         |
       OH        OH
```

Pyrophosphate

```
     OH   OH   OH
     |    |    |
O = P — C — P = O
     |    |    |
     OH  CH₃  OH
```

Etidronate (Ethane-1-hydroxy-1,1-diphosphonate)

```
     OH   CI   OH
     |    |    |
O = P — C — P = O
     |    |    |
     OH   CI   OH
```

Clodronate (Dichloromethane diphosphonate)

```
     OH   OH   OH
     |    |    |
O = P — C — P = O
     |    |    |
     OH  CH₂  OH
          |
         CH₂
          |
         NH₃
```

Pamidronate (3-amino-1-hydroxypropylidene-1,1-diphosphonate)

Fig. 7.1. Structural formulae of commonly used bisphosphonates in relation to pyrophosphate.

examination of osteoclasts from animals given bisphosphonates has shown shrinkage of the ruffled border (the site of osteoclastic bone resorption) and abnormalities of lysosomes, including inhibition of lysosomal enzyme function (Fleisch 1988). Pamidronate may also prevent the recruitment of osteoclast progenitors (Boonekamp et al. 1987).

In the clinic, bisphosphonates may be generally regarded as "osteoclast poisons". They are safe, have minimal side effects and are not metabolised in man. Between 25% and 40% of an intravenous dose is excreted early on through the kidney and the remainder is taken up by bone. It has been estimated that the half life of bisphosphonates in bone is very long, probably greater than two years. All bisphosphonates, however, suffer from poor oral bioavailability and in humans we have shown that pamidronate has an absorption between 0.1% and 0.8% (Dodwell et al. 1990).

Bisphosphonates have been shown to have therapeutic effects in many common diseases affecting the skeleton; when used in Paget's disease of bone, a condition characterised by abnormal osteoclast activity, pamidronate reduces pain and the radiological and biochemical parameters of abnormal bone turnover. However, within the practice of oncology the established place of the bisphosphonates is in the treatment of the hypercalcaemia of malignancy. Discussion of the pathophysiology and treatment of this condition is outside the scope of this chapter (see Chap. 8), but the efficacy of therapy with bisphosphonates in the treatment of tumour-induced hypercalcaemia provided impetus to investigate their effects on the abnormal bone turnover and increased osteolysis of skeletal metastases (Tables 7.4, 7.5).

In 1983 Jung et al. studied the effects of dichloromethylene bisphosphonate (clodronate) on calcium balance in 10 normocalcaemic patients with advanced metastatic bone disease or myeloma. There was a marginal decrease in bone resorption in the treated group and, although this study was not designed to test symptomatic effect, the authors reported encouraging results in terms of pain relief in some of their patients and also reversal of paralysis in 1 patient with extensive destruction of the lumbar spine.

Siris et al. (1983) treated 10 women who had skeletal metastases from breast cancer with oral clodronate (3.2 g daily) in a placebo-controlled, double-blind, cross-over study. All had elevated hydroxyproline excretion and 8 of 10 were hypercalcaemic or hypercalciuric. Eight patients had moderate to severe bone pain. Significant reductions in calcium and hydroxyproline excretion were seen during clodronate treatment periods when compared to pre-study or placebo periods. An analgesic effect was also noted in the majority of patients. There were no adverse effects.

Elomaa et al. (1983) were the first to perform a long-term controlled trial of a bisphosphonate in patients with osteolytic bone metastases. Thirty-four normo-calcaemic women with skeletal metastases from breast cancer were randomly allocated to receive treatment with oral clodronate (1.6 g daily) or placebo for 3–9 months. There was a fall in the urinary hydroxyproline and calcium excretion in treated patients compared to placebo. New bone metastases were more common and analgesic requirements were higher in the placebo group. Hormonal and cytotoxic therapy were uncontrolled between the treatment and control groups. After further follow-up (Elomaa et al. 1985) it was reported that the incidence of new metastases and pathological fracture was significantly decreased in the clodronate-treated group despite similar development of soft tissue metastases in both groups. Eleven patients in the clodronate group were alive at 2 years in comparison with 4 from the control group (p<0.005). However, unusually, the majority of deaths in the control group were from hypercalcaemia. It was also reported that new bone metastases developed after withdrawal of clodronate indicating that the drug had no long-term effect on the prevention of further bone metastases.

In the largest randomised study to date, Van Holten-Verzantvoort et al. (1987) reported the results of a multi-centre trial using oral pamidronate in 131 women with osteolytic metastases from breast cancer. Specific anti-tumour therapy was left at the discretion of the clinician and was variable between treatment groups. At a median follow-up of 14 months there was a significant reduction in the incidence of pathological fracture, hypercalcaemia and severe bone pain in the pamidronate-treated group. The need for radiotherapy for skeletal bone pain was more than halved. At the original protocol dose of 600mg daily there was a drop-out rate of 25% because of nausea and vomiting. Because of this the dose of pamidronate was decreased to 300mg daily and the drop-out rate was reduced to 8%.

If the events related to skeletal morbidity i.e., hypercalcaemia, changes of systemic medication, radiotherapy, fracture or surgery are added, the cumulative sum of complications is highly significantly reduced in the pamidronate-treated group (Fig. 7.2). However, this apparent decrease in morbid events has not so far translated into a survival benefit. In a later report (Cleton et al. 1989) fewer patients in the pamidronate arm had radiological evidence of disease progression at 6 and 12 months compared to control. This trial provides compelling evidence of the beneficial effects of pamidronate in skeletal metastases.

A number of investigators have now reported the use of intravenous pamidronate alone for the treatment of patients with breast cancer and skeletal metastases. Morton et al. (1988) reported a study of 16 women with progressive bone metastases from breast cancer who were given intravenous pamidronate (30mg weekly for 4 weeks then 30mg fortnightly for a further 5 months) as sole therapy. All patients had progressed on hormone treatment. At each visit serum calcium, albumen and phosphate were measured and a fasting urine sample for calcium/creatinine and hydroxyproline/creatinine ratios was collected. Pain was scored on a linear analogue scale and plain radiology was repeated 3 monthly. Evidence of sclerosis was seen in 4 patients (an example is given in Fig. 7.3) and in a further 4 patients disease remained stable for greater than 6 months. Parallel falls in 2 tumour markers were seen in 3 patients (2 who had evidence of sclerosis and 1 whose disease was radiologically stable). There was a marked fall in calcium excretion and, in particular, those patients who responded had the lowest level (Fig. 7.4). In 3 patients calcium excretion rose after an initial fall and this was predictive of disease progression within bone (Fig. 7.4). No consistent effects on urine hydroxyproline excretion were seen and there was no change in alkaline phosphatase or osteocalcin levels. There was a significant

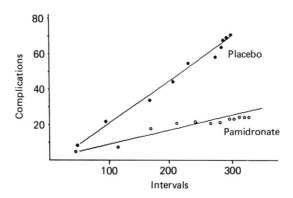

Fig. 7.2. Cumulative number of "skeletal events" (pain, pathological fracture and hypercalcaemia) in patients treated with pamidronate (*open circles*) and control (*filled circles*). (By courtesy of O.L.M. Bijvoet.)

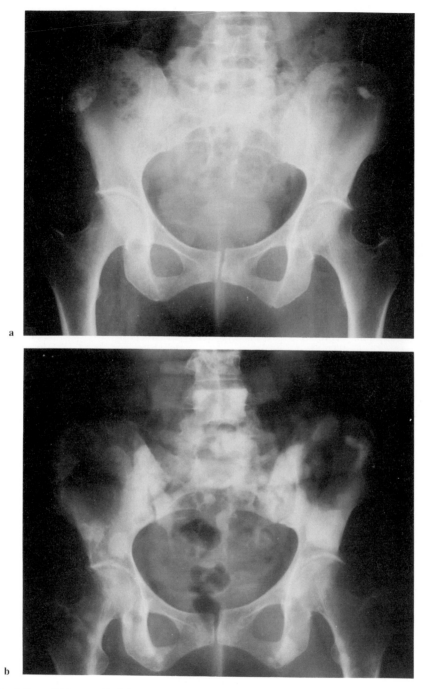

Fig. 7.3. **a** Widespread lytic bone metastases in a patient with breast cancer. **b** Sclerosis of previous lytic metastases after therapy for 6 months with intravenous pamidronate.

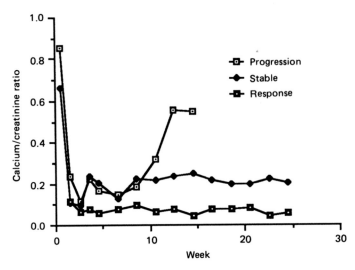

Fig. 7.4. Median calcium : creatinine ratios in patients treated with intravenous pamidronate according to category of response (in bone).

improvement in patients' perception of pain expressed as a percentage of a linear analogue scale. However, improvement in pain did not necessarily correlate with radiological response and as such a placebo effect cannot can be excluded. Similar phase II trials of intravenous pamidronate in skeletal breast cancer (Coleman et al. 1988 and Lipton et al. 1990) have confirmed these encouraging results.

More recently, interest has focused on the use of bisphosphonates in the treatment of prostate cancer metastatic to the skeleton. This followed the recognition that bone resorption is substantially increased in the presence of predominantly osteoblastic metastases (Percival et al. 1987; Urwin et al. 1985; Galasko 1976).

Most experience with bisphosphonates in prostate cancer has, however, been restricted to studies with etidronate. Carey and Lippert (1988) used oral etidronate to palliate pain in 12 patients suffering from skeletal metastases, all of whom had failed endocrine therapy. Ten patients (83%) had a subjective response to treatment with a reduction in narcotic use and pain intensity as measured on a visual analogue scale. Percival et al. (1985) also reported improvement in a patient with paraplegia from prostate metastases. However, in a careful randomised prospective, double-blind, placebo-controlled study, Smith (1989) saw no difference in the symptomatic response rate or analgesic requirements of a group of 57 patients with hormone-refractory metastatic prostatic cancer and bone pain between treatment and placebo groups.

Studies with second-generation bisphosphonates in prostate cancer are scanty. Adami et al. (1985) reported short-lived relief of bone pain in a small group of patients treated with clodronate. Pamidronate was recently shown to have a useful analgesic effect in an isolated case report of a patient with hormone-resistant prostate cancer (Masud and Slevin 1989), and Pelger et al. (1989) have demonstrated beneficial metabolic effects in patients with metastatic prostate cancer given pamidronate. Clarke et al. (unpublished data) have demonstrated significant improvements in pain, mobility and analgesic requirements in 10 of 18 patients with painful progressive metastatic prostate cancer given intravenous pamidronate. Consistent falls in calcium excretion were seen, whereas urinary hydroxyproline excretion showed a less consistent pattern, suggesting the presence of more than one osteolytic destructive mechanism. Deteriorating bone scans also showed evidence of stabilisation and reversal of increasing tumour marker levels suggested a direct or indirect anti-tumour action of pamidronate in this group of patients.

As multiple myeloma is a disease which is characterised by widespread lytic bone destruction where osteoclast activation is implicated in the pathogenesis (Garrett et al. 1987) it is a good candidate for treatment with inhibitors of bone resorption. In this regard Delmas et al. (1982) reported beneficial effects on morbidity due to myelomatous bone destruction in a small uncontrolled study of oral clodronate.

More recently, Merlini et al. (1990) performed a controlled study in patients with myeloma using intravenous clodronate. All patients had symptomatic bone pain and hypercalciuria. Sixty-eight consecutive patients were assigned on alternating dates to a group with supportive clodronate treatment with chemotherapy or with chemotherapy alone. In each group 30 patients were assessable. Pain was measured by visual analogue scale and routine radiographic follow-up was employed. There was a significantly superior analgesic effect in the clodronate treated group with a reduction of bone pain in almost all patients (27 of 30). The number of new osteolytic foci and the pathological fracture rate were also significantly reduced in the clodronate-treated group. The authors also noted osteosclerotic repair of a number of rib and humeral fractures and partial repair of a wide osteolytic lesion in the pelvis in clodronate-treated patients. Comparative reductions in paraprotein levels were, however, not reported. Once again, this study confirmed the ability of bisphosphonates to reduce calcium excretion significantly. Toxicity was minimal and median survival of the clodronate-treated group was 45 months compared with 30 months for those treated only with chemotherapy. This result, however, was not statistically significant. The study may be criticised in that the biochemical parameters of bone turnover were only assessed in clodronate-treated patients and the effect of chemotherapy alone on these parameters is, therefore, not known. Also, placebo injections were not given and the contribution of clodronate treatment to pain relief was obscured. The pronounced placebo effect of intravenous infusions and the importance of placebo-control when assessing pain was demonstrated by the study of Ralston et al. (1989b). Patients with erosive rheumatoid arthritis were treated with repeated intravenous infusions of pamidronate or placebo. No effect on joint destruction was seen, but there was a pronounced analgesic effect in both groups of patients.

It could also be argued that bisphosphonate treatment was not given optimally in Merlini's study (mean interval between courses was 4 months) as the incidence of hypercalcaemia was not reduced compared to control and calcium excretion (and by inference osteoclastic bone resorption) only suppressed intermittently.

Gallium Nitrate

Recently, gallium nitrate (a bone-seeking agent with potent effects on osteoclastic bone resorption) has been shown to be highly effective in the treatment of tumour-induced hypercalcaemia (Warrell et al. 1988). Its powerful inhibition of bone resorption has led investigators to use this agent in the treatment of bone metastases. Warrell et al. (1987) evaluated its effect on biochemical parameters of bone turnover in 22 patients with bone metastases. Significant reductions in hydroxyproline excretion were seen and serum ionised calcium and phosphate levels declined significantly. There was an increase in immunoreactive parathyroid hormone and activated vitamin D. The effect on bone pain was, however, not evaluated. In a small study, Scher et al. (1987) treated 23 patients suffering from hormone-resistant prostate cancer with an intravenous infusion of gallium nitrate over 7 days. Two patients achieved short partial remissions but 7 had a reduction of bone pain. Again, the biochemical indices of bone turnover showed a signicant reduction of bone resorption.

Gallium nitrate is a potential new therapeutic agent for the treatment of osteolysis and is currently being investigated in both hypercalcaemia and bone metastases. However, the need for slow intravenous infusions may detract from its use.

Conclusions and Prospects

It is clear that for many patients with skeletal metastases there is little in terms of currently available systemic anti-tumour treatment; this statement applies particularly to patients with squamous cell lung cancer, hypernephroma and melanoma. It is likely that the development of more effective cytotoxic agents for the treatment of these solid tumours will enable us to palliate these groups of patients with bone metastases more effectively. More objective criteria and improved radiological techniques are required in order that the results of systemic treatment on bone metastases can be better evaluated. Tumour markers may be a useful tool in this regard if used in conjunction with other criteria. It is equally important that future studies take account of quality of life and psychological well-being for this group of patients and do not merely report response and survival data.

Of the available "resorption inhibitors" bisphosphonates are the most active drugs in this area and are currently the subject of numerous clinical studies. It should be stated that despite the many encouraging reports of the usefulness of these agents in skeletal disease they are not yet established as standard therapy and the results of large-scale controlled trials are awaited.

As well as studies in patients with established bone lesions, which we have discussed, bisphosphonates may have a preventive role. It has been shown (Galasko 1976) that osteoclastic bone destruction is important during the early phase of the development of skeletal metastases whereas direct bone tumour interactions may be responsible for the latter stages of this process.

Studies are now underway to assess the role of bisphosphonates, particularly pamidronate, given to women with advanced breast cancer but no evidence of skeletal disease radiographically, and also after primary surgery for women at a high risk of skeletal recurrence. Long-term controlled studies will, however, be required to determine any preventive effect.

Bisphosphonates may also have a role in the prevention of osteoporosis.

Reid et al. (1988), have shown that steroid induced loss of vertebral mineral density may be prevented by concurrent administration of oral pamidronate. The widespread use of adjuvant chemotherapy or ovarian ablation for pre-menopausal women with poor-risk breast cancer is likely to lead to an increased incidence of symptomatic osteoporosis in later life. Bisphosphonate drugs may, therefore, have wider applicability than their role in the treatment of established skeletal metastases. A problem with currently available bisphosphonates is poor oral bioavailability and at the present time more effective drugs with greater oral absorption are under development.

The development of more specific agents to inhibit the progression of skeletal metastases is hindered by our lack of knowledge concerning the control of both physiological and pathological bone cell biology and particularly the role of autocrine and paracrine processes in osteoclast recruitment and function and osteoblast activity. A greater understanding of the role of cytokines in normal and pathological circumstances will enable us to develop more specific agents to improve our treatments of this condition.

Acknowledgement. We wish to thank Miss Maria Middleton and Mrs Jean Miller for their secretarial skills.

References

Adami S, Salvagno G, Guarrera G, Bianchi G, Dorizzi R, Rosini S (1985) Dichloromethylene diphosphonate in patients with prostatic carcinoma metastatic to the skeleton. J Urol 134: 1152–1154

Alexieva-Figuschi J, van Gilse HA, Hop WCJ, Phoa CH, Blonk-vd. Wijst J, Treurniet RE (1980) Progestin therapy in advanced breast cancer: megestrol acetate – an evaluation of 160 treated cases. Cancer 46:2369–2372

Alonso-Munoz MC, Ojeda-Gonzalez MB, Beltram-Fabregat M et al. (1988) Randomized trial of tamoxifen versus aminoglutethimide and versus combined tamoxifen and aminoglutethimide in advanced postmenopausal breast cancer. Oncology 45:350–353

Bamberger MH, Lowe FC (1988) Ketoconazole in initial management and treatment of metastatic prostate cancer to spine. Urology 32:301–303

Belanger A, Labrie F, Dupont A, Brochu M, Cusan L (1988) Endocrine effects of combined treatment with an LHRH agonist in association with flutamide in metastatic prostate carcinoma. Clin Invest Med 11:321–326

Blackledge GRP, Latief T, Mould JJ, Spooner D, Morrison M (1986) Phase II evaluation of megestrol acetate in previously treated patients with advanced breast cancer: relationship of response to previous treatment. Eur J Cancer Clin Oncol 22:1091–1094

Blomqvist C, Elomaa I, Porkka L, Karonen SL, Lamberg-Allardt C (1988) Evaluation of salmon calcitonin treatment in bone metastases from breast cancer – a controlled clinical trial. Bone 9:45–51

Bonneterre J, Coppens H, Mauriac L et al. (1985) Aminoglutethimide in advanced breast cancer: clinical results of a French multicentre randomized trial comparing 500 mg and 1 g daily. Eur J Cancer Clin Oncol 21:1153–1158

Boonekamp PM, Lowik CWGM, van de Wee-Pals LJA, et al. (1987) Enhancement of the inhibitory action of APD on the transformation of osteoclast precursors into resorbing cells after dimethylation of the amino group. Bone Miner 2:29–42

Bosl GJ, Gluckman R, Geller NL et al. (1986) VAB-6 – an effective chemotherapy regimen for patients with germ cell tumours. J Clin Oncol 4:1493-1496

Brule G (1978) Co-operative clinical study of 178 patients treated with 'Nolvadex'. In: The hormonal control of breast cancer. ICI Ltd Pharmaceuticals Division Alderley Park, Macclesfield, Cheshire, p 35–39

Brunner KW, Sonntag RW, Alberto P, Senn HJ, Martz G, Obrecht P, Maurice P (1977) Combined chemo- and hormonal therapy in advanced breast cancer. Cancer 39:2923–2933

Canney PA, Priestman TJ, Griffiths T, Latief TN, Mould JJ, Spooner D (1988) Randomizing trial comparing aminoglutethimide with high-dose medroxyprogesterone acetate in therapy for advanced breast carcinoma. J Nal Cancer Inst 80:1147–1151

Carey PO, Lippert MC (1988) Treatment of painful prostatic bone metastases with oral etidronate disodium. J Urol 32:403–407

Carmo-Pereira J, Oliveira Costa F, Henriques E, Cantinho-Lopes MG, Godinho F, Sales-Luis A (1988) Primary chemotherapy with mitoxantrone and prednisone in advanced breast carcinoma. A phase II study. Eur J Cancer Clin Oncol 24:473–476

Ceci G, Passalaqua R, Bisagni G, Bella M, Coccini G (1985) Aminoglutethimide in advanced breast cancer. Tumori 71:483–489

Cleton FJ, van-Holten-Verzantvoort AT, Zwinderman A et al. (1989) Long-term bisphosphonate treatment of bone metastases in breast cancer patients – effects on morbidity and quality of life. In: Burckhardt P (ed) Disodium pamidronate (APD) in the treatment of malignancy-related disorders. Hans Huber Publishers, Toronto, pp 113–120

Coleman RE, Rubens RD (1987) The clinical course of bone metastases from breast cancer. Br J Cancer 55:61–66

Coleman RE, Woll PJ, Miles M, Rubens R (1988) 3-amino 1, 1 hydroxypropyledine bisphosphonate (APD) for the treatment of bone metastases from breast cancer. Br J Cancer 58:621–625

Davies J, Trask C, Souhami RL (1979) Effect of mithramycin on widespread painful bone metastases in cancer of the breast. Cancer Treat Rep 63:1835–1838

Delmas PD, Charhon S, Chapuy MC, Vignon E, Briancon D, Edouard C, Meunier PJ (1982) Long-term effects of dichloromethylene diphosphonate (C12MDP) on skeletal lesions in multiple myeloma. Metab Bone Dis Rel Res 4:163–168

De Lena M, Brandi M, Logroscino A, Lorusso V, Paradiso A, Maiello E (1988) Intravenous administration of cyclophosphamide, methotrexate and 5-fluorouracil in metastatic breast cancer. A pilot study. Tumori 74:57–63

Di Costanzo F, Gori S, Tonato M, Buzzi F, Crino L, Grignani F, Davis S (1986) Vindesine and mitomycin C in chemotherapy refractory advanced breast cancer. Cancer 57:904–907

Dodwell DJ, Howell A, Morton A et al. (1990) Biochemical effects, anti-tumour activity and pharmacokinetics of oral and intravenous pamidronate (APD) in the treatment of skeletal breast cancer. 31st Annual Meeting ACP/BACR meeting 1990 abstract no.8.11 page 92

Eagen RT, Hahn RG, Myers RP (1978) Adriamycin versus 5-fluorouracil and cyclophosphamide in the treatment of metastatic prostate cancer. Cancer Treat Rep 60:115–117

Elomaa I, Blomqvist C, Grohn P, Porkka L, Kairento AL, Selander K, Lamberg-Allardt C, Holmstrom T (1983) Long-term controlled trial with diphosphonate in patients with osteolytic bone metastases. Lancet i:146–148

Elomaa I, Blomqvist C, Porkka L et al. (1985) Diphosphonates for osteolytic metastases. Lancet i:1155-1156

Elomaa I, Taube T, Blomqvist C, Rissanen P, Rannikka S, Alfthan O (1988) Aminoglutethimide for advanced prostatic cancer resistant to conventional hormonal therapy. Eur Urol 14:104–106

Fidler M (1981) Incidence of fracture through metastases in long bones. Acta Orthop Scand 52:623–627

Fleisch H (1988) Bisphosphonates – mechanisms of action. In: Burckhardt P (ed) Disodium pamidronate (APD) in the treatment of malignancy-related disorders. Hans Huber Publishers, Toronto, pp 21–35

Fon GT, Wong WS, Gold RH, Kaiser LR (1981) Skeletal metastases of melanoma: radiographic, scintigraphic and clinical review. AJR 137:103–108

Frytak S, McLead RA, Gunderson LL, Pritchard DJ, Unni KK (1988) Metastatic bone disease: lung cancer. In: Sim FH (ed) Diagnosis and management of metastatic bone disease. Multidisciplinary approach. Raven Press, New York, pp 265–271

Galasko CSB (1976) Mechanisms of bone destruction in the development of skeletal metastases. Nature 263:507–508

Galasko CSB (1986) Local complications of skeletal metastases. In: Skeletal metastases. Butterworths & Co, London, pp 125–155

Garrett IR, Durie BGM, Nedwin GE et al. (1987) Production of the bone-resorbing cytokine lymphotoxin by cultured myeloma cells N Engl J Med 317:526–532

Gennari C, Agnusdei D (1988) Calcitonin in bone pain management. Curr Ther Res 44:712–721

Gennari C, Francini G, Chierichetti SM, Nami R, Gonelli S, Piolini M (1989) Salmon calcitonin treatment in bone metastases. Curr Ther Res 45:804–812

Gregory EJ, Cohen S, Oines DW, Mims CH (1985) Megestrol acetate therapy for advanced breast cancer. J Clin Oncol 3:155–160

Harmsen HJ Jr, Porsius AJ (1988) Endocrine therapy of breast cancer. Eur J Cancer Clin Oncol 24:1099–1116

Harris AL, Cantwell BMJ, Carmichael J, Dawes P, Robinson A, Farndon J, Wilson R (1989) Phase II study of low dose aminoglutethimide 250 mg/day plus hydrocortisone in advanced post-menopausal breast cancer. Eur J Cancer Clin Oncol 25:1105–1111

Henderson IC, Allegra JC, Woodcock T, Wolff T, Bryan S, Cartwright K, Dukart G, Henry D (1989) Randomized clinical trial comparing mitoxantrone with doxorubicin in previously treated patients with metastatic breast cancer. J Clin Oncol 7:560–571

Hayward JL, Carbone PP, Heuson JC, Humaoka S, Segaloff A, Rubens RD (1977) Assessment of response to therapy in advanced breast cancer. Eur J Cancer 13:89–95

Hitchins RN, Philip PA, Wignall B, et al. (1988) Bone disease in testicular and extragonadal germ cell tumours. Br J Cancer 55:793–796

Hoffken K, Kempf H, Miller AA, Miller B, Schmidt CG, Faber P, Kley HK (1986) Aminoglute-thimide without hydrocortisone in the treatment of postmenopausal patients with advanced breast cancer. Cancer Treat Rep 70:1153–1157

Hortobagyi GN, Buzdar AU, Frye D, et al. (1985) Oral medroxyprogesterone acetate in the treatment of metastatic breast cancer. Breast Cancer Res Treat 5:321–326

Howell A, Mackintosh J, Jones M, et al. (1988) The definition of the "no change" category in patients treated with endocrine therapy and chemotherapy for advanced carcinoma of the breast. Eur J Cancer Clin Oncol 24:1567–1572

Jackson IM, Matthews MJ, Diver JMJ (1989) LHRH analogues in the treatment of cancer. Cancer Treat Rev 16:161–172

Johansson JE, Andersson SO, Beckman KW, Lingardh G, Zador G (1987) Clinical evaluation of flutamide and estramustine as initial treatment of metastatic carcinoma of prostate. Urology 29:55–59

Johnson DE, Appelt G, Samuels ML et al. (1976) Metastases from testicular carcinoma – a study of 78 autopsied cases. Urology 8:234–239

Johnson DE, Babaian RJ, Von-Eschenbach AC, Wishnow KI, Tenney D (1988) Ketoconazole therapy for hormonally refractory metastatic prostate cancer. Urology 31:132–134

Jung A, Chantraine A, Donath D, Van Ouwenaller C, Turnill D, Mermillod B, Kitler ME (1983) Use of dichloromethylene diphosphonate in metastatic bone disease. N Engl J Med 308:1499–1501

Kaye SB, Woods RL, Fox RM, Coates AS, Tattersall MHN (1982) Use of aminoglutethimide as second-line endocrine therapy in metastatic breast cancer. Cancer Res 42:3445–3447

Labrie F, Dupont A, Belanger A et al. (1982) New hormonal therapy in prostatic carcinoma: combined treatment with an LHRH agonist and an antiandrogen. Clin Invest Med 5:267–275

Leone BA, Romero A, Rabinovich et al. (1988) Stage IV Breast Cancer: clinical course and survival of patients with osseous versus extraosseous metastases at initial diagnosis. The GOCS (Grupo Oncologico Cooperativo Del Sur) experience. Am J Clin Oncol 11:618–622

Lerner HJ, Band PR, Israel L, Leung BS (1976) Phase II study of tamoxifen; report of 74 patients with stage IV breast cancer. Cancer Treat Rep 60:1431–1435

Lipton A, Harvey H, Givanie et al. (1990) Disodium pamidronate (APD)-dose seeking study in patients with breast and prostate cancer. In: Rubens R (ed) The Management of bone metastases and hypercalcaemia by osteoclast inhibition. Hogrefe and Huber, Toronto/Lewiston New York/Bern/Stuttgart

Lipton A, Harvey HA, Santen RJ et al. (1982) Randomized trial of aminoglutethimide versus tamoxifen in metastatic breast cancer. Cancer Res 42:3434–3436

Lundgren S, Gunderson S, Klepp R, Lonning PE, Lund E, Kvinnsland S (1989) Megestrol acetate versus aminoglutethimide for metastatic breast cancer. Breast Cancer Res Treat 14:201–206

Lyss AP (1987) Systemic treatment for prostate cancer. Am J Med 83:1120–1128

Manni A, Santen RJ, Boucher AE et al. (1986) Hormone stimulation and chemotherapy in advanced prostate cancer: interim analysis of an ongoing randomized trial. Anticancer Res 6:309–314

Mansi JL, Berger U, Easton D, et al. (1987) Micrometastases in bone marrow in patients with primary breast cancer: evaluation as an early predictor of bone metastases. Br Med J 295:1093–1096

Marks SC, Popoff SN (1988) Bone cell biology: the regulation of development, structure and function in the skeleton. Am J Anat 183:1–44

Masud T, Slevin ML (1989) Pamidronate to reduce bone pain in a normocalcaemic patient with disseminated prostatic carcinoma. Lancet i:1021–1022

Mattsson W, von Eyben F, Hallsten L, Bjelkengren G (1982) A phase II study of combined 5-fluorouracil and mitomycin C in advanced breast cancer. Cancer 49:217–220

Mauriac L, Coste P, Richaud P, Lamarche P, Mage P, Bonichon F (1988) Clinical study of an LHRH agonist (ICI 118.630, Zoladex) in the treatment of prostatic cancer. Am J Clin Oncol 11:8117–8119

McNeil BJ (1984) Value of bone scanning in neoplastic disease. Semin Nucl Med 14:277–284

Merlini G, Parrinello GA, Piccinini L et al. (1990) Long-term effects of parenteral dichloro-methylene bisphosphonate (CL2MBP) on bone disease of myeloma patients treated with chemotherapy. Haematol Oncol 8:23–30

Minton MJ, Knight RK, Rubens RD, Hayward JL (1981) Corticosteroids for elderly patients with breast cancer. Cancer 48:883–887

Morton AR, Cantrill JA, Pillai GV et al. (1988) Sclerosis of lytic bone metastases after disodium aminohydroxypropylidene bisphosphonate (APD) in patients with breast carcinoma. Br Med J 297:772–773

Mouridsen HT, Ellemann K, Mattsson W, Palshof T, Daehnfeldt JL, Rose C (1979) Therapeutic effect of tamoxifen versus tamoxifen combined with medroxyprogesterone acetate in advanced breast cancer in postmenopausal women. Cancer Treat Rep 63:171–175

Murray RML, Pitt P (1981) Medical adrenalectomy in patients with advanced breast cancer resistant to anti-oestrogen treatment. Breast Cancer Res Treat 1:91–95

Muss HB, Howard V, Richards R 2d et al. (1981) Cyclophosphamide versus cyclophosphamide, methotrexate and 5-fluorouracil in advanced prostatic cancer: a randomized trial. Cancer 47:1949–1953

Muss HB, Richards F, Jackson DV et al. (1982) Vincristine, doxorubicin, and cyclophosphamide versus low-dose intravenous cyclophosphamide, methotrexate and 5-fluorouracil in advanced breast cancer. Cancer 50:2269–2274

Muss HB, Case D, Cooper MR, Richards F 2d, Spurr CL, Resnick MI, Zekan P, Nelson EC, Puckett JB, Pope E et al. (1985) Cytotoxic chemotherapy and androgen priming in patients with advanced carcinoma of the prostate. A phase II trial of the Piedmont Oncology Association. Am J Oncol 8:394–400

Neri B, Bartalucci S, Pieri A et al. (1989) Complete androgen blockade as treatment for advanced prostate cancer: clinical response and side effects. Anticancer Res 9:13–16

Parvinen L-M, Numminen S (1985) Chemotherapy in advanced breast carcinoma. Comparison between doxorubicin-cyclophosphamide and cyclophosphamide-methotrexate-5-fluorouracil-vincristine-prednisone. Acta Radiol Oncol 24:391–394

Pavone-Macaluso M, De-Voogt HJ, Viggiano G, Barasolo E, Larddennois B, De-Pauw M, Sylvester R (1986) Comparison of diethylstilbestrol, cyproterone acetate and medroxyprogester-one acetate in the treatment of advanced prostatic cancer: final analaysis of a randomized phase III trial of the European Organization for Research on Treatment of Cancer Urological Group. J Urol 136:624–631

Pelger RCM, Lycklama AAB, Nijeholt A, Papapoulos SE (1989) Short term metabolic effects of pamidronate in patients with prostatic carcinoma and bone metastases. Lancet ii:865

Percival RC, Watson ME, Williams JL, Kanis JA (1985) Carcinoma of the prostate: remission of paraparesis with inhibitors of bone resorption. Postgrad Med J 61:551–553

Percival RC, Urwin GH, Harris S, Yates AJP, Williams JL, Beneton M, Kanis JA (1987) Biochemical and histological evidence that carcinoma of the prostate is associated with increased bone resorption. Eur J Surg Oncol 13:41–49

Perry MC, Kardinal CG, Korzun AH, Ginsberg S, Raich PC et al. (1987) Chemohormonal therapy in advanced carcinoma of the breast: cancer and leukemia group B protocol 8081. J Clin Oncol 5:1534–1545

Ralston SH, Gallacher SJ, Patel U et al. (1989a) Comparison of three intravenous bisphosphonates in cancer-associated hypercalcaemia. Lancet ii:1180–1182

Ralston SH, Hacking L, Willocks L, Bruce F, Pitkeathly DA (1989b) Clinical, biochemical and radiographic effects of aminohydroxypropylidine bisphosphonate treatment in rheumatoid arthritis. Ann Rheum Dis 48:396–399

Reid IR, Heap SW, King AR, Ibbertson HK (1988) Two-year follow up of bisphosphonate (APD) treatment in steroid osteoporosis. Lancet ii:1144

Ribeiro G (1977) In: Proceedings of the symposium on hormonal aspects of breast cancer therapy, Tel Aviv. ABIC Ltd, Chemical and Pharmaceutical Industries.

Roth A, Kolaric K (1986) Analgesic activity of calcitonin in patients with painful osteolytic metastases of breast cancer. Results of a controlled randomized study. Oncology 43:283–287

Rubens RD, Tinson CL, Coleman RE et al. (1988) Prednisolone improves the response to primary endocrine treatment for advanced breast cancer. Br J Cancer 55:626–630

Scher HI, Yagoda A (1987) Bone metastases: pathogenesis, treatment and rationale for use of resorption inhibitors. Am J Med 82:(Suppl 2a):6–27

Scher HI, Curley T, Geller N, et al. (1987) Gallium nitrate in prostate cancer: evaluation of antitumor activity and effects on bone turnover. Cancer Treat Rep 71:887–893

Scott WW, Johnson DE, Schmidt JE et al. (1987) Chemotherapy of advanced prostatic carcinoma with cyclophosphamide or 5-fluorouracil: results of first national randomized study. J Urol 114:909–911

Sharp JG, Mann SL, DeBoer J, et al. (1989) Long-term culture as a method of detection of occult tumor cells in bone marrow and blood. J In Vitro Cell Develop Biol 25: meeting abstract no.105

Sherry MM, Greco FA, Johnson DH, Hainsworth JD (1986) Metastatic breast cancer confined to the skeletal system. An indolent disease. Am J Med 81:381–386

Siris ES, Hyman GA, Canfield RE (1983) Effects of dichloromethylene diphosphonate in women with breast carcinoma metastatic to the skeleton. Am J Med 74:401–406

Smith IE, Macaulay V (1985) Comparison of different endocrine therapies in management of bone metastases from breast carcinoma. J R Soc Med 78:15–17

Smith IE, Fitzharris BM, McKinna JA et al. (1978) Aminoglutethimide in treatment of metastatic breast carcinoma. Lancet ii:646–649

Smith IE, Harris AL, Morgan M et al. (1981) Tamoxifen versus aminoglutethimide in advanced breast carcinoma: a randomised cross-over trial. Br Med J 283:1432–1434

Smith JR (1989) Palliation of painful bone metastases from prostate cancer using sodium etidronate: results of a randomized, prospective, double-blind, placebo-controlled study. J Urol 141:85–87

Smith PH, Suciu S, Robinson MR et al. (1986) A comparison of the effect of diethystilbestrol with low dose estraumustine phosphate in the treatment of advanced prostatic cancer: final analysis of a phase III trial of the European Organization for Research on Treatment Of Cancer. J Urol 136:619–623

Sogani PC, Vagaiwala MR, Whitmore WF Jr. (1984) Experience with flutamide in patients with advanced prostatic cancer without prior endocrine therapy. Cancer 54:744–750

Solowat MS (1984) Newer methods of hormonal therapy for prostate cancer. Urology 24 (Suppl 5):30–38

Stoll BA (1983) Natural history, prognosis, and staging of bone metastases. In: Stoll BA, Parbhoo S (eds) Bone metastases: monitoring and treatment. Raven Press, New York, pp 1–4

Stoll BA (1985) Mechanisms in endocrine therapy of bone metastases. J R Soc Med 78 (Suppl 9): 11–14

Tofe AJ, Francis MD, Harvey WJ (1975) Correlation of neoplasms with incidence and localisation of skeletal metastases. J Nucl Med 16:986–989

Trillet V, Revel D, Combaret V et al. (1989) Bone marrow metastases in small cell lung cancer: detection with magnetic resonance imaging and monoclonal antibodies. Br J Cancer 60:83–88

Twycross RG, Fairfield S (1982) Pain in far-advanced cancer. Pain 14:303–310

Urwin GH, Percival RC, Harris MNC, Beneton JK, Williams JL, Kanis JA (1985) Generalised increase in bone resorption in carcinoma of the prostate. Br J Urol 57:721–723

Valavaara R, Pyrhonen S, Heikkinen M et al. (1988) A new antioestrogenic compound, for treatment of advanced breast cancer. Phase II study. Eur J Cancer Clin Oncol 24:785–790

van Holten-Verzantvoort AT, Bijvoet OLM, Hermans J et al. (1987) Reduced morbidity from skeletal metastases in breast cancer patients during long-term bisphosphonate (APD) treatment. Lancet ii:983–985

Van Veelen H, Willemse PHB, Tjabbes T, Scweitzer JH, Sleijfer DT (1986) Oral high-dose medroxyprogesterone acetate versus tamoxifen. Cancer 58:7–13

Warrell RP Jr, Alcock NW, Bockman RS (1987) Gallium nitrate inhibits accelerated bone turnover in patients with bone metastases. J Clin Oncol 5:292–298

Warrell RP Jr, Israel R, Frisone M, Snyder T, Gaynor JJ, Bockman RS (1988) Gallium nitrate for acute treatment of cancer-related hypercalcaemia. A randomized double-blind comparison to calcitonin. Ann Intern Med 108:669–674

Whitehouse JMA (1985) Site-dependent response to chemotherapy for carcinoma of the breast. J R Soc Med 78 (Suppl 9):18–22

Williams SD, Birch R, Einhorn LH et al. (1987) Treatment of disseminated germ-cell tumours with cisplatin, bleomycin and either vinblastine or etoposide. N Engl J Med 316:1435–1440

Worgul TJ, Santen RJ, Samojlik E et al. (1983) Clinical and biochemical effect of aminoglutethimide in the treatment of advanced prostatic carcinoma. J Urol 129:51–55

8   Pathogenesis and Management of Cancer-Associated Hypercalcaemia

S.H. Ralston

Pathogenesis of Cancer-Associated Hypercalcaemia

Introduction

Hypercalcaemia is the most common metabolic complication of malignant disease, occurring in about 5%–10% of cancer patients overall (Fisken et al. 1980). Although hypercalcaemia can occur with virtually any tumour, some cancers cause hypercalcaemia more frequently than others: squamous cancers and uro-epithelial cancers, for example, are common causes of hypercalcaemia, as are breast cancers and myeloma. Conversely, adenocarcinomas of the intestine seldom cause hypercalcaemia (Mundy and Martin 1982). These differences are interesting in that they reflect the ability of some tumours to release humoral factors which cause hypercalcaemia by their effects at regulatory sites of calcium homeostasis in bone, intestine and kidney.

Classification

For many years, it was considered that in most cancer patients, hypercalcaemia arose as the result of excessive release of skeletal calcium by bone metastases – so-called metastatic hypercalcaemia (Mundy and Martin 1982). In the relatively small group of patients without bone lesions, hypercalcaemia was attributed to the systemic release of humoral hypercalcaemic factor(s), "humorally mediated hypercalcaemia" (Mundy and Martin 1982). It is now clear that such a classification is oversimplistic; first, no significant correlation exists between the extent of bone metastases and serum calcium values in cancer patients (Ralston et al. 1982); second, biochemical evaluation reveals evidence of an underlying humoral aetiology in the majority of hypercalcaemic cancer patients, irrespective of the presence of bone lesions (Stewart et al. 1980; Ralston et al. 1984a);

third, evaluation of patients with metastatic bone disease has shown that the amounts of calcium released by metastases alone are insufficient to precipitate hypercalcaemia unless normal homeostatic mechanisms for the excretion of calcium are also impaired (Ralston et al. 1984a). These data indicate that in the vast majority of cases, humoral factors are probably responsible for hypercalcaemia, both in the presence and in the absence of metastatic bone disease.

Mediators of Hypercalcaemia

Hypercalcaemia may theoretically arise as the result of increased release of calcium from bone, reduced excretion of calcium by the kidney or excessive absorption of calcium by the intestine. In the search for putative humoral mediators of cancer-associated hypercalcaemia, most attention has focused on factors which increase bone resorption (Mundy and Martin 1982). Recently, however, it has become evident that factors which alter the renal handling of calcium are equally as important as bone resorbing factors in most cases (Ralston et al. 1984a).

Substances which have been implicated in the pathogenesis of cancer-associated hypercalcaemia are discussed below.

Bone-Resorbing Factors

Prostaglandins

Prostaglandins of the E series were invoked as humoral hypercalcaemic factors shortly after their bone-resorbing properties were discovered (Klein and Raisz 1970). Initial investigations showed that cultured cells from certain animal tumours associated with hypercalcaemia produced large amounts of prostaglandins and that the in vitro bone-resorbing activity associated with such tumours was blocked by inhibitors of prostaglandin synthetase (Tashjian 1975). While these early results seemed to point to a causal role for prostaglandins in the pathogenesis of hypercalcaemia, infusions of prostaglandin E_2 (the most potent bone resorber) failed to cause hypercalcaemia in experimental animals (except at massive doses) (Franklin and Tashjian 1975, Beliel et al. 1973), probably because it was rapidly broken down in the pulmonary circulation to metabolites with weak bone-resorbing effects (Anggard and Samuelsson 1964). Moreover, clinical studies showed a poor correlation with circulating prostaglandin levels and serum calcium values in cancer patients (Robertson et al. 1976) and, with a few exceptions (Seyberth et al. 1975), prostaglandin synthetase inhibitors were unsuccessful in the treatment of hypercalcaemia or osteolytic bone lesions in vivo (Brenner et al. 1982). Subsequent investigations have revealed that normal bone, in common with other normal tissues and tumours unassociated with hypercalcaemia, produce prostaglandins in appreciable amounts (Greaves et al. 1980). Thus, while prostaglandins may play an important role in the local regulation of bone turnover, they are unlikely to be involved as circulating humoral mediators of hypercalcaemia.

Prostaglandin-Stimulating Factors

The inhibitory effect of indomethacin on the in vitro bone-resorptive activity of certain tumour extracts stimulated further research into the possible role of tumour-associated bone-resorbing factors which acted by stimulating endogenous production of prostaglandins by bone. It is now clear that several factors, including tranforming growth factors, epidermal growth factor and platelet-derived growth factor, stimulate bone resorption by such a mechanism (Tashjian et al. 1985). In retrospect, one of these factors could have accounted for the prostaglandin-mediated bone-resorbing activity released by the tumours studied by Minkin et al. (1981). More recently, Bringhurst and his colleagues have isolated a novel prostaglandin-stimulating bone-resorbing factor from a transitional-cell bladder tumour which had been associated with hypercalcaemia in vivo (Bringhurst et al. 1986).

Of the growth factors which stimulate endogenous prostaglandin production by bone, both epidermal growth factor and transforming growth factors alpha and beta (TGFα, TGFβ) have been shown to cause hypercalcaemia when infused into experimental animals (Tashjian et al. 1986). Systemic calcium-elevating properties have not yet been demonstrated for the factor described by Bringhurst. It is at present unclear whether any of the above factors are released systemically in amounts sufficient to cause bone resorption or hypercalcaemia in vivo. The response of some patients' hypercalcaemia to indomethacin treatment (Seyberth et al. 1975) suggests, however, that in some patients at least, hypercalcaemia may arise as the result of prostaglandin-mediated pathways.

Growth Factors

Growth factors are a group of peptides produced by both normal and malignant tissues which were initially identified by their ability to stimulate cell replication in tissue culture systems (Patt and Houck 1983). Of relevance to the pathogenesis of cancer-associated hypercalcaemia is the ability of many growth factors to stimulate bone resorption in vitro (Mundy et al. 1984). As mentioned previously, growth factors appear to stimulate bone resorption by a prostaglandin-dependent mechanism in some experimental systems (Tashjian et al. 1985; Raisz et al. 1983), whereas in others non-prostaglandin-mediated pathways are involved (Mundy et al. 1985).

Bone-resorbing activity associated with a number of human and animal tumours has been found to co-elute with TGFα- and TGFβ like activity in vitro, leading to the suggestion that these factors may be potentially important as humoral mediators of hypercalcaemia (Mundy et al. 1984, 1985). Since transforming growth factors and epidermal growth factor are present in breast carcinomas (Travers et al. 1988) – tumours associated with both hypercalcaemia and bone metastases – it is clear that the TGFs are potentially important local osteolytic agents. While these substances do possess calcium-elevating activity when infused into mice (Tashjian et al. 1986), there is no information on whether or not they are released systemically by human tumours in amounts sufficient to cause bone resorption or hypercalcaemia.

Lymphokines

Cytokines produced by cells of the immune system, including interleukin-1 alpha and beta (IL-1α, IL-1β) and tumour necrosis factors alpha and beta (TNF), possess among a variety of other biological effects (Duff 1989), potent bone-resorbing properties (Gowen et al. 1983; Bertolini et al. 1986). Current evidence indicates that both groups of cytokines may be important in the pathogenesis of bone resorption and hypercalcaemia associated with haematological tumours such as myeloma and some cases of lymphoma (Garrett et al. 1987; Mundy et al. 1974; Yamamoto et al. 1989). These factors almost certainly comprise the bone-resorbing activity previously isolated from activated peripheral blood leucocytes and lymphoid myeloma cell lines which was known as OAF – "osteoclast-activating factor" (Mundy et al. 1974).

Both IL-1 and TNF are capable of stimulating bone resorption and hypercalcaemia when infused systemically into experimental animals (Garrett et al. 1987; Sabatini et al. 1988). However, in myeloma at least, they probably act on a mainly local basis, since histological studies have shown little evidence of increased osteoclastic activity at sites uninvolved by tumour (Battaille et al. 1986). While IL-1 and/or TNF are largely responsible for accelerated bone resorption in myeloma, it should be emphasised that the occurrence of hypercalcaemia is determined mainly by the co-existence of renal impairment due to the nephrotoxic effect of Bence–Jones protein, rather than the number of osteolytic lesions per se (Durie et al. 1981).

IL-1 and TNF have been implicated in the pathogenesis of bone resorption and hypercalcaemia associated with solid tumours also; certain squamous carcinoma cell lines have been found to produce IL-1α (Sato et al. 1988; Fried et al. 1989) and this cytokine appears to account for most of the in vitro bone-resorbing activity associated with such tumours (Fried et al. 1989). It is at present unclear to what extent this cytokine is released systemically by these tumours; infusion of IL-1-α-neutralising antibodies into animals bearing tumours which produced both IL-1 alpha and PTH-related peptide (PTHrP) did not correct the hypercalcaemia, whereas infusion of PTHrP antibodies did (Sato et al. 1989). Although solid tumours have not yet been shown to produce TNF, there is good evidence to suggest that many tumours indirectly enhance TNF release by cells of the immune system (Body et al. 1989; Yonenda et al. 1989) and that this sequence of events may be responsible in part for the cachexia associated with cancer (Tracey et al. 1989). Circulating immunoreactive TNFα levels have recently been found to be elevated in about 60% of unselected patients with tumour-associated hypercalcaemia (Body et al. 1989), suggesting that TNF could partly be responsible for systemic increases in bone resorption and inhibition of bone formation (Stewart et al. 1982; McDonnell et al. 1982) in some tumours. Whether such a mechanism could alone account for the occurrence of hypercalcaemia in solid tumours is doubtful; in rheumatoid arthritis where production of TNF and IL-1 are also increased (Duff 1989), hypercalcaemia does not occur and osteolysis is largely restricted to periarticular bone near the site of cytokine release – the inflamed joint.

Vitamin-D Metabolites

Active metabolites of vitamin D have predominantly been implicated in the pathogenesis of hypercalcaemia associated with malignant lymphomas. Since

1985, there have been several reports of patients with lymphoma-associated hypercalcaemia in whom serum 1,25-dihydroxycholecalciferol (1,25-DHCC) levels were markedly raised in the presence of depressed parathyroid hormone (PTH) levels (Davies et al. 1985; Breslau et al. 1984; Rosenthal et al. 1985). The hypercalcaemia in these patients was due to increased bone resorption, usually combined with moderate renal failure and, in a few cases, increased intestinal calcium absorption (Breslau et al. 1984).

In this situation, the tumour itself is the source of the 1,25-DHCC; cultured lymphoma cells and human T-cell lymphoma virus-1 (HTLV-1) transformed lymphocytes have both been shown to be capable of producing 1,25-DHCC from 25-HCC in vitro (Fetchick et al. 1986; Mudde et al. 1985). In vivo, the excessive synthesis of 1,25-DHCC is unregulated, mainly dependent on the concentration of the precursor (25-HCC) and abolished by effective treatment of the primary tumour, consistent with extra-renal synthesis of the metabolite (Davies et al. 1985).

Vitamin-D metabolites seem less important in the hypercalcaemia associated with solid tumours, although one case of a hypercalcaemic patient with small-cell lung cancer has been reported in which there was excessive production of 1,24R-DHCC by the tumour – a novel metabolite with biological activity comparable to that of 1,25-DHCC (Shigeno et al. 1985). The detectable or raised 1,25-DHCC levels which are seen in about 50% of patients with other solid tumours (Ralston et al. 1984b, 1987; Yamamoto et al. 1987), are not associated with increased intestinal calcium absorption (Ralston et al. 1987) and appear to be due to the stimulatory effect of PTH-related peptides on renal 1,25-DHCC production (Ralston et al. 1984b; Ralston et al. 1987).

Parathyroid Hormone-Like Factors

Parathyroid Hormone

Similarities have long been recognised between the syndrome of cancer-associated hypercalcaemia and primary hyperparathyroidism; both conditions are characterised by hypophosphataemia due to reduced renal tubular reabsorption of phosphate (Lafferty 1966; Stewart et al. 1980; Ralston et al. 1984a), increased nephrogenous excretion of cyclic adenosine monophosphate (NcAMP) (Stewart et al. 1980),increased renal tubular reabsorption of calcium (Ralston et al. 1984c) and a systemic increase in osteoclastic activity (Stewart et al. 1982, McDonnell et al. 1982). Because of these similarities, excessive production of ectopic PTH by tumour tissue was, not unnaturally, one of the first suggested mechanisms of humoral hypercalcaemia in malignancy (Lafferty 1966). Most workers, however, have failed to find evidence of true ectopic PTH production in tumours associated with hypercalcaemia (Skrabanek et al. 1980). Clinical studies using a variety of radio-immunoassays directed at various portions of the molecule have shown that PTH concentrations are low or undetectable in serum samples and tumour tissue from patients with cancer-associated hypercalcaemia (Stewart et al. 1980). Moreover, messenger RNA encoding for PTH has also been found to be absent from human and animal tumours associated with the syndrome (Simpson et al. 1983). While instances of true ectopic PTH production probably do occur, this appears to be an extremely rare event (Yoshimito et al. 1989).

Parathyroid Hormone-Related Peptides

With the exclusion of PTH as a mediator of cancer-associated hypercalcaemia, attention turned to the possible role of factors which mimicked the effects of parathyroid hormone at the end-organ level. Several groups isolated substances from human tumours associated with hypercalcaemia which stimulated activity of adenylate cyclase in bone and kidney cells in vitro (Strewler et al. 1983; Stewart et al. 1983; Rodan et al. 1983). Although these factors were distinct from PTH, their biological effects were competitively inhibited by synthetic PTH-receptor blockers, indicating that they were capable of binding to and activating the PTH receptor in vitro. Studies using a sensitive cytochemical bioassay technique on plasma samples from hypercalcaemic cancer patients also demonstrated PTH-like activity (Goltzman et al. 1981), confirming that the putative PTH-like factor(s) were not only released in vitro, but were also present in the systemic circulation in vivo.

Following extensive studies one such factor was purified to homogeneity, sequenced, cloned and expressed (Moseley et al. 1987; Suva et al. 1987). Sequencing data revealed a striking similarity between this factor and PTH with regard to the amino-terminal sequence, with 8 out of the first 13 amino acids identical. Because of this, and the functional similarities with PTH, the factor was named parathyroid-hormone related protein (PTHrP). Away from the amino terminal region, PTHrP and PTH are quite distinct and are encoded by different genes. It is of interest that despite the limited sequence homology, immune sera raised against even the amino-terminal of PTH react poorly with PTHrP, and vice versa, so explaining the paradox of PTH-like bioactivity in patients with cancer-associated hypercalcaemia with the absence of PTH immunoreactivity in serum or tumour tissue.

PTHrP-like factors have now been isolated from a number of tumours associated with malignant hypercalcaemia, including bladder cancers, squamous lung cancers, renal cortical cancers and breast cancers (Strewler et al. 1987; Ikeda et al. 1988). While different forms of PTHrP with molecular weights in the range 6–18 kD have been described, this seems to be due to variations in splicing of the messenger RNA and/or intracellular processing and cleavage of the peptide, rather than PTHrP gene duplications (Martin and Suva 1988).

Current evidence suggests that PTHrP is probably the most important mediator of hypercalcaemia in patients with solid tumours. Immunoreactive PTHrP values are raised in the majority of hypercalcaemic cancer patients (Henderson et al. 1989; Burtis et al. 1989) and infusions of synthetic PTHrP fragments can reproduce most of the biochemical abnormalities found clinically, including hypercalcaemia, phosphaturia, increased NcAMP excretion, increased renal tubular calcium reabsorption, increased osteoclastic bone resorption and increased 1,25-DHCC synthesis (Kemp et al. 1987; Horiuchi et al. 1987; Yates et al. 1988). While the stimulatory effect of PTHrP on 1,25-DHCC is at slight variance with the variable 1,25-DHCC levels seen clinically (Ralston et al. 1984b), the discrepancy can probably be explained on the basis of extraneous factors which act to suppress 1,25-DHCC production in some patients. These include: severe hypercalcaemia, renal impairment (Horiuchi et al. 1987), low levels of precursor 25-HCC (Ralston et al. 1984b) and co-production by the tumour of factors which specifically inhibit 1,25-DHCC synthesis (Fukomoto et al. 1989).

Although PTHrP is probably the major mediator of hypercalcaemia in cancer, other factors may also be involved; recently it has been shown that hypercalcaemia induced in experimental animals by transplantation of PTHrP-producing tumours is incompletely reversed by infusion of PTHrP antibodies (Kukreja et al. 1988). This suggests that, in some circumstances, other calcium-elevating factors released by the tumour in vivo may act in combination with PTHrP to cause hypercalcaemia (Mundy et al. 1985; Ralston et al. 1989a). Such factors may be important not only in the pathogenesis of hypercalcaemia, but also in explaining the depressed bone formation which occurs in advanced hypercalcaemia of malignancy (Stewart et al. 1982; McDonnell et al. 1982; Ralston et al. 1989a).

While PTHrP is present in many tumours from patients who are normocalcaemic (Danks et al. 1988), some go on to develop hypercalcaemia at a later date, with tumour progression (Ralston SH, Danks JA, Martin TJ, unpublished data). This indicates that mere production of PTHrP in situ by the tumour is not the only factor of importance in the development of hypercalcaemia; the peptide must also be released from tumour cells in quantities sufficient to exert its systemic effects on bone and kidney.

Apart from its importance as a mediator of cancer-associated hypercalcaemia, PTHrP also plays an important physiological role in the control of foetal calcium homeostasis (Rodda et al. 1988), lactation (Budayr et al. 1989) and keratinocyte function (Meredino et al. 1986). For a more complete discussion of these aspects of PTHrP effects, the reader is referred to a recent review by Martin and Suva (1988).

Mechanisms of Hypercalcaemia: Summary

Different mechanisms and mediators of hypercalcaemia are involved in the pathogenesis of hypercalcaemia in different tumour types and even within the same tumour type. These are summarised in Table 8.1 and discussed briefly below.

In myeloma, hypercalcaemia is invariably associated with increased bone resorption due to widespread osteolytic bone lesions (Mundy and Martin 1982) and renal impairment (Durie et al. 1981), probably due to the effects of Bence–Jones protein on the kidney. The immune-related cytokines TNFβ and IL-1 appear to be the predominant osteolytic mediators (Garrett et al. 1987; Yamamoto et al. 1989).

In lymphoma, various mechanisms may contribute to the hypercalcaemia; local release of IL-1 and TNF as described above (Mundy et al. 1974), excessive production of 1,25-DHCC (Breslau et al. 1984; Davies et al. 1985, Rosenthal et al. 1985), or, in HTLV-1 associated adult T-cell lymphomas/leukaemia, production of PTHrP (Fukomoto et al. 1988; Motokura et al. 1988). Lymphomas associated with increased 1,25-DHCC levels appear to be the only type of malignancy in which elevated intestinal calcium absorption plays a significant role in the pathogenesis of hypercalcaemia (Breslau et al. 1984; Ralston et al. 1987).

Table 8.1. Principal mediators of hypercalcaemia in malignancy, by tumour type

Tumour	Bone metastases	Factor[a]	Pathophysiology		Kidney	
			Bone	Gut	Tubule	GFR[b]
Myeloma	+++	TNF IL-1	+++	−	−	+++
Lymphoma	+/−	1,25 "OAF"	++	+	−	++
(HTLV-1)		PTHrP	+++	−	+++	+/−
Solid tumours (except breast cancer)	+/−	PTHrP	+++	−	+++	+/−
		?PG-S	+++	−	?	+/−
Breast cancer	+++	PG GFs Cath-D	+++	−	−	++
	+/−	PTHrP	+++	−	+++	+/−

[a] Abbreviations: IL-1, interleukin-1; TNF, tumour necrosis factor; OAF, osteoclast-activating factor; PTHrP, PTH-related protein; PG-S, prostaglandin stimulating factor; PG, prostaglandin; GF, growth factors; Cath-D, cathepsin D.
[b] Alterations in GFR are due to non-specific effects of sodium depletion or other tumour product, rather than the putative humoral factors (see text and Fig. 8.1).

Table 8.2. Symptoms of hypercalcaemia

Gastro-intestinal tract	Kidney	Central nervons system	General
Anorexia	Polyuria	Obtundation[a]	Malaise
Nausea	Polydipsia	Confusion[a]	Fatigue
Vomiting[a]	Dry mouth	Depression	
Constipation		Coma[a]	
		Lowered pain threshold?	

[a] Generally associated with severe hypercalcaemia (serum calcium >3.50 mmol/l).

In solid tumours *other* than breast carcinoma, PTHrP is the principal cause of hypercalcaemia (Martin and Suva 1988; Ralston 1987) although, in some cases, interactions between other bone-resorbing factors and PTHrP may also contribute (Martin and Suva 1988). Some patients with solid tumours who have clinical evidence of humorally-mediated hypercalcaemia (absent or few bone metastases) and who do not exhibit biochemical evidence of PTHrP excess, may respond clinically to treatment with inhibitors of prostaglandin synthetase (Seyberth 1975). Here, prostaglandin-stimulating factors may be involved in the pathogenesis of hypercalcaemia (Bringhurst et al. 1986).

In breast cancer, a tumour generally associated with predominantly local osteolytic hypercalcaemia, evidence can be found for PTHrP-mediated hyper-calcaemia in approximately 50%–60% of cases (Isales et al. 1987; Percival et al.

1985). In the remainder, local osteolysis is probably the main pathogenic mechanism, combined with other factors such as sodium depletion (Hosking et al. 1981) and immobilisation (Ralston et al. 1989a). The mediators of local osteolysis in breast cancer are unclear, but may comprise PTHrP (Ikeda et al. 1988), the transforming growth factors (Travers et al. 1988), prostaglandins (Greaves et al. 1980), cathepsin D (Wo et al. 1989), or some combination of the above.

Management of Cancer-Associated Hypercalcaemia
Clinical Assessment

Cancer-associated hypercalcaemia seldom presents a diagnostic problem; the tumour is usually obvious at the bed-side or is already known about by the time hypercalcaemia develops. Occasionally, however, hypercalcaemia may be the presenting feature of an occult tumour. In such cases, the diagnosis can usually be made fairly quickly on the basis of the typical biochemical findings of low or undetectable PTH levels, low albumin levels and a tendency to hypochloraemic alkalosis (Boyd and Ladenson 1984).

Clinically, cancer-associated hypercalcaemia tends to present in one of three ways; with mild hypercalcaemia (serum calcium less than 3.0 mmol/l) which is discovered on an incidental basis in an apparently asymptomatic patient; with moderate hypercalcaemia (3.0–4.0 mmol/1) which is usually associated with some symptoms (Warwick et al. 1961) (Table 8.2); and with severe hypercalcaemia (greater than 4.0 mmol/l) which is almost always symptomatic and is rapidly fatal if not treated as a matter of urgency. These differing presentations demand different forms of management.

Indications for Treatment

The main aims of antihypercalcaemic therapy in cancer patients are to improve symptoms and hence to improve the quality of life; survival may be little affected since most patients have advanced and/or untreatable tumours by the time hypercalcaemia presents (Ralston et al. 1990).

The presence of symptoms which may conceivably be related to hypercalcaemia is an indication for treatment, no matter how advanced the tumour appears to be. Although it is often difficult to decide whether such symptoms are due to the hypercalcaemia, or other effects of the tumour, there is little to be lost and much to be gained by a therapeutic trial of antihypercalcaemic therapy.

When hypercalcaemia is controlled, symptoms are much relieved and a high proportion of patients (60%–70%) improve enough to be discharged from in-patient hospital care (Ralston et al. 1990).

It is at present unclear whether patients with mild and genuinely asymptomatic hypercalcaemia should be treated; further studies in this area are necessary.

Principles of Medical Management

At the outset, it should be emphasised that the only effective way of controlling hypercalcaemia in the long-term is to treat the tumour itself. Having said this, only a minority of hypercalcaemic cancer patients can be offered such treatment, which emphasises the clinical importance of medical antihypercalcaemic therapy. A wide variety of agents have been used in the treatment of hypercalcaemia (Table 8.3). Most act by inhibiting osteoclastic bone resorption, and/or enhancing urinary excretion of calcium. Restriction of dietary calcium and/or vitamin D is seldom effective in cancer-associated hypercalcaemia except in the rare instances (e.g., lymphoma) where 1,25-DHCC levels are elevated (Breslau et al. 1984; Davies et al. 1985). Even here, however, therapy also needs to be given to counteract the generally more important renal and skeletal components of hypercalcaemia (Rosenthal et al. 1985).

The treatment of choice depends on the severity of hypercalcaemia and the clinical condition of the patient.

Specific Management Problems

Life-threatening Hypercalcaemia

In patients who present acutely with life-threatening hypercalcaemia (i.e., serum calcium 4.00 mmol/l or above), one must act to reduce serum calcium values quickly.

Clinically, these patients are usually unwell and often confused; they are almost invariably sodium-depleted and as a result have markedly reduced urinary excretion of calcium due to impaired GFR and increased sodium-linked calcium reabsorption in the proximal renal tubule (Hosking 1983). In patients with PTHrP-mediated hypercalcaemia, urinary calcium excretion may be further impaired by humorally mediated increases in distal tubular reabsorption of calcium (Ralston et al. 1984c) (Fig. 8.1).

Table 8.3. Drugs used in the treatment of cancer-associated hypercalcaemia

	Action on bone resorption	Action on renal calcium excretion	Other mechanism
Saline	−	+++	−
Diuretics + saline	−	+++	−
Calcitonin	++	+++	−
Mithramycin	+++	+?	Anti-tumour?
Bisphosphonates	+++	−	−
Gallium	+++	−	Anti-tumour?
Phosphate	+	−	Physico-chemical[a]
Steroids	+/−?	?	Anti-tumour

[a] Forms insoluble complexes with calcium in bone and soft tissues.

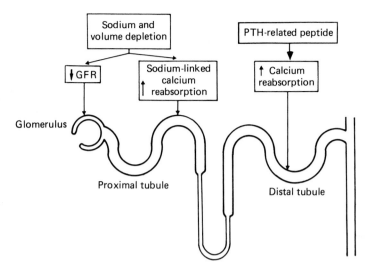

Fig. 8.1. Abnormalities of renal calcium handling in cancer-associated hypercalcaemia. Impaired GFR and increased sodium-linked calcium reabsorption in the proximal renal tubule are a non-specific feature of many types of hypercalcaemia and can generally be reversed or improved by sodium repletion. Increased distal tubular calcium reabsorption in the context of malignancy is thought to be due to PTHrP, whereas in hyperparathyroidism a similar abnormality occurs as the result of PTH excess.

Initially, a calcium diuresis is induced by restoring the extracellular fluid deficit with intravenous saline 4–6 l daily (Hosking et al. 1981). While this alone may reduce serum calcium values by 0.30–0.50 mmol/l over the first 48 h or so, not all patients respond adequately (Ralston et al. 1985) and in these subjects additional therapy is needed. Calcitonin is a useful drug in this situation; it has acute inhibitory effects on osteoclastic bone resorption and renal tubular calcium reabsorption (Hosking and Gilson 1984; Ralston et al. 1985), which lower serum calcium values within 2 h of starting therapy (Wisneski et al. 1978). Although calcitonin's inhibitory effect on bone resorption is transient, due to down-regulation of receptors on osteoclasts, the renal tubular effect is more sustained (Ralston et al. 1985) and in practice, the drug can usually control hypercalcaemia adequately until other more potent osteoclast inhibitors have taken effect. The combination of calcitonin and bisphosphonates has been particularly successful in this situation (Ralston et al. 1986).

When calcitonin is ineffective, intravenous phosphate is the treatment of choice; this lowers blood calcium within minutes of infusion due to the formation of insoluble calcium/phosphate complexes in bone and soft tissues (Herbert et al. 1966). Although the duration of effect is brief (24–48 h on average), phosphates, like calcitonin, can buy time for other agents to take effect. Intravenous phosphate should be given slowly (40 mmol/l 4 h) and therapy should be avoided if possible in patients with pre-existing hyperphosphataemia and renal impairment; many cases have been described when too rapid or inappropriate administration of phosphate has resulted in clinical deterioration or death due to acute renal failure or hypotension (Breuer and LeBauer 1967).

An alternative way of treating severe hypercalcaemia is by forced saline diuresis (Suki et al. 1970). High doses of loop diuretics (frusemide 80–100 mg

1–2 hourly) are used to induce a sodium-linked calcium diuresis and the urinary electrolyte losses are replaced with large quantities of intravenous fluids (approxiamtely 750 ml/h). Over a 24–48-h period, this regimen gave an average reduction of 0.80 mmol/l in serum calcium, but has the drawback that it requires central venous pressure monitoring and frequent measurements of serum and urinary electrolytes. Because of this, it is considered by many clinicians to be too intensive for routine use in cancer patients in whom the primary aims of therapy are palliative. Although commonly used, diuretics are not indicated in patients who are being given moderate quantities of saline; there is no evidence that they potentiate the response and they can make things worse by causing volume depletion.

Moderate Hypercalcaemia

In this situation, a rapid reduction in serum calcium is seldom necessary; it is sufficient to start treatment with moderate quantities of intravenous saline (2–3 l daily) in order to correct possible volume depletion and, at the same time, to give drug therapy to try and inhibit bone resorption to control hypercalcaemia in the longer term.

The agents of first choice in the longer-term control of hypercalcaemia are probably the bisphosphonates (Fleish 1982); these compounds, which are synthetic analogues of the naturally occurring pyrophosphate, share a common "core" structure of P–C–P atoms (Fig. 8.2) which adsorb to hydroxyapatite crystals and serve to concentrate the drugs in bone. When the bisphosphonate-containing bone is resorbed by the osteoclasts, the drug is liberated within the cytoplasm and inhibits cellular activity by mechanisms which are at present unclear. The potency with which different bisphosphonates inhibit bone resorp-

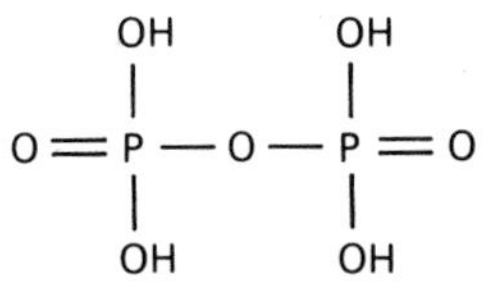

$$
\begin{array}{ccc}
\text{OH} & & \text{OH} \\
| & & | \\
\text{O}=\text{P}-\text{O}-\text{P}=\text{O} & & \text{Pyrophosphoric acid} \\
| & & | \\
\text{OH} & & \text{OH}
\end{array}
$$

$$
\begin{array}{ccc}
\text{OH} & \text{R}' & \text{OH} \\
| & | & | \\
\text{O}=\text{P}-\text{C}-\text{P}=\text{O} & & \text{Bisphosphonic acid} \\
| & | & | \\
\text{OH} & \text{R}'' & \text{OH}
\end{array}
$$

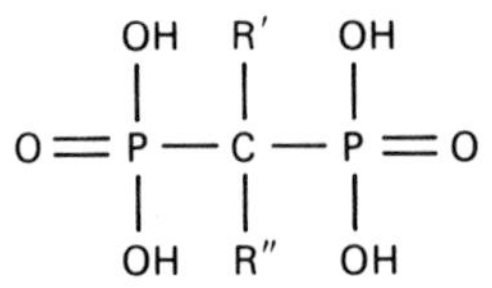

Etidronate: $R'=CH_3$, $R''=OH$
Clodronate: $R'=Cl$, $R''=Cl$
Pamidronate: $R'=NH_2-(CH_2)2$, $R''=OH$

Fig. 8.2. Structure of pyrophosphate and bisphosphonates. Pyrophosphate is a naturally occurring inhibitor of calcium phosphate crystallisation from which the bisphosphonates were derived.

tion varies with the structure of the side chain (Fleish 1982). Of the compounds which are currently available for clinical use, amino-substituted bisphosphonates such as pamidronate (aminohydroxy-propylidene bisphosphonate; APD; AHPrBP) are most potent followed by clodronate (dichloromethylene bisphosphonate ClMBP) and etidronate (hydroxyethylene bisphosphonate; EHDP; EHBP). The differences in potency may partly be explained by preferential inhibitory effects of the aminobisphosphonates on the formation of osteoclasts from precursors or the accession of the mature cells to bone (Boonekamp et al. 1987).

Currently, etidronate pamidronate and clodronate are licensed in the UK for the treatment of cancer-associated hypercalcaemia although at the time of writing, only etidronate is available in the USA.

Since all bisphosphonates are rather poorly absorbed from the gastrointestinal tract the intravenous form is preferable for the acute treatment of hypercalcaemia.

Intravenous etidronate is given by slow infusion, 7.5 mg/kg body weight/day for three consecutive days (Hasling et al. 1987); continued treatment for up to 5 days does not seem to improve the calcium-lowering response (Kanis et al. 1987). Previous high-dose regimens of 500–1000 mg daily (Jung 1972) are no longer used because of concern about the risk of acute renal failure (Bounameaux et al. 1983). Like all bisphosphonates, etidronate has a relatively slow onset of action. In patients who have previously been rehydrated, 2–3 days may elapse before calcium values drop appreciably (Ralston et al. 1989b; Kanis et al. 1987), although the apparent rate of response will obviously be faster when the fluids are commenced at the same time. Treatment is partially effective in most cases and serum calcium values generally fall to a nadir of 2.8–2.9 mmol/l at about 4–6 days. Although total serum calcium values have been reported to fall to normal in 75%–90% of patients (Hasling et al. 1987), the albumin-adjusted levels (which more accurately reflect the physiologically important ionised calcium fraction) are normalised in only 25%–30% of cases (Kanis et al. 1987; Ralston et al. 1989b). The failure of etidronate fully to correct hypercalcaemia is often due to PTHrP-mediated increases in renal tubular reabsorption of calcium, which is manifested by finding persistent hypercalcaemia in the presence of normal or only slightly raised fasting urinary calcium/creatinine values (an index of bone resorption) (Ralston et al. 1988).

The effect of intravenous etidronate lasts about 10–12 days (Ringerberg and Ritch 1987; Ralston et al. 1989b); it has been reported that the duration of remission may be extended up to 30 days by giving oral etidronate 20 mg/kg per day from day 4 of treatment (Ringerberg and Ritch 1987), although our experience with the oral preparation has been disappointing (Ralston et al. 1989b). Both oral and intravenous etidronate cause mild hyperphosphataemia due to the direct effect of the drug on renal tubular phosphate reabsorption, but this does not appear to be of clinical importance.

Clodronate is a slightly more potent inhibitor of bone resorption than etidronate in vitro, but, at the doses used clinically, the drugs have similar calcium-lowering effects (Jung 1972; Ralston et al. 1989b). Various dose regimens of clodronate have been used, ranging from single infusions of 500–600 mg over 6 h (Adami et al. 1987; Bonjour et al. 1988) to repeated daily infusions of between 300 mg and 500 mg to a total of over 3 g (Jung et al. 1972; Adami et al. 1987). Current evidence suggests that there is little to choose between these regimens, and the single dose is, of course, more convenient. The time-course of response to clodronate is similar to that of etidronate, although the effect lasts a little longer (12–14 days). In our experience (Ralston et al. 1989b), approximately 40% of patients are rendered normocalcaemic by a single dose of 600 mg, which is similar to that reported by others (Adami et al. 1987). An oral form of clodronate is available and is effective in some cases (Chapuy et al. 1980; Adami et al. 1987). Like etidronate, clodronate is well-tolerated; there has, however, been one report of acute renal failure in a patient who was given 19.9 g of the drug over a 30-day period (Bounameaux et al. 1983); lower doses do not appear to carry this risk.

Pamidronate appears to be superior to etidronate and clodronate in the treatment of hypercalcaemia, at least at the doses metioned above (Ralston et al. 1989b), owing to its greater potency in inhibiting bone resorption (Boonekamp et al. 1987). Many therapeutic regimens of pamidronate have been used ranging from repeated daily doses of 15 mg to a total of 150 mg, to single infusions of between 5 mg and 90 mg (Sleeboom et al. 1983; Ralston et al. 1985; Thiebaud et al. 1986a; Coleman and Rubens 1987; Morton et al. 1988; Ralston et al. 1988; Nussbaum et al. 1989). The optimal dose remains a subject of debate; although many patients respond adequately to doses of between 15 mg and 30 mg (Ralston et al. 1987; Coleman and Rubens 1987), doses of between 60 mg and 90 mg may be needed in some patients with severe hypercalcaemia and in patients whose hypercalcaemia has recurred or has been resistant to other agents (Thiebaud et al. 1986a; Nussbaum et al. 1989).

The time course of response to pamidronate is similar to that of the other bisphosphonates, although control of hypercalcaemia is better and the response more prolonged (20–30 days) (Morton et al. 1988; Ralston et al. 1988, 1989b). In a recent randomised comparative study, serum calcium levels (Fig. 8.3) and urinary calcium excretion (Fig. 8.4) at nadir were significantly lower with 30 mg pamidronate than with standard doses of etidronate and clodronate (Ralston et al. 1989b).

Like other bisphosphonates, pamidronate is well tolerated, although a transient pyrexia may be encountered after the first dose. This is seldom clinically significant in patients with malignancy, but inexplicably, may be associated with malaise and rigors in patients with benign disease (Gallacher et al. 1989). Renal impairment has not been reported. Although oral pamidronate has been successfully used in the treatment of hypercalcaemia (Thiebaud et al. 1986b), it is poorly tolerated due to gastro-intestinal upset, and most workers now use the intravenous preparation.

Of the other osteoclast inhibitors available for longer-term control of hypercalcaemia, mithramycin is effective (Perlia et al. 1970), but is limited by its potential for serious toxicity manifested by thrombocytopenia, hepatic dysfunction, renal tubular damage and gastro-intestinal upset (Brown and Kennedy 1965). It appears to work primarily by a cytotoxic effect on osteoclasts, but may also inhibit renal tubular reabsorption of calcium by mechanisms which are unclear (Ralston et al. 1985). Although mithramycin is usually safe on one or two occasions, the risk of toxicity is cumulative with repeated doses and because of this, it has largely been superseded by the bisphosphonates in the long-term control of hypercalcaemia. Calcitonin, either alone, or in combination with corticosteroids, is less effective than pamidronate in the treatment of cancer-associated hypercalcaemia (Ralston et al.1985), and on the basis of published

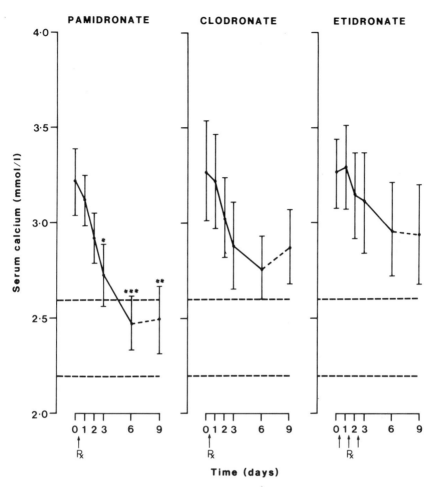

Fig. 8.3. Effect of three intravenous bisphosphonates on serum calcium; pamidronate was given as a single intravenous infusion of 30 mg, clodronate as a single intravenous infusion of 600 mg and etidronate as three consecutive daily infusions of 7.5 mg/kg body weight. All three bisphosphonates caused serum calcium to fall significantly from base-line, although the response was slightly more rapid with pamidronate (significant at 24 h) than with clodronate and etidronate (significant at 48 h). At the nadir, on day 6, serum calcium values were significantly lower in the pamidronate group and this difference was sustained up to day 9. Values given are means ± 95% confidence intervals. *p<0.05, **p<0.01, ***p<0.001 for differences between pamidronate and the other groups. Reproduced with permission from Ralston et al. (1989b).

data also appears to be less effective than the other bisphosphonates. In view of this, calcitonin is probably best reserved for the acute situation, although further work on the combination of calcitonin and bisphosphonates would be of interest in patients with PTHrP-mediated increases in renal tubular calcium reabsorption who respond incompletely to bisphosphonates alone (Ralston et al. 1985).

Gallium nitrate has recently been used successfully in the treatment of cancer-associated hypercalcaemia (Warrell et al. 1988). Like mithramycin, this drug seems to act by a cytotoxic effect on osteoclasts, but is less toxic systemically. Comparative studies indicate that intravenous gallium nitrate is

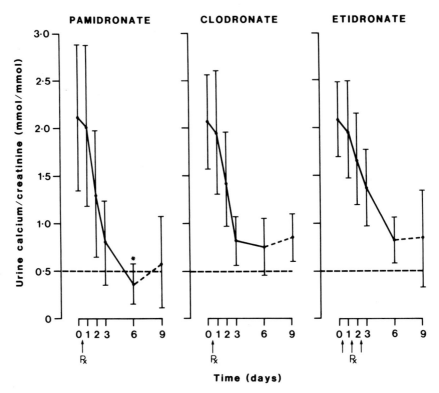

Fig. 8.4. Effect of intravenous bisphosphonates on bone resorption as reflected by fasting urinary calcium/creatinine ratio. All three bisphosphonates caused a significant fall in urinary calcium/creatinine ratio from raised base-line levels, reflecting the importance of increased bone resorption in the pathogenesis of hypercalcaemia and its suppression in the response to bisphosphonate therapy. As was the case with serum calcium, urinary calcium/creatinine values at nadir were significantly lower in the pamidronate group than in other treated groups. Values given are means ±95% confidence intervals. *p<0.05 for difference between pamidronate and other groups. Reproduced with permission from Ralston et al. (1989b).

superior to calcitonin in the treatment of cancer-hypercalcaemia with an efficacy similar to that of the bisphosphonates (Warrell et al. 1988). Its only significant drawback is the requirement for a continuous intravenous infusion over 5 days, although other more convenient ways of administering the drug may be found in the future.

Maintaining Normocalcaemia

The ideal drug for the long-term control would be effective orally and well tolerated. Regrettably, none of the currently available antihypercalcaemic agents possess these attributes. Corticosteroids are widely used and well tolerated but are generally ineffective unless the tumour itself is steroid-responsive (e.g., myeloma, lymphoma) (Thallasinos and Joplin 1970). Inorganic phosphate is effective when given orally but is poorly tolerated because of gastro-intestinal upset (Thallasinos and Joplin 1968).

While oral bisphosphonates such as clodronate and pamidronate have been used in the long-term control of hypercalcaemia, they are limited by gastro-intestinal intolerance (pamidronate) (Thiebaud et al. 1986b) and limited efficacy in solid tumours (clodronate) (Adami et al. 1987). Etidronate, although reasonably well tolerated, has limited efficacy in our experience (Ralston et al. 1989b). In view of this, an alternative way of controlling hypercalcaemia in the long-term is with repeated infusions of bisphosphonates on a day-patient basis; pamidronate is particularly suited to this type of regimen in view of its long duration of effect. Intermittent infusions of between 30 mg and 60 mg pamidronate every 2–3 weeks (Ralston et al. 1988; Morton et al. 1988) are generally effective initially, although with tumour progression, the hypercalcaemia may become partially resistant (Ralston et al. 1988).

References

Adami S, Bolzicci GP, Rizzo A et al. (1987) The use of dichloromethylene bisphosphonate and aminobutane bisphosphonate in hypercalcaemia of malignancy. Bone Miner 2:395–404

Anggard E, Samuelsson B (1964). Metabolism of prostaglandin E1 in the guinea pig lung: The structure of two metabolites. J Biol Chem 239:4097–4102

Battaille R, Chappard D, Alexandre C, Dessauw P, Sany J (1986) Interest of bone histomor-phomeric analysis in monoclonal gammopathy. Br J Cancer 53:805–810

Beliel OM, Singer FR, Coburn JW (1973). Prostaglandins: effect on plasma calcium concentration. Prostaglandins 3:237–241

Bertolini DR, Nedwin GE, Brown TS, Smith DD, Mundy GR (1986). Stimulation of bone resorption and inhibition of bone formation in vitro by human tumour necrosis factors. Nature 319:576–578

Body JJ, Dumon JC, Glibert F, Nejai S, Fernandez G (1989) Increased production of TNF alpha in tumor-associated hypercalcaemia. J Bone Miner Res 4 (Suppl):s253 (abstract)

Bonjour JP, Phillipe J, Guelpa G, Bisetti A, Rizzoli R, Jung A, Rosini S, Kanis JA (1988) Bone and renal components in intravenous hypercalcemia of malignancy and response to a single infusion of clodronate. Bone 9:123–130

Boonekamp PM, Lowik CWGM, van der Wee Pals LJA, van Wijk-van Lennep MML, Thesing CW, Bijvoet OLM (1987). Enhancement of the inhibitory action on the transformation of osteoclast precursors into bone resorbing cells after demethylation of the amino group. Bone Miner 2:39–42

Bounameaux H, Schifferli J, Montani JP, Jung A, Chatelanat F (1983) Renal failure associated with intravenous diphosphonates. Lancet i:471

Boyd JC, Ladenson JH (1984). Value of laboratory tests in the differential diagnosis of hypercalcaemia. Am J Med 77:863–872

Brenner DE, Harvey HA, Lipton A, Demers L (1982) A study of prostaglandin E2, parathormone and response to indomethacin in patients with hypercalcemia of malignancy. Cancer 49:556–561

Breslau NA, McGuire JL, Zerwekh JE, Frenkel EP, Pak CYC (1984) Hypercalcaemia associated with increased serum calcitriol levels in three patients with lymphoma. Ann Intern Med 100:1–7

Breuer RI, LeBauer J (1967). Caution in the use of phosphates in the treatment of severe hypercalcemia. J Clin Endocrinol 27:695–698

Bringhurst FR, Bierer BE, Godeau F, Neyhard N, Varner V, Segre GV (1986) Humoral hypercalcemia of malignancy: release of a prostaglandin-stimulating bone resorbing factor in vitro by human transitional carcinoma cells. J Clin Invest 77:456–464

Brown JH, Kennedy BJ (1965). Mithramycin in the treatment of disseminated testicular neoplasms. N Engl J Med 272:111–118

Budayr AA, Halloran BP, King JC, Diep D, Nissenson RA, Strewler GJ (1989) High levels of parathyroid hormone-like protein in milk. J Bone Miner Res 4 (Suppl):s138 (abstr).

Burtis WJ, Brady TG, Wu TL, Ersbak J, Stewart AF (1989). Rapid immunoradiometric assay (IRMA) for parathyroid hormone-like protein (PTHLP). J Bone Miner Res 4 (Suppl):s310 (abstr)

Chapuy MC, Meunier PJ, Alexandre C (1980). Effects of disodium dichloromethylene diphosphon-
    ate on hypercalcemia produced by bone metastases. J Clin Invest 65:1243–1247
Coleman RE, Rubens RD (1987) 3-amino-1,1-hydroxypropylidene bisphosphonate (APD) for
    hypercalcaemia of breast cancer. Br J Cancer 56:465–469
Danks JA, Ebeling PR, Hayman J, Chou ST, Moseley JM, Dunlop J, Kemp BE, Martin TJ (1988)
    Parathyroid hormone-related protein of cancer: immunohistochemical localisation in cancers and
    in normal skin. J Bone Miner Res 4:273–278
Davies M, Hayes ME, Mawer EB, Lumb GA (1985) Abnormal vitamin D metabolism in Hodgkin's
    lymphoma. Lancet ii:1186–1188
Duff GW (1989). Peptide regulatory factors in non-malignant disease. Lancet i:1432–1435
Durie BJM, Salmon SE, Mundy GR (1981). Relation of osteoclast activating factor production to
    the extent of metastatic bone disease in myeloma. Br J Cancer 47:21–30
Fetchick DA, Bertolini DR, Sarin PS, Weintraub ST, Mundy GR, Dunn JD (1986). Production of
    1,25 dihydroxyvitamin D by human T-cell lymphotrophic 1 virus transformed lymphocytes. J Clin
    Invest 78:592–596
Fisken RA, Heath DA, Bold AM. Hypercalcaemia – a hospital survey. QJ Med 1980;196:405–418
Fleish H (1982). Bisphosphonates: mechanisms of action and clinical applications. In: Peck WA (ed)
    Bone and mineral research, vol 1. Amsterdam, Excerpta Medica, pp 319–357
Franklin RB, Tashjian AH (1975). Intravenous infusions of prostaglandin E2 raises plasma calcium
    in the rat. Endocrinology 97:240–243
Fried RM, Voelkel EF, Rice RH, Levine L, Gaffney EV, Tashjian AH (1989) Two squamous cell
    carcinomas not associated with humoral hypercalcemia produce a potent bone resorption
    stimulating factor which is interleukin-1 alpha. Endocrinology 125:742–751
Fukomoto S, Matsumoto T, Ikeda K, et al. (1988) Clinical evaluation of calcium metabolism in adult
    T-cell leukaemia/lymphoma. Arch Intern Med 148:921–925
Fukomoto S, Matsumoto T, Yamoto H et al. (1989) Supression of serum 1,25 dihydroxyvitamin D in
    humoral hypercalcemia of malignancy is caused by elaboration of a factor that inhibits renal
    1,25-dihydroxyvitamin D production. Endocrinology 124:2057–2062
Gallacher SJ, Ralston SH, Patel U, Boyle IT (1989) Side effects of pamidronate. Lancet ii:42–43
Garrett IR, Durie BJM, Nedwin GE et al. (1987) Production of lymphotoxin – a potent bone
    resorbing cytokine – by cultured myeloma cells. N Engl J Med 317:526–532
Goltzman D, Stewart AF, Broadus AE (1981). Malignancy-associated hypercalcemia: evaluation
    with a cytochemical bioassay for parathyroid hormone. J Clin Endocrinol Metab 53:899–904
Gowen M, Wood DD, Ihrie EJ, McGuire MKB, Russell RGG (1983) An interleukin-1 like factor
    stimulates bone resorption in vitro. Nature 306:378–380
Greaves M, Ibbotson KJ, Atkins D, Martin TJ (1980) Prostaglandins as mediators of bone
    resorption in renal and breast tumours. Metabolism 58:201–210
Hasling C, Charles P, Mosekilde L (1987) Etidronate disodium in the management of malignancy-
    associated hypercalcemia. Am J Med 82 (Suppl 2A):51–54
Henderson JE, Shustik C, Kremer R, Rabbani SA, Hendy GN, Goltzman D (1989) Immunoreactive
    parathyroid hormone-like peptide in the plasma of patients with malignancy and with
    hyperparathyroidism. J Bone Miner Res 4 (Suppl):s323 (abstr)
Herbert LA, Lemann J, Peterson JR, Lennon EJ (1966) Studies of the mechanism by which
    phosphate lowers serum calcium concentration. J Clin Invest 45:1866–1894
Horiuchi H, Caulfield MP, Fisher JE et al. (1987) A similarity of synthetic peptide from human
    tumor to parathyroid hormone in vivo and in vitro. Science 238:1566–1568
Hosking DJ, Cowley A, Bucknall CA (1981) Rehydration in the treatment of severe hypercal-
    caemia. Q J Med 200:473–478
Hosking DJ (1983). Disequilibrium hypercalcaemia. Br Med J 286:326–327
Hosking DJ, Gilson D (1984) Comparison of the renal and skeletal actions of calcitonin in the
    treatment of severe hypercalcaemia of malignancy. Q J Med 211:359–369
Ikeda K, Mangin M, Dreyer B et al. (1988) Identification of transcripts encoding a parathyroid
    hormone-like peptide in messenger RNA's from a variety of human an animal tumors associated
    with hypercalcaemia of malignancy. J Clin Invest 81:2010–2014
Isales C, Carcangui ML, Stewart AF (1987) Hypercalcaemia in breast cancer: a re-evaluation. Am J
    Med 82:1143–1147
Jung A (1972) Comparison of two parenteral diphosphonates in hypercalcemia of malignancy. Ann
    Intern Med 29:923–930
Kanis JA, Urwin GH, Gray RES et al. (1987) Effects of intravenous etidronate disodium on skeletal
    and calcium metabolism. Am J Med 82 (Suppl 2A):55–70
Kemp BE, Moseley JM, Rodda CP et al. (1987) Parathyroid hormone-related protein of

malignancy: active synthetic fragments. Science 237:1568–1570

Klein DC, Raisz LG (1970) Prostaglandins: stimulation of bone resorption in tissue culture. Endocrinology 80:1436–1440

Kukreja SC, Shavin DH, Wimbiscus S, Ebeling PR, Wood WI, Martin TJ (1988) Antibodies to parathyroid hormone-related protein lower serm calcium in athymic mouse models of malignancy-associated hypercalcaemia. J Clin Invest 82:1798–1802

Lafferty FW (1966) Pseudohyperparathyroidism. Medicine 45:247–260

Martin TJ, Suva LJ (1988) Parathyroid hormone-related protein: a novel gene product. Bailliere's Clin Endocrinol Metab 2:1003–1029

McDonnell GD, Dunstan CR, Evans RA et al. (1982) Quantitative bone histology in the hypercalcaemia of malignant disease. J Clin Endocrinol Metab 55:1066–1072

Meredino TJ, Insogna KL, Milstone LM, Broadus AE, Stewart AF (1986). A parathyroid hormone-like protein from cultured human keratinocytes. Science 231:388–390

Minkin C, Fredericks RS, Porkess S et al. (1981) Bone resorption and humoral hypercalcemia of malignancy: stimulation of bone resorption in vitro by tumour extracts is inhibited by prostaglandin synthetase inhibitors. J Clin Endocrinol Metab 53:941–947

Morton AR, Cantrill JA, Craig AE, Howell A, Davies M, Anderson DC (1988) Single versus daily intravenous aminohydroxypropylidene bisphosphonate (APD) for the hypercalcaemia of malignancy. Br Med J 296:811–814

Moseley JM, Kubota M, Diefenbach-Jagger H et al. (1987) Parathyroid hormone-related protein purified from a human lung cancer cell line. Proc Natl Acad Sci USA 84:5048–5052

Motokura T, Fukomoto S, Takahashi S, Watanabe T, Matsumoto T, Igarashi T, Ogata E (1988) Expression of parathyroid hormone-related protein in a human T-cell lymphoma lymphotrophic virus type 1 infected cell. Biochem Biophys Res Comm 154:1182–1188

Mudde AH, Van der Berg H, Breedveld FC, Nijweide PJ, Papapoulos SE, Bijvoet OLM (1985) Lymphoma-associated hypercalcaemia. In vitro demonstration of 1,25 dihydroxyvitamin D3 production. Calcif Tissue Int 38 (Suppl):s36 (abstr)

Mundy GR, Luben RA, Raisz LG, Oppenheim JJ, Buell DN (1974) Bone resorbing activity in supernatants from lymphoid cell lines. N Engl J Med 290:867–871

Mundy GR, Martin TJ (1982) Hypercalcaemia of malignancy: pathogenesis and management. Metabolism 31:1247–1277

Mundy GR, Ibbotson KJ, D'Souza SM, Simpson EL, Jacobs JW, Martin TJ (1984) The hypercalcemia of cancer: clinical implications and pathogenic mechanisms. N Engl J Med 310:1718–1726

Mundy GR, Ibbotson KJ, D'Souza SM (1985) Tumor products and the hypercalcemia of malignancy. J Clin Invest 76:391–394

Nussbaum SR, Mallette L, Gagel R et al. (1989) Single dose treatment of hypercalcemia of malignancy with aminohydroxypropylidene bisphosphonate (APD). J Bone Miner Res 4 (Suppl):s313 (abstr)

Patt LM, Houck JC (1983) Role of polypeptide growth factors in normal an abnormal growth. Kidney Int 23:603–610

Percival RC, Yates AJP, Gray RES et al. (1985) Mechanisms of hypercalcaemia in carcinoma of the breast. Br Med J 291:776–779

Perlia CP, Gubisch NJ, Wolter J, Edelberg D, Dederick MM, Taylor SG (1970) Mithramycin treatment of hypercalcemia. Cancer 1970; 25:389–394

Raisz LG, Simmons HA, Sandberg AL, Canalis E (1983). Direct stimulation of bone resorption by epidermal growth factor. Endocrinology 23:603–610

Ralston SH (1987) The pathogenesis of humoral hypercalcaemia of malignancy. Lancet ii:1443–1446

Ralston SH, Fogelman I, Gardner MD, Boyle IT (1982) Hypercalcaemia and metastatic bone disease: is there a causal link? Lancet i:903–905

Ralston SH, Fogelman I, Gardner MD, Boyle IT (1984a) Relative contribution of humoral and metastatic factors to the pathogenesis of hypercalcaemia in malignancy. Br Med J 288:812–813

Ralston SH, Cowan RA, Robertson AG, Gardner MD, Boyle IT (1984b) Circulating vitamin D metabolites and hypercalcaemia of malignancy. Acta Endocrinol 106:556–563

Ralston SH, Fogelman I, Gardner MD, Dryburgh FJ, Cowan RA, Boyle IT (1984c) Hypercalcaemia of malignancy: evidence for a non-parathyroid humoral mediator with an effect on renal tubular calcium handling. Clin Sci 66:187–191

Ralston SH, Gardner MD, Dryburgh FJ, Jenkins AS, Cowan RA, Boyle IT (1985) Comparison of aminohydroxypropylidene diphosphonate, mithramycin and corticosteroids/calcitonin in treatment of cancer-associated hypercalcaemia. Lancet ii:907–910

Ralston SH, Alzaid AA, Gardner MD, Boyle IT (1986) Treatment of cancer-associated hypercalcaemia with combined aminohydroxypropylidene bisphosphonate and calcitonin. Br Med J 292:1549–1550

Ralston SH, Cowan RA, Gardner MD, Fraser WD, Marshall E, Boyle IT (1987) Comparison of intestinal calcium absorption and circulating 1,25-dihydroxyvitamin D levels in malignancy-associated hypercalcaemia and primary hyperparathyroidism. Clin Endocrinol 26:281–291

Ralston SH, Alzaid AA, Gallacher SJ, Gardner MD, Cowan RA, Boyle IT (1988) Clinical experience with aminohydroxypropylidene bisphosphonate (APD) in the management of cancer-associated hypercalcaemia. Q J Med 258:825–834

Ralston SH, Boyce BF, Cowan RA, Gardner MD, Fraser WD, Boyle IT (1989a) Contrasting mechanisms of hypercalcemia in patients with early and advanced humoral hypercalcemia of malignancy. J Bone Miner Res 4:103–111

Ralston SH, Gallacher SJ, Patel U, Campbell J, Boyle IT (1990) Cancer associated hypercalcaemia; morbidity and mortality: experience in 126 patients. Ann Intern Med 112:499–504

Ralston SH, Gallacher SJ, Patel U, Dryburgh FJ, Fraser WD, Cowan RA, Boyle IT (1989b) Comparison of three intravenous bisphosphonates in cancer-associated hypercalcaemia. Lancet ii:1180–1183

Ringerberg QS, Ritch PS (1987) Efficacy of oral administration of etidronate disodium in maintaining normal serum calcium levels in previously hypercalcemic cancer patients. Clin Ther 9:1–7

Robertson RB, Baylink DJ, Metz SA, Cummings KB (1976) Plasma prostaglandin E in patients with cancer with and without hypercalcaemia. J Clin Endocrinol Metab 43:1330–1335

Rodan G, Insogna KL, Vignery A et al. (1983) Factors associated with humoral hypercalcaemia of malignancy stimulate adenylate cyclase in osteoblastic cells. J Clin Invest 72:1151–1515

Rodda CP, Kubota M, Heath JA et al. (1988) Evidence for a novel parathyroid hormone-related protein in fetal lamb parathyroid glands and sheep placenta: Comparisons with a similar protein implicated in humoral hypercalcaemia of malignancy. J Endocrinol. 117:261–271

Rosenthal N, Insognal KL, Godsall JW, Smaldone L, Waldron JA, Stewart AF (1985) Elevations in circulating 1,25-dihydroxyvitamin D in three patients with lymphoma-associated hypercalcaemia. J Clin Endocrinol Metab 60:29–33

Sabatini M, Boyce BF, Aufdemorte T, Bonewald L, Mundy GR (1988) Infusions of recombinant interleukin-1 alpha and beta cause hypercalcemia in normal mice. Proc Natl Acad Sci USA 85:5235–5239

Sato K, Fuji Y, Kasono K, Tsushima T, Shizume K (1988) Production of interleukin-1 alpha and a parathyroid hormone-like factor by a squamous cell carcinoma of the oesophagus (EC-GI) derived from a patient with hypercalcemia. J Clin Endocrinol Metab 67:592–621

Sato K, Fuji Y, Kashara T et al. (1989) Treatment by anti-PTH related protein antibody and anti-interleukin-1 antibody of hypercalcemia in nude mice transplanted with squamous cell carcinoma producing PTHrP and IL-1 alpha. J Bone Miner Res 4 (Suppl):s310 (abstr)

Seyberth HW, Segre GV, Morgan JL, Sweetman BJ, Potts JT, Oates JA (1975) Prostaglandins as mediators of hypercalcemia in certain types of cancer. N Engl J Med 273:1278–1283

Shigeno C, Yamamoto I, Dokoh S et al. (1985) Identification of 1,24R-dihydroxyvitamin D3-like bone resorbing lipid in a patient with cancer-associated hypercalcaemia. J Clin Endocrinol Metab 61:761–768

Simpson EL, Mundy GR, D'souza SM, Ibbotson KJ, Bockman R, Jacobs JW (1983) Absence of parathyroid hormone messenger RNA in non-parathyroid tumors associated with hypercalcemia. N Engl J Med 309:325–330

Skrabanek P, McPartlin D, Powell DM (1980) Tumour hypercalcaemia and ectopic hyperparathyroidism. Medicine 59:262–282

Sleeboom HP, Bijvoet OLM, Van Oosteroom AT, Gleed JH, O'Riordan JLH (1983) Comparison of intravenous (3-amino-1-hydroxypropylidene)-1, 1-bisphosphonate and volume repletion in tumour induced hypercalcaemia. Lancet ii:239–243

Stewart AF, Horst RL, Deftos LJ, Cadman EC, Lang R, Broadus AE (1980) Biochemical evaluation of patients with cancer-associated hypercalcemia: evidence for humoral and non-humoral groups. N Engl J Med 303:1377–1383

Stewart AF, Vignery A, Silvergate A et al. (1982) Quantitative bone histomorphometry in humoral hypercalcemia of malignancy: uncoupling of bone cell activity. J Clin Endocrinol Metab 55:219–227

Stewart AF, Insogna KL, Goltzman D, Broadus AE (1983) Identification of adenylate cyclase stimulating activity in extracts of tumor associated with humoral hypercalcemia of malignancy. Proc Natl Acad Sci USA 80:1454–1459

Stewart AF, Insogna KL, Goltzman D, Broadus AE. Suva LJ, Winslow GA, Moseley JM et al.

(1987) A parathyroid hormone-related protein implicated in malignant hypercalemia: cloning and expression. Science 237:893–896

Strewler GJ, Williams RD, Nissenson RA (1983) Human renal carcinoma cells produce hypercalcaemia in the nude mouse and a novel protein recognised by parathyroid hormone receptors. J Clin Invest 71:769–774

Strewler GJ, Stern PH, Jacobs JW et al. (1987) Parathyroid hormone-like protein from renal carcinoma cells: structural and functional homology with parathyroid hormone. J Clin Invest 80:1803–1807

Suki WN, Yium JJ, Von Minden M, Saller-Hebert C, Eknoyan C, Martinez-Maldonado M (1970) Acute treatment of hypercalcemia with furosemide. N Engl J Med 283:836–840

Suva LJ, Winslow GA, Moseley JM et al. (1987) A parathyroid hormone-related protein implicated in malignant hypercalemia: cloning and expression. Science 237:893–896

Tashjian AH (1975). Tumor humors and the hypercalcemia of cancer. N Engl J Med 293:1317–1318

Tashjian AH, Levine L (1978). Epidermal growth factor stimulates prostaglandin production and bone resorption in cultured mouse calvariae. Biochem Biophys Res Comm 85:966–972

Tashjian AH, Voelkel EH, Lazzaro M et al. (1985) Alpha and beta human transforming growth factors stimulate prostaglandin production and bone resorption in cultured mouse calvariae. Proc Natl Acad Sci USA 82:4535–4538

Tashjian AH, Voelkel EF, Lloyd W, Derynck R, Winkler ME, Levine L (1986) Actions of growth factors on plasma calcium. J Clin Invest 78:1405–1409

Thallasinos N, Joplin GF (1968) Phosphate treatment of hypercalcaemia due to carcinoma. Br Med J iv:14–19

Thallasinos N, Joplin GF (1970) Failure of corticosteroid therapy to correct the hypercalcaemia of malignant disease. Lancet ii:537–539

Thiebaud D, Jaeger PH, Jaquet AF, Burckhardt P (1986a) A single day treatment of tumour induced hypercalcaemia by intravenous aminohydroxypropylidene bisphosphonate. J Bone Miner Res 1:555–562

Thiebaud D, Portmann L, Jaeger P et al. (1986b) Oral versus intravenous AHPrBP (APD) in the treatment of hypercalcemia of malignancy. Bone 7:247–253

Tracey KJ, Vlassara H, Cerami A (1989). Cachectin/tumour necrosis factor. Lancet i:1122–1126

Travers MT, Barrett-Lee PJ, Berger U, et al. (1988) Growth factor expression in normal, benign and malignant breast tissue. Br Med J 296:1621–1624

Warrell RP, Israel R, Frisone M, Snyder T, Gaynor JJ, Bockman RS (1988) Gallium nitrate for acute treatment of cancer-related hypercalcemia. Ann Intern Med 108:669–674

Warwick OH, Yendt ER, Olin JS (1961). The clinical features of hypercalcemia associated with malignant disease. J Canad Med Ass 23:719–723

Wisneski LA, Croom WP, Silva OL, Becker KL (1978) Salmon calcitonin in hypercalcemia. Clin Pharmacol Ther 24:219–222

Wo G, Bonewald LF, Oreffo R, Chirgwin JM, Capony F, Rochefort H, Mundy GR (1989) Evidence that lysosomal procathepsin D secreted by human breast cancer cells activates osteoclasts. J Bone Miner Res 5:s322 (abstr)

Yamamoto I, Kitamura N, Aoki J et al. (1987) Circulating 1,25 dihydroxyvitamin D concentrations in patients with renal cell carcinoma hypercalcaemia are rarely suppressed. J Clin Endocrinol Metab 64:175–179

Yamamoto I, Kawano M, Sone T, Iwato K, Shigeno C, Kuramoto A (1989) Production of interleukin-1 beta, a potent bone resorbing cytokine, by human myeloma cells. J Bone Miner Res 5:s254 (abstr)

Yates AJP, Guttierez GE, Smolens P et al. (1988) Effects of a synthetic peptide of a parathyroid hormone-related protein on calcium homeostasis, renal tubular calcium reabsorption and bone metabolism in vivo and in vitro. J Clin Invest 81:932–938

Yonenda T, Alsina M, Chavez J, Bonewald L, Mundy GR (1989) Hypercalcemia in a human tumor is due to tumor necrosis factor production by host immune cells. J Bone Miner Res 4 (Suppl):s324 (abstr)

Yoshimito K, Yamasaki R, Sakai H et al. (1989) Ectopic production of parathyroid hormone by small cell lung cancer in a patient with hypercalcemia. J Clin Endocrinal Metab 68:976–981

9 Radiotherapy in the Management of Bone Metastases

P.J. Hoskin

Irradiation was first used in the treatment of bone metastases only a few months after the discovery of x-rays by Roentgen in 1895 and the first report of the effective pain relief in bone metastases was in 1907 following irradiation of pelvic metastases from carcinoma of the breast (Leddy 1930). Since these early observations radiation has become established as a highly effective treatment for painful bone metastases.

Principles of External Beam Irradiation

Most treatments for bone pain will involve the use of an external beam of ionising radiation. This may be produced in the form of gamma rays from a radioactive source, usually cobalt (^{60}Co) or caesium (^{137}Cs), or as x-rays produced by the bombardment of a high-atomic-weight target such as tungsten by high energy electrons.

Low and intermediate energy (orthovoltage) x-ray beams interact with matter by different processes from those of high energy megavoltage x-ray beams. As a result of this, bone which has a high atomic weight relative to soft tissue will receive relatively higher absorbed doses of irradiation when treated with orthovoltage beams than with megavoltage beams. The ratio of energy absorption in bone to soft tissue is of the order of 2 : 1 for a 250 KeV x-ray beam whilst no differential effect is seen for a beam of 2 MeV (Meredith and Massey 1977).

Radiotherapy Treatment Techniques for Bone Metastases

In the treatment of bone metastases by external beam irradiation two principle techniques are used: localised external beam treatment for single sites and wide field irradiation (hemibody irradiation) where there are multiple involved symptomatic sites.

The principles of using a localised external beam treatment are that a beam arrangement of suitable penetration to give an even dose of radiation to the affected bone is required and, secondly, that the area to be treated is accurately defined and localised.

Many bones, in particular the ribs, skull, clavicle, scapula and sternum are relatively superficial and an orthovoltage beam of 250–300KeV will give sufficient penetration adequately to treat the affected area. Such beams are directed using steel or lead-lined applicators attached to the head of the machine. Various sizes of applicator are available to suit the required area to be treated and the position can be marked on the skin with indelible pen or small tattoos.

For more deeply seated bones such as long bones, pelvis and spine a megavoltage beam will be required to achieve sufficient penetration; in the pelvis and long bones opposing beams are most commonly employed to attain an even dose across the volume to be treated. With such areas localisation using surface anatomy is unreliable and under optimal conditions a treatment simulator will be used. This machine, which reproduces the treatment beam and patient position, emits x-rays of diagnostic quality and can take radiographs giving an accurate view of the area treated by a given beam position. Once the correct beam position is defined the entry points are marked on a patient's skin together with a permanent record using small tattoos at the beam centre and corners. Using these landmarks the megavoltage treatment machine can reproduce the position as defined by the simulator, enabling accurate localisation of the painful area within the x-ray beam. This also facilitates matching of radiation fields should an adjacent area require treating at a future date avoiding potentially hazardous overlap of irradiated areas.

The treatment of larger areas of the body is technically more complex. This is partly because most treatment machines are designed to treat areas of up to 30 or 40 cm^2 and also because the dose absorbed will vary across a large volume of varying thickness. These factors, together with the use of the machine under non-standard conditions, means that routine calibrations or dosimetry cannot be readily used. Although purpose-built machines are available most patients requiring hemibody irradiation will be treated using a standard cobalt machine or linear accelerator but with the distance from the machine to the patient increased from the usual 80–100 cm to 2–3 m. This enables a sufficiently large field size to be obtained. The most satisfactory way of checking dosimetry in this situation is by direct measurement of the radiation dose on the body surface with radiation-sensitive monitors such as lithium fluoride chips or by using diode monitors.

Biological Effects of Ionising Radiation

The biological effect of the x-ray or gamma ray is to cause, along its path, ionisation which will result in both direct and indirect damage to nuclear DNA.

The consequence of this damage is impairment of DNA synthesis, abnormal mitosis and cell death when the cell attempts to divide.

The effects on normal tissue are spared relative to tumour by delivering radiation in small daily treatments rather than as a single dose. The overall biological effect will depend on the total dose of radiation administered and also the time over which it is given and the number of individual treatments used to reach the final dose. By dividing the treatment into a number of small daily fractions a bigger overall biological dose may be delivered to the tumour without exceeding the radiation tolerance of surrounding normal tissues. From this general principle have arisen a number of dose fractionation schedules in common clinical use for the treatment of bone metastases. These range from relatively low doses given as a single fraction to lengthy regimens of daily treatment over 4 or 5 weeks which attempt to deliver a high overall tumour dose. There is confusion over the relative efficacy of these different schedules. This may be principally because, despite a number of proposals, there is no universally accepted means of converting a given dose fractionation schedule into a standard unit of biological radiation activity which is applicable to a given tumour type or normal tissue type.

Pathological Changes after Bone Irradiation

Bone irradiation can result in a number of pathological changes in the bone, ranging from none or only mild atrophy to osteitis, necrosis and sarcomatous change.

Only relatively small doses of irradiation will result in inhibition of bone growth with single doses as low as 4 Gy resulting in permanent shortening of a growing bone in young children. Fractionated irradiation of the epiphyseal plate to doses of 10–12 Gy in daily fractions of 1.8 Gy will result in growth impairment. In a different context, radiation has been used to prevent heterotopic bone formation following total hip arthroplasty which is reported to occur in 10%–15% of patients undergoing this operation. Post-operative radiotherapy using doses as low as 10 Gy in 10 daily fractions appears effective in suppressing this excessive bone growth (Anthony et al. 1987).

In man the effect of bone irradiation has been studied at post mortem and in vivo using radio-isotope kinetic studies. The initial microscopic changes following irradiation of a bone containing metastases are of degeneration and necrosis of the tumour cells, followed by collagen proliferation. A fibrous stroma rich in capillaries is formed followed by a period of osteoblastic activity in which woven bone is laid down. This is then gradually replaced by lamellar bone and intratrabecular stroma gives way to bone marrow tissue. Remineralisation of bone following irradiation has been demonstrated both radiographically and by strontium (^{85}Sr) and calcium (^{47}Ca) kinetic studies. Calcification in lytic areas occurs with relatively small doses of irradiation in the order of 20–30 Gy following a period of 3–6 weeks with maximum recalcification at 2 months from the time of irradiation. These changes are in contrast to the effect of irradiation on normal bone when histological examination of bone surrounding an area of invasion by metastatic tumour shows no significant changes, and spectrophotometry following radical irradiation to the pelvis shows no appreciable change in bone mineral content (Matsubayashi et al. 1981; Garmatis and Chu 1978; Dalen and Edsmyr 1974).

Clinical Use of Radiotherapy for Bone Metastases

The possible indications for irradiation in the management of bone metastases are shown in Table 9.1.

Bone Pain

The most common clinical problem from bone metastases is pain. Radiotherapy remains the treatment of choice for localised metastatic bone pain in the majority of patients. There may, however, be several causes of bone pain as a result of bone invasion by a metastasis, some of which may be less responsive to irradiation than others. These are shown in Table 9.2. The important emotional component to metastatic pain which may considerably modify pain perception in the cancer patient must also be taken into account in the management of bone pain. It is also important to consider that not all bone pain in the patient with metastatic cancer is due to bone metastases and, particularly in weight-bearing areas such as the hip and spinal column, degenerative joint disease and osteoporosis are common conditions.

Accurate localisation and diagnosis with supporting radiographs or isotope bone scans are therefore important before recommending irradiation. In selected cases CT scanning or magnetic resonance imaging may give further valuable information in defining the involved area, particularly in sites such as

Table 9.1.   Possible indications for irradiation in the management of bone metastases

1.   Palliative treatment
      a) Bone pain
      b) Nerve or spinal cord compression
      c) Pathological fracture
2.   Prophylaxis
      a) Nerve or spinal cord compression
      b) Pathological fracture

Table 9.2.   Possible mechanisms for bone pain from bone metastases

Bone invasion and local destruction
Pathological fracture or vertebral collapse
Nerve root compression
Muscle spasm
Soft tissue infiltration
Periostitis
Joint instability

the spinal column where extensive bone disease can be identified by the use of isotope scanning or magnetic resonance imaging, despite normal radiographs.

Localised Bone Pain

A review of the current literature shows a large number of retrospective and non-randomised studies and three prospective randomised studies reporting the efficacy of local irradiation for bone pain. Overall, response rates of around 85% are reported, with complete responses in around half of patients. The details of treatment technique and dose vary considerably between different centres and no particular approach appears to be superior in terms of pain relief (Hoskin 1988).

Histology of the primary tumour does not appear to influence the likelihood of response. The survival of patients treated for bone metastases is often poor with median survival generally of <1 year for primary tumours other than breast cancer. In those studies where long-term follow-up is reported, patients who respond appear consistently to maintain pain relief for many months or even years. These are, however, only small numbers of patients out of the total treated, predominantly those with primary tumours of breast and prostate.

The Radiation Therapy and Oncology Group (RTOG) has reported results of a prospective randomised study of 1016 treatments for metastatic bone pain using a variety of dose fractionation schedules ranging from 15 Gy delivered in 1 week to 40.5 Gy in 15 fractions over 3 weeks. An overall response rate of 90% was observed and approximately half of responders maintained pain relief until death, with a median duration of pain relief in complete responders of 12–15 weeks and in "minimal" responders 20–28 weeks. The initial report of this study found no difference in efficacy between the different dose fractionation schedules when the patients were analysed in two separate groups depending upon whether single metastases or multiple sites were present (Tong et al. 1982). More recent analysis, in which both groups of patients were analysed together and including a more detailed pain assessment with analgesic requirements, has found a significant association between the number of fractions given and complete response. A complete response rate of 55% was seen after 40.5 Gy in 15 daily fractions and only 28% after 25 Gy in 5 daily fractions (p= 0.0003) (Blitzer 1985). Another prospective randomised study of 57 treatments comparing 24 Gy in 6 fractions over 3 weeks with 20 Gy in 2 fractions over 1 week has shown no difference in response rates which were around 50% in each arm (Madsen 1983).

The Royal Marsden Hospital has reported results of a prospective randomised study comparing a single fraction of 8 Gy to a fractionated course of 30 Gy in 10 daily fractions (Price et al. 1986). No difference was seen between the two dose fractionation arms for either rate of onset of pain relief (Fig. 9.1) or duration of pain relief (Fig. 9.2).

Overall, the weight of evidence from retrospective and prospective studies suggests that there is no clear dose–response effect for pain relief after local irradiation of bone metastases. Two exceptions to this case are the re-analysis of the RTOG study (Blitzer 1985) and a recent non-randomised study (Arcangeli et al. 1989) in which total doses greater than 40 Gy are claimed to be more effective than lower doses.

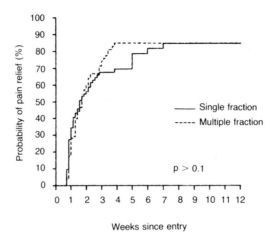

Fig. 9.1. Onset of pain relief after radiotherapy to painful bone metastases. (from Price et al. (1986), with permission of the editor and publisher of *Radiotherapy and Oncology*.)

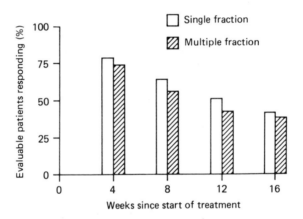

Fig. 9.2. Duration of pain relief after radiotherapy to painful bone metastases. (from Price et al. (1986), with permission of the editor and publisher of *Radiotherapy and Oncology*.)

Two recent studies have reported significant response rates after single fractions of only 4 Gy to painful bone metastases (Price et al. 1988; Karstens et al. 1989) and this, taken together with the poor correlation between response and histological types of tumour and the observation of early responses occurring within 24 hours of low-dose irradiation, further supports the hypothesis that prolonged high-dose treatments are unnecessary for pain relief.

Bone Pain in Multiple Sites

Where there are multiple scattered sites of painful bone metastases, wide field hemibody irradiation is preferable to treating each site individually with local irradiation. Using single fractions of 6–7 Gy to the upper hemibody and 6–8 Gy to the lower hemibody, pain relief is reported in around 75% of patients. This can be very rapid, occurring in many patients within 24–48 h of treatment. In a series from the Royal Marsden Hospital, patients with multiple myeloma or metastatic prostate carcinoma responded similarly with a response rate of 82% (Hoskin et al. 1989).

Hemibody irradiation is inevitably more toxic than localised external beam irradiation which is in general associated with minimal side effects. This is an important consideration in the setting of a palliative treatment in patients with widespread disease. Virtually all patients receiving lower hemibody irradiation suffer mild acute gastro-intestinal toxicity, usually in the form of nausea and diarrhoea 12–24 h following treatment. This is minimised by intensive premedication with intravenous hydration, steroids and anti-emetics and can generally be readily controlled with appropriate medication following treatment. More severe symptoms, however, may occur in up to 25% of patients. Other acute toxicities include alopecia following upper hemibody irradiation and bone marrow depression which is seen in about 10% of patients receiving a single half-body treatment, but in most patients who have sequential treatment of upper and lower hemibodies.

The most serious toxicity following hemibody irradiation is the development of pneumonitis after upper hemibody irradiation. This is both total dose and dose-rate dependent but occasional cases are still reported despite the use of moderate doses around 6 Gy corrected for the reduced density in lung and using low dose-rates to protect the lung. Radiation pneumonitis following hemibody irradiation is difficult to treat and usually fatal.

Hemibody irradiation therefore is highly effective with rapid pain relief maintained for most patients until death, but against this must be balanced the greater toxicity and small chance of life-threatening complications such as neutropenia and pneumonitis. Bone pain recurring following wide field irradiation may be treated with local irradiation without detriment to the patient and with good result.

An alternative to hemibody irradiation is the use of systemic radio-isotopes to deliver ionising radiation to multiple sites of bone metastases. This depends upon selective uptake of the isotope at the involved site and may be achieved in one of two ways. Firstly, in the particular instance of carcinoma of the thyroid, the majority of differentiated carcinomas will concentrate radioactive iodine. The administration of ^{131}I to patients with bone metastases from iodine-concentrating differentiated thyroid cancer will, therefore, enable the selective administration of radioactive iodine to involved sites. Unfortunately, a retrospective evaluation suggests that this is not a particularly effective form of treatment for bone pain: in one series pain relief was seen in only 2 of 21 patients with bone metastases from thyroid cancer (Brown et al. 1984).

In other tumours, bone-seeking isotopes have been employed in an attempt to concentrate radioactive isotope at sites of active bone turnover. Two isotopes in particular have been evaluated: radioactive phosphorus (^{32}P) and strontium (^{89}Sr). A number of small studies, the first being reported over 30 years ago (Kenney et al. 1941), have claimed efficacy for ^{32}P given intravenously to patients with multiple bone metastases. However, this technique has not acquired widespread popularity, principally because it is in general associated with considerable bone marrow suppression. More recently, ^{89}Sr has emerged as a potentially useful treatment. It is preferentially concentrated in areas of osteoblastic activity and delivers a smaller dose of radiation to the bone marrow producing 1.4 MeV beta particles with a range of only a few millimetres as it decays to yttrium. A further potential advantage is that it has a relatively long physical half life of 50.5 days and is retained at sites of osteoblastic bone metastases so that high absorbed doses to local sites may be delivered (Robinson 1986). Response rates from a number of small prospective studies suggest that it may be as effective as hemibody irradiation in terms of pain relief, with minimal clinical toxicity, although the largest of these studies (Robinson 1986) found bone marrow suppression in 80% of patients. Preliminary results of a prospective randomised placebo-controlled trial also confirm that ^{89}Sr is an active agent for bone pain superior to placebo in its analgesic effects (Lewington and Jenkins 1989).

Pathological Fracture

Pathological fracture due to metastatic cancer may take two principal forms; fractures which are amenable to surgical fixation, such as those involving the shaft of a long bone, and those which cannot be fixed surgically including fractures of the ribs, girdle bones and vertebral collapse especially where multiple vertebrae are involved with tumour. In the former case, surgical fixation will be the treatment of choice although in selected patients where there is advanced disease, pre-existing immobility or poor general health, surgery may be contra-indicated and local irradiation remains a valuable palliative tool. In patients who undergo surgical fixation, local irradiation is commonly given post-operatively. This is on the basis that metastatic tumour remaining in the bone may progress, causing further local pain and loosening of the surgical fixation. Conventionally, fields covering the entire length of a prosthesis or intramedullary nail are used because of the potential risk of dissemination through the marrow cavity occurring during the operative procedure. The role of radiotherapy in this post-operative setting has not been subjected to critical prospective evaluation and it is likely that many patients, particularly those receiving specific systemic anticancer therapy and those who have a relatively short prognosis, do not require post-operative irradiation.

For bones where surgical fixation is not possible, such as the pelvis, ribs and scapula, local irradiation is the treatment of choice, achieving both pain relief and bone healing. An example of the results from irradiating a fracture through a large lytic lesion in the ilium of a patient with metastatic breast cancer is shown in Fig. 9.3.

The optimum management of vertebral collapse is less clear. Where local bone pain is present or neurological compression occurs local irradiation is indicated, although in the latter case initial surgical fixation may be more appropriate, particularly when a single vertebra is involved. Where vertebral collapse is asymptomatic and particularly where several levels are involved, either deferring treatment until symptoms arise or the use of systemic therapy may be more acceptable.

There are few published data on the results of irradiation for pathological fracture. One retrospective analysis of 27 pathological fractures in various sites reports pain relief in 67% and remineralisation in 33% after 40–50 Gy delivered in 4–5 weeks (Rieden et al. 1986).

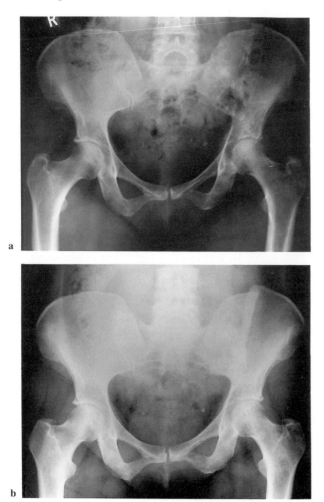

Fig. 9.3.a,b. Pathological fracture of ilium due to secondary breast carcinoma before (**a**) and after (**b**) radiotherapy.

Spinal Nerve Root and Cord Compression

Spinal cord compression may be due to blood-borne extradural or intradural metastases but is also associated with direct invasion of the spinal cord by metastases from a vertebral body. These may take the form of a lytic lesion in the vertebral body with an associated soft tissue mass causing local destruction or, at a more advanced stage, vertebral collapse may occur. Early diagnosis is essential in this condition and a major determinant of outcome. Confirmation of the precise anatomical site of the compression is obtained using myelography. This is recommended even where the apparent level may be obvious clinically as multiple levels of disease are not infrequently found on more detailed investigations and there is then a need for more extensive treatment fields than may be expected from the clinical findings. More recently, magnetic resonance imaging has been used as an alternative to myelography; it has the advantage of being non-invasive and demonstrating considerably more detail of the bone disease than myelography. This is demonstrated in Fig 9.4. However, a retrospective analysis of 12 patients having both myelography and magnetic resonance imaging before radiotherapy for spinal cord compression has failed to demonstrate any significant impact of using magnetic resonance imaging upon the treatment volume chosen (Graham et al. 1989). Conventionally, the volume to be treated will encompass the site of compression defined at myelography with a margin of two vertebral bodies above and below this level. A single megavoltage field directed on the spinal column with the treatment simulator should be used to define the vertebral levels (see p. 172).

Both radiotherapy and decompressive surgery are effective in the initial management of cord compression. An extensive review of the literature (Findlay 1984) has failed to demonstrate any advantage for surgery over radiotherapy in patients with a previously confirmed diagnosis of malignancy, and for most patients, therefore, initial treatment with high-dose steroids and local irradiation is appropriate. Surgery is reserved for those patients in whom spinal cord compression is the initial form of presentation of their malignancy in order to obtain a histological diagnosis and in those who deteriorate whilst receiving irradiation. There may, in addition, be a subgroup with extensive vertebral collapse and spinal instability in whom surgical decompression combined with stabilisation is the best initial management.

The outcome of treatment depends primarily upon the speed of diagnosis and neurological status at the initiation of treatment. Radiotherapy is superior to surgery in achieving pain relief, reported in 76% of patients treated with primary

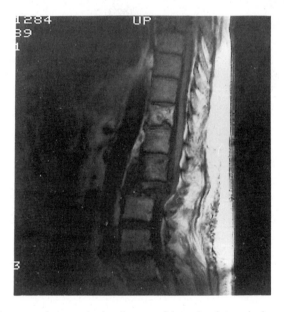

Fig. 9.4. MRI demonstrating vertebral collapse and intrusion into spinal canal from secondary breast carcinoma.

radiotherapy and only 36% of patients having laminectomy alone. The addition of radiotherapy to surgery achieved pain relief in 67%. Between one-third and one-half of patients will be ambulant following treatment, predominantly those who present whilst still ambulant, and 20%–25% will suffer significant neurological deterioration during treatment, whether by surgery with or without radiotherapy or by radiotherapy alone (Findlay 1984).

Nerve roots may be compressed by bone metastases in the vertebrae, affecting either the cauda equina or peripheral nerve roots, and in the skull, affecting the cranial nerves. Cauda equina compression should be treated in the same way as spinal cord compression, with urgent investigation and treatment in order to prevent weakness in the lower limbs and deterioration of sphincter control. Peripheral nerve root compression presents with nerve root pain and weakness in the associated myotome. Vertebral destruction or collapse may be seen on a plain radiograph while computed tomograms or magnetic resonance imaging may show earlier stages of the process when plain films are normal despite troublesome symptoms.

Extensive metastatic infiltration of the skull base, resulting in cranial nerve lesions, is well recognised particularly in asssociation with bone metastases from primary breast cancer. The fifth, sixth and seventh cranial nerves are the most commonly affected but others may also be involved. Standard x-ray views of the skull may be insufficient to detect metastases in this site but coned views or tomograms of the skull base will give further information. CT scanning is also valuable in this site, as shown in Fig. 9.5 demonstrating extensive skull base infiltration in a patient with prostatic carcinoma presenting with involvement of the fifth, sixth, seventh and eighth cranial nerves. Where disease is localised to the skull base, parallel opposed megavoltage fields are used to irradiate this

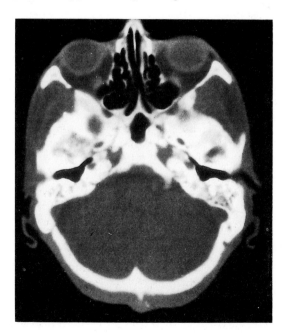

Fig. 9.5.   Skull base infiltration by secondary prostatic carcinoma.

area. Treatment may be facilitated by using a plastic head shell to immobilise the patient and enable more accurate, reproducible localisation of the treatment fields. This is an important consideration in this area to prevent damage to the surrounding normal structures which are sensitive to irradiation, in particular the eye.

Retrospective analyses of the results of skull base irradiation for metastases causing cranial nerve palsies report symptom improvement in between 50% and 78% of patients. Response is maintained until death in around 80% of responders and median survival from diagnosis of this condition was between 10 and 20 months, depending on the primary tumour type (Vikram and Chu 1979; Hall et al. 1983).

Prophylactic Irradiation

Bone metastases present to the clinician either as bone pain, pathological fracture or neurological involvement. However, in many patients asymptomatic bone metastases may be present and be found incidentally, usually as a result of radiographic skeletal survey or isotope bone scan during routine staging procedures. In most common tumours such as lung, breast and prostate there will be no curative treatment and systemic therapy will be reserved until symptoms arise. The role of local irradiation in such a situation remains unclear but two indications for prophylactic irradiation of bone metastases may be considered.

1. *Prevention of Pathological Fracture.* The presence of a lytic deposit causing cortical erosion in a long bone carries a threat of pathological fracture particularly when a weight-bearing area is involved. Fig. 9.6 shows the progression of a lytic deposit from carcinoma of the breast, resulting in spontaneous fracture through an area of cortical destruction. In such cases internal fixation is indicated as the initial procedure of choice, followed by post-operative radiotherapy. There is controversy as to whether local irradiation to such areas can prevent pathological fracture. Some studies have recommended early surgical intervention for all patients with "high risk" metastases, particularly lytic femoral metastases larger than 2.5 cm involving the cortex or associated with pain, or any lesion causing destruction of more than 50% of the cortex (Beals et al. 1971; Harrington 1986). Other studies have cast doubt upon this commonly held view and a risk of fracture of only 5% after prophylactic irradiation of such lesions has been demonstrated (Cheng et al. 1980). This may reflect changing patterns in the use of systemic treatment in addition to the response to irradiation. It is of interest that this study found that solitary lytic deposits were at less risk of pathological fracture than diffuse lytic involvement characterised by mottled x-ray appearances, particularly in the region of the femoral neck where surgical intervention at an early stage is still recommended.

2. *Prevention of Neurological Symptoms.* Irradiation of asymptomatic metastases to prevent spinal cord or nerve compression is an even more difficult area since, unlike pathological fracture, there are no criteria using current imaging techniques which will predict the likelihood of progressive neurological symptoms from a vertebral collapse or area of vertebral destruction. Magnetic

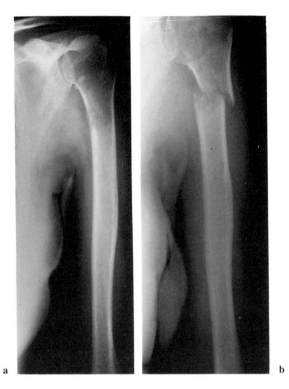

Fig. 9.6.a,b. Lytic deposit in humerus from secondary breast carcinoma (**a**) progressing to spontaneous pathological fracture (**b**).

resonance imaging has demonstrated metastases in the vertebral body which can be seen at an early stage of encroachment upon the spinal canal, as shown in Fig. 9.4. Prospective evaluation of the natural history of such lesions may enable patients with incipient cord or cauda equina compression to be identified and treated with local irradiation before symptoms develop. Such imaging techniques are not currently available routinely and prophylactic irradiation of all vertebral metastases in order to prevent a small number of neurological sequelae cannot be recommended.

It may, however, be possible to define a group of patients with vertebral metastases who have a high risk of subsequent neurological complications in whom prophylactic spinal irradiation could be valuable. A retrospective study in small cell lung cancer found a 4% incidence of cord compression. Predictors of spinal cord compression in this group were local back pain associated with a positive bone scan in the spine and cerebral metastases with a positive bone scan; the incidence of cord compression in these two groups was 36% and 25% respectively (Goldman et al. 1989). Further studies to correlate the results of imaging and clinical features with the risk of cord compression are required in an attempt to define more clearly those patients who would benefit from prophylactic treatment.

Conclusion

Bone metastases are a cause of considerable morbidity for many cancer patients. Radiotherapy is an effective palliation for bone pain with overall response rates consistently greater than 80%, is the treatment of choice for most patients with neurological complications from a bone metastasis and will enable pain relief and healing after pathological fracture. It may also have a role in the prevention of neurological complications and pathological fracture by prophylactic treatment of asymptomatic metastases. Future studies should attempt to define more clearly those patients who may benefit from selected prophylactic irradiation as well as continuing to address the as yet unresolved question of the optimum dose-fractionation radiation schedules in these different clinical circumstances.

References

Anthony P, Keys H, McCollister CE, Rubin P, Lush C (1987) Prevention of heterotopic bone formation with early postoperative irradiation in high risk patients undergoing total hip arthroplasty: comparison of 10.00 Gy vs 20.00 Gy schedules. Int J Radiat Oncol Biol Phys 13:365–369

Arcangeli G, Micheli A, Arcangeli G, Giannarelli D, La Pasta O, Trollis A et al. (1989) The responsiveness of bone metastases to radiotherapy: the effect of site, histology and radiation dose on pain relief. Radiother Oncol 14:95–101

Beals RK, Lawton GD, Snell WE (1971) Prophylactic internal fixation of the femur in metastatic breast cancer. Cancer 28:1350–1354

Blitzer PH (1985) Reanalysis of the RTOG study of the palliation of symptomatic osseous metastasis. Cancer 55:1468–1472

Brown AP, Greening WP, McCready VR, Shaw HJ, Harmer CL (1984) Radioiodine treatment of metastatic thyroid carcinoma: the Royal Marsden Hospital experience. Br J Radiol 57:323–327

Cheng DS, Seitz CB, Eyre HJ (1980) Nonoperative management of femoral, humeral and acetabular metastases in patients with breast carcinoma. Cancer 45:1533–1537

Dalen N, Edsmyr F (1974) Bone mineral content of the femoral neck after irradiation. Acta Radiol Ther Phys Biol 14:139–144

Findlay GFG (1984) Adverse effects of the management of spinal cord compression. J Neurol Neurosurg Psychiatry 47:761–768

Garmatis CJ, Chu F (1978) The effectiveness of radiation therapy in the treatment of bone metastases from breast cancer. Radiology 16:235–237

Goldman JM, Ash CM, Souhami RL, Geddes DM, Harper PG, Spiro SG, Tobias JS (1989) Spinal cord compression in small cell lung cancer: a retrospective study of 610 patients. Br J Cancer 59:591–593

Graham JD, Hoskin PJ, Williams M (1989) The influence of MRI on the treatment of spinal cord compression. Br J Cancer 61:183

Hall SM, Buzdar AV, Blumenschein GR (1983) Cranial nerve palsies in metastatic breast cancer due to osseous metastasis without intracranial involvement. Cancer 52:180–184

Harrington KD (1986) Impending pathological fractures from metastatic malignancy: evolution and management. American Academy of Orthopaedic Surgeons instructional course lectures 35:357–381

Hoskin PJ (1988) Scientific and clinical aspects of radiotherapy in the relief of bone pain. Cancer Surv 7:69–86

Hoskin PJ, Ford HT, Harmer CL (1989) Hemibody irradiation for metastatic bone pain. Clin Oncol 1:41–42

Karstens JH, Schnabel B, Amman J (1989) Management of metastatic bone pain: preliminary results with single fraction (4 Gy) radiotherapy. Onkologie 12:41–42

Kenney J, Marinelli L, Woodard H (1941) Tracer studies with radioactive phosphorus in malignant neoplastic disease. Radiology 37:683–687

Leddy ET (1930) Roentgen treatment of metastasis to the vertebrae and bones of the pelvis from carcinoma of the breast. Am J Roentgenol Radiat Ther 24:657–672

Lewington VJ, Jenkins JD (1989) Strontium-89 therapy in disseminated prostatic carcinoma. Abstract 86, Proc British Assoc of Urological Surgeons

Madsen EL (1983) Painful bone metastasis: efficacy of radiotherapy assessed by the patients: a randomised trial comparing 4 Gy x 6 versus 10 Gy x 2. Int J Radiat Oncol Biol Phys 9:1775–1779

Matsubayashi T, Koga H, Nishiyama Y, Tominaga S, Sourada T (1981) The reparative process of metastatic bone lesions after radiotherapy. Jpn J Clin Oncol 11:253–249

Meredith WJ, Massey JB (1976) Fundamental physics of radiology. John Wright & Sons, Bristol

Price P, Hoskin PJ, Easton D, Austin D, Palmer SG, Yarnold JR (1986) Prospective randomised trial of single and multifraction radiotherapy schedules in the treatment of painful bony metastases. Radiother Oncol 6:247–255

Price P, Hoskin PJ, Easton D, Austin D, Palmer SG, Yarnold JR (1988) Low dose single fraction radiotherapy in the treatment of metastatic bone pain. Radiother Oncol 12:297–300

Reiden K, Kober B, Mende U, zum Winkel K (1986) Strahlentherapie pathologischer Frakturen und frakturgefährdeter Skelettläsionen. Strahlenther Onkol 162:742–749

Robinson RG (1986) Radionuclides for the alleviation of bone pain in advanced malignancy. Clinics in Oncol 5:39–49

Tong D, Gillick L, Hendrickson F (1982) The palliation of symptomatic osseous metastases: final results of the study by the Radiation Therapy Oncology Group. Cancer 50:893–899

Vikram B, Chu F (1979) Radiation therapy for metastases to the base of the skull. Radiology 130:465–468

10   Isotope Therapy For Bone Metastases

Susan E.M. Clarke

Introduction

Therapy using radioactive labelled tracer molecules is at present an area of considerable interest and research. The principle of using a tracer molecule to target radiotherapy to a tumour has been well established with the use of iodine-131 in the treatment of follicular thyroid cancer and phosphorus-32 to treat polycythaemia rubra vera (Seidlin et al. 1946; O'Mara 1978).

Targeted radiotherapy has several theoretical advantages over external beam radiotherapy. The radiation dose is delivered to the tumour alone and normal tissue is spared unnecessary radiation. On theoretical grounds there should, therefore, be no limit to the amount of radiation administered or to the number of times it is used, unlike conventional radiotherapy. Given an adequate blood supply, the radiation dose should be evenly administered throughout the tumour volume and the intracellular uptake of the therapeutic radiopharmaceutical ensures that the radiation dose is deposited close to the tumour cell nucleus.

Despite these theoretical advantages, the present use of therapeutic radio-pharmaceuticals is extremely limited. The problems that are being encountered and their possible solutions will be discussed in this chapter.

Characteristics of Radionuclides Used For Therapy

The radionuclides that are suitable for therapy have very different characteristics to those that are generally selected for diagnostic purposes. In diagnostic imaging the main requirement is for single-energy gamma-emitting radionuclides, whereas in therapy gamma radiation is of minor therapeutic importance

Table 10.1. Nuclides suitable for therapy

Radionuclide	Half life (days)	e_{max} (MeV)	Max. gamma Energy (keV)
^{131}I	8.1	0.60	364
^{32}P	24.5	0.25	—
^{90}Y	2.7	2.27	—
^{153}Sm	1.9	0.81	103
^{89}Sr	52.0	1.49	—
^{186}Re	3.7	1.07	137

but adds significantly to the irradiation of tissues other than the target. A small percentage of gamma radiation (less than 10%) in the energy range of 100–200 keV serves the purpose of visualising uptake of the radionuclides in the tumour prior to therapy and facilitates pharmacokinetic and dosimetric information to be obtained from which the optimum dose can be calculated.

Radionuclides which are considered suitable for therapy may be divided into three main categories:

1. Beta emitters
2. Alpha emitters
3. Electron capture and internal conversion decaying radionuclides

These three categories of radionuclides will be discussed.

Beta-emitting Radionuclides

Beta-particle-emitting radionuclides such as phosphorus-32 and iodine-131 have been used for many years as therapeutic agents. Beta particles are effective in therapy since they deposit their ionising radiation within a short range, thereby avoiding radiation damage to non-target tissue. Beta emitters may be divided into those with low ranges of less than 200 μm such as osmium-191 and gold-199 and medium-range beta emitters, mean range 200 μm–1 mm, such as rhenium-186 and iodine-131. Finally long-range beta emitters can be used with a mean range of greater than 1 mm such as phosphorus-32, yttrium-90 and rhenium-188. It is important that the radionuclide to be used in therapy is carrier-free, that is, it contains no non-radioactive forms of the nuclide. The production of carrier-free beta-emitting radionuclides is complex and involves an (n,8) reaction, followed by a beta minus decay and chemical separation. The need for high flux reactors and enriched target materials to produce most of the beta-emitting radionuclides renders their production expensive and this is one factor that is limiting research into their therapeutic role.

Alpha-emitting Radionuclides

Alpha particles are highly suited for therapy. They have an extremely short range (50–90 μm) and a high linear energy transfer (LET) of about 80 keV per micron. Potential alpha-emitting radionuclides are limited to astatine-211 and bismuth-212 since most alpha emitters have complex decay schemes with unsuitable daughter nuclides. Both astatine-211 and bismuth-212 have relatively short half lives which may limit their efficacy in therapy. They can, however, being halogens, be used to label proteins and enzymes (Andres et al. 1986) although the carbon–astatine bond has been shown to be relatively unstable.

Electron Capture and Internal Conversion Decaying Radionuclides

In both electron capture and internal conversion, an inner shell electron vacancy is created in the atom which is filled from an outer shell with the release of auger electrons or low energy x-rays. These low-energy particles deposit a high dose of energy but have a very short range (less than 1 μm) and are only of therapeutic significance if the source is attached or very close to target DNA. Examples of nuclides with potentially useful auger electron cascades are gallium-67, rubidium-97, iodine-123 and caesium-129. All these nuclides are prepared by irradiation with charged particles in a carrier-free form. Their biological efficacy because of their extremely short range remains a matter of uncertainty.

The Criteria for Selection

Given the large number of potentially suitable nuclides for therapy, certain factors must be taken into consideration when assessing the suitability of a radionuclide. The half life of the nuclide must be long enough for adequate accumulation of the radiopharmaceutical within the target tissue to take place and a significant radiation dose to be delivered. The half life must not be too long, however, as the rate of delivery of the dose will be too low.

The chemistry of the nuclide is also a factor that must be considered. The ideal radionuclide will be of a chemical form that will permit incorporation of the radionuclide into complex molecules such as aromatic ring structures.

The radionuclide should also have a low gamma yield to reduce unwanted radiation to non-target tissues. A low percentage of suitable gamma photons, however, have the advantage of enabling target localisation to be checked and dosimetric calculations to be performed by standard gamma camera imaging. The decay product of the radionuclide must be stable or long-lived to avoid unwanted irradiation to other tissues.

The radionuclide should, ideally, be readily obtainable and inexpensive to prepare. Unfortunately, the requirement for high flux reactors and enriched targets in the production of many beta-emitting radionuclides results in high production costs. Iodine-131, however, remains inexpensive and readily available. The development of generators to produce some therapeutic radionuclides is being explored at present.

Radiobiology

Since most radiobiology research is being performed using external beam radiation in vitro, there remains a considerable amount of uncertainty as to the effects of low-dose radiation and low-dose rate radiation.

It is well established that different types of ionising radiation differ in their effectiveness in damaging the biological system. Relative biological effectiveness depends largely on the spatial pattern of energy deposition. The hit-size weighting model postulates that below a certain level of local energy deposition no response is detected.

It is now accepted that cellular DNA is the primary target for ionising radiations. Radiation with a high LET causes more irreparable damage than at with a low LET. High LET radiation, that is alpha particles, approximately 3.5 MeV exhibit a killing efficiency for human cells in culture between 0.14 and 0.2. With the use of more energetic alpha particles this value may approach 1.0 (Todd et al. 1985). Cells that survive ionising radiation may be arrested in a given phase of the cell cycle such as G_1 or G_2 and lose their cloning capacity or show other signs of impaired function.

With low LET and low dose irradiation, initial damage may be modified by post-irradiation cellular processes such as repair or enhanced damage expression. Cells can, to some extent, protect themselves against the effect of radiation and repair radiogenic damage. The enzyme superoxide dismutase has been shown to confer irradiation resistance to *Drosophila melanogaster* and may also be important in mammalian systems (Peng et al. 1986).

DNA repair following potentially lethal damage is readily observed with the use of x-rays, but rarely and only in late G_1 phase after exposure to high LET radiation. DNA repair in mammalian cells appears to be dose-dependent (Goodhead 1985).

It is important to remember that the hundreds of different cell lines in the mammalian organism have different characteristics with regard to radiation sensitivity. Bergonie and Tribondeau have stated that the sensitivity of certain cell types or tissues is directly proportional to their mitotic activity. Immature stem cells, whether quiescent or in proliferation, are usually radiosensitive whilst differentiated cells are more or less radioresistant. The need, therefore, to target the tumour stem cells is obviously essential. The radiosensitivity of cells may be increased using the "oxygen-effect" due to oxygen-derived radical production.

Dosimetry

The established method for calculating a tumour radiation dose from internally administered radioisotopes is by the MIRD schema. The method consists of calculating the radiation dose to the tumour target from two sources. The first source is the tumour target tissue itself and the second source is tissues adjacent to the tumour. Problems arise using the schema to calculate tumour dose, however, as the assumption is made that the distribution of the radiopharmaceutical within the tumour is uniform. The second source is only relevant if the radiopharmaceutical is a gamma emitter since the short path length of beta and alpha particles theoretically localises the non-target component of radiation to the non-target tissue.

A further source of error when calculating dose using MIRD schedules is the site of binding of the radiopharmaceutical within the tumour. The MIRD data do not distinguish between the uniform distribution of a non-specific radiopharmaceutical, one that binds to surface membrane of the cell and a radiopharmaceutical that crosses the cell membrane and is internalised. If the tumour cell

DNA is the target for cell inactivation at therapeutic doses, the dose to the cell nucleus is a more appropriate dose to calculate than the dose to the tumour as a whole. The mean dose to the tumour cell nuclei from a radiopharmaceutical bound to the cell membrane will obviously differ significantly from that from a radiopharmaceutical that is distributed uniformly in the tissue spaces or from that of a radiopharmaceutical that crosses the cell membrane and is bound in the site of the plasma close to the cell nucleus.

Attempts have been made to measure variations in tumour dose using micro-dosimetric analysis. Griffiths et al. (1988) have used miniature thermo luminescent dosimeters (TLD) implants to measure variations in tumour dose. Fisher (1985) has applied micro-dosimetric analysis for the case of alpha emitters to radioimmunotherapy. Humm and Cobb (1990) have also used micro dosimetric analysis and demonstrated that the energy deposition in a tumour cell nucleus from a membrane bound radiopharmaceutical such as radiolabelled antibody may be several times greater than that estimated with the assumption of uniform source distribution.

When deciding on the radionuclide to be used in therapy, information about the distribution of the pharmaceutical within the tumour is, therefore, vital. A pharmaceutical that is distributed in a heterogeneous manner throughout the tumour, such as an antibody, favours the choice of a larger range beta-emitting radionuclide. A pharmaceutical that is internally localised within the tumour cell should ideally be labelled with an alpha-emitting radionuclide or an electron capture and internal conversion-decaying radionuclide.

Mechanisms for Localisation

There are various mechanisms used to localise radionclides for therapy within a tumour (Table 10.2).

Internal localisation of a radionuclide within a tumour can only occur if the radiopharmaceutical is able to cross the cell membrane of the tumour and then is bound within the cell cytoplasm or to the cellular DNA. Iodine-131 is internally localised by well differentiated follicular thyroid carcinoma cells. The degree of

Table 10.2. Mechanisms for localising radiopharmaceuticals for therapy

Intracellular binding	Metabolic pathway, e.g., Iodine-131, ^{131}I-MIBG
	DNA binding, e.g., bleomycin
Membrane binding	Antigen/antibody, e.g., ^{131}I-antimelanoma antibody
	Hormone/receptor, e.g., ^{131}I-vinyloestradiol
Tumour capillary bed blockade	e.g., Yttrium[9]-90 microspheres
Surrounding normal tissue localisation	Bone uptake for bone metastases, e.g., [153]Sm-EHDP
	Intracavitary administration, e.g., ^{131}I-HMFGI

uptake depends on the extent to which the malignant cell continues to exhibit the metabolic features of the normal thyroid follicular cell. Metaiodobenzyl-guanidine, a guanethidene analogue, is another agent that has been developed to localise in neuroectodermally derived cells that have become neoplastic but retain their ability to take up amine precursors. When labelled with iodine-131 in therapeutic doses, significant intracellular radiation doses are delivered to those neuroectodermally derived tumours. Both these radiopharmaceuticals achieve intracellular localisation by incorporation into metabolic pathways.

Another mechanism for intracellular localisation is to utilise the DNA-binding ability of certain chemicals. The DNA-binding ability of bleomycin is due to the bithiazole and sidechain amine. Studies using radiolabelled bleomycin have been disappointing, however, as the tumour to non-tumour ratio is significantly reduced following radiolabelling (Beer et al. 1986).

Binding to the cell membrane of the tumour is another mechanism for localising radionuclides for therapeutic purposes. The main areas currently being investigated are the utilisation of tumour-specific antigens on cell membranes of tumours. Antibodies to many membrane-located antigens have been derived and, following radiolabelling, tumours have been imaged and early results of therapy have been reported. The main problem, however, is one of specificity as a majority of tumour antigens that have been isolated have been found to be tumour-associated rather than tumour-specific. Binding of anti-bodies to other tissues that also express the antigen, therefore, occurs with resultant unwanted radiation doses to non-tumour tissue. In addition, as the antibodies are raised in mice to human antigens, non-specific accumulation of the labelled antibodies occurs in liver, spleen and bone marrow, again resulting in undesirable radiation doses to these organs. The potential use for radiolabelled antibodies for tumour therapy will be discussed later in the chapter. Another theoretical method for localising radionuclides to the cell membrane is by taking advantage of the receptors such as oestrogen receptors present on the surfaces of some tumour cells. Vinyloestradiol has been successfully labelled with [123]I- and ^{131}I-iodine with no change in receptor binding observed after radiolabelling (Beer et al. 1986). Considerable work is required in this area before radiolabelled substances with receptor affinity become therapeutically useful.

Finally localisation of a radiopharmaceutical within or adjacent to a tumour may be achieved even though no specific tumour uptake or binding of the pharmaceutical has occurred. The radiopharmaceutical may be introduced directly into the capillary bed of the tumour in the form of radiolabelled microspheres. Microspheres are 10 μm in diameter and embolise the tumour when they are delivered into the capillary bed. The degree of degradability of the microsphere and the rate at which it degrades must be modified, taking into account the half life of the radionucliude. Yttrium-90 glass microspheres have been administered via the hepatic artery to patients with hepatic metastases and partial response reported (Shapiro et al. 1989). Tumour serum albumin microspheres labelled with yttrium-90 have also been successfully prepared.

Therapy doses of a radionuclide may also be localised close to the tumour by utilising uptake mechanisms in adjacent non-tumour tissue. A number of different radiopharmaceuticals have been developed for therapy of bone metastases that are taken up into bone such as strontium-89, rhenium-186 EHDP, yttrium-90 EDTMP, samarium-153 EDTMP and phosphorus-32 EHDP

(Pecker 1942; Ketring 1987; Carichner et al. 1989: Potsaid et al. 1976). Uptake of phosphorus-32 into marrow is also utilised in the treatment of polycythaemia rubra vera (O'Mara 1978).

Finally, localisation of therapeutic radiopharmaceuticals may be achieved using regional administration of the agent. Yttrium-90, gold-198 and phosphorus-32 have been used in colloidal form for intracavity therapy. The use of short-range beta particles emitted from the colloid in contact with the affected tissue surface gives a high radiation dose to the affected tissue, with resultant palliation of malignant effusions. Recently, antibodies labelled with beta emitters have been used to treat ascites from ovarian cancer following intraperitoneal administration (Stewart et al. 1987).

The Use of Radionuclides for Therapy

Although many alpha- and beta-emitting radionuclides exist, relatively few have been evaluated clinically. The following radionuclides have been included as some promising results in therapy have been reported (Table 10.2).

Iodine-131

Historically, iodine-131 was one of the first radionuclides to be used in therapy. Iodine-131 is a beta emitter, half life 8.1 days with a maximum particle energy (e_{max}) of 0.60 MeV. In addition, iodine-131 emits several gamma photons, the highest with a keV of 637. Its metabolic incorporation into follicular thyroid carcinoma cells results in the intracellular deposition of its radiation dose. Its successful use in therapy is well established with dramatic resolution of soft tissue and bone metastases. Its main disadvantages in treating follicular thyroid cancer are the unwanted gamma photon emissions, which significantly increase the whole-body radiation dose and necessitate isolation of the patient immediately post-therapy to prevent unwanted radiation doses to staff and family. A further, though less significant, disadvantage is the uptake of iodine-131 by the salivary glands which may result in parotitis and a dry mouth after treatment.

Phosphorus-32

Like iodine-131, phosphorus-32 has been used in therapy for many years. It has a long half life of 14.3 days, an e_{max} of 1.7 MeV and no unwanted gamma emissions. After intravenous administration, phosphorus-32 localises in the bone marrow and trabecular and cortical bone. Phosphorus-32 has been used in various forms in therapy. Early studies utilised colloidal ^{32}P-therapy (Hill et al. 1962). Later studies used phosphorus-32 diphosphonates (Hall et al. 1975; Francis et al. 1976).

Yttrium-90

Yttrium-90 is a pure beta emitter, with a half life of 2.7 days and a high maximum energy of 2.3 MeV. Since the early 1970s, yttrium-90 has been used in the silicate, citrate, ferric hydroxide and resin forms (Bowen et al. 1975) and is currently chiefly used as the colloidal silicate (Dunscombe and Ramsey 1980). Recently, reports have been published exploring the use of ^{90}Y-EDTMP, ^{90}Y-antibodies and ^{90}Y-labelled glass microspheres in therapy (Shapiro et al. 1989).

Samarium-153

Samarium-153 is a radiolanthide with a relatively short half life of 46.3 h and a low maximum energy of 0.81 MeV. It also emits a 103-keV gamma photon which may be used for imaging. Samarium-153 can now be produced in high yield and high specific activity by neutron activation of enriched samarium-152. Samarium-153 complexes of citrate, nitrate and biologically active molecules such as transferrin and bleomycin have been studied as potential tumour-seeking compounds (Hisada and Ando 1973). Boniface et al. (1989) recently successfully labelled samarium-153 to an IgG monoclonal antibody K-1-21 purified from ascites. Samarium-153 EDTMP has recently been developed and is being used in the treatment of prostatic bone metastates (Gorckler et al. 1987).

Strontium-89

Strontium-89 has a long half life of 50.5 days and a beta-particle energy of 1.49 MeV. Reports of the use of strontium-89 appeared in the literature as early as 1942 (Pecker 1942). More recently, interest has been revived and several clinical trials of the use of strontium-89 in palliating bone pain in patients with prostatic metastases have been undertaken with promising results (Carrelta et al. 1989; Lewington et al. 1988).

Rhenium-186

Rhenium-186 has similar chemical properties to technetium-99m. It is a beta-emitting radionuclide with a maximum beta energy of 1.07 MeV and a 9% abundant gamma ray of 137 keV which could be used for imaging. Its half life is 3.7 days. Ketring et al. (1987) investigated the use of rhenium-186 as a label for EHDP. Recently, rhenium-186 has been complexed to pentavalent DMSA (Blower et al. 1990) for potential use in therapy of medullary thyroid cancer (Allen et al. 1990).

Radiopharmaceuticals for Therapy

In recent years, two main areas of research have proved fruitful in the development of radiopharmaceuticals suitable for therapy. The first area of research was the development in Ann Arbor, Michigan of the guanethidine analogue ^{131}I-metaiodobenzylguanidine, which has been used successfully in both the diagnosis and treatment of neuroectodermally derived tumours. The second has been the intensive development of radiolabelled antibodies to tumour-specific and tumour-associated antigens.

[131]I-Metaiodobenzylguanidine

Wieland et al. (1980) successfully imaged the dog adrenal medulla using the paraisomer of an arylacyl guanidine. Since then the labelled guanethidine noradrenaline analogue ^{131}I-metaiodobenzylguanidine (mIBG) has been used to image phaeochromocytoma, neuroblastomas, carcinoid tumours, medullary thyroid carcinomas and other neuroectodermally derived tumours.

Since 80% of phaeochromocytomas take up mIBG, its use in the treatment of patients with recurrent malignant phaeochromocytoma has been attempted with some success (Marchandise et al. 1985). Doses of up to 11 GBq (300 mCi) have been used and some dramatic results have been reported.

More than 90% of neuroblastomas take up mIBG and since uptake is often marked and retention prolonged, ^{131}I-mIBG has been used in therapy in a significant number of children with bone and soft tissue metastases. Although most children treated have been clinically Stage IV with no response or relapse following chemotherapy, complete remissions have been achieved in a few cases and nearly half the reported cases have experienced partial remission (Hoefnagel et al. 1987).

In 1984, Fischer et al. described uptake of ^{131}I-mIBG in a patient with a midgut carcinoid tumour. Since then reports in the literature indicate that more than 50% of carcinoids are able to concentrate ^{131}I-mIBG. There appears no relation between the urinary excretion of 5-hydroxy indolacetic acid (5-HIAA) and the degree of MIBG uptake. Therapy has been undertaken, with limited success, with palliative response being achieved in patients with large volume tumours.

Therapy in other neuroectodermally derived tumours, such as medullary thyroid cancer and paragangliomas, has been attempted but palliative results only have been reported, with relief of bone pain being one of the significant responses recorded (Poston et al. 1985; McEwan et al. 1987; Clarke et al. 1987; Baulieu et al. 1988; Van Gils et al. 1989; Hoefnagel et al. 1986).

Monoclonal Antibodies

The concept of the "magic bullet" proposed by Ehrlich in 1906 proved particularly attractive to those involved in treating patients with tumours. Ehrlich originally conceived the target-seeking antibody that would deliver therapy through immune substances. In the last decade significant advances have been made in the isolation of tumour-specific antigens with the development of antibodies to these antigens. Initially, however, results obtained with monoclonal antibodies were disappointing due to non-specific tumour binding of the antibodies. In the 1960s some success in tumour imaging was obtained using iodine-131 antifibrin to image a number of different tumours (McCardle et al. 1966). In 1975 a breakthrough came with the introduction by Kohler and Milstein of a technique for the production of monoclonal antibodies by using the hybridoma technique in which lymphocytes from the spleen of a mouse immunised with tumour cells are fused with myeloma cells. The splenic lymphocytes secrete a number of tumour-specific antibodies and fusion with the myeloma cell line results in a hybridoma clone which will continue to produce significant quantities of antibody (Milstein 1980).

Antibodies are immunoglobulins that are produced by plasma cells in response to an antigenic stimulus. Tumour antigens are large molecules of 100 daltons or more which are expressed by the tumour cell. Immunoglobulins possess specific binding regions that recognise distinct sites called determinants or epitopes on the antigen surface.

Immunoglobulins are classified as IgE, IgM, IgE, IgA or IgD according to their structure and function. IgG type antibodies are the main class used in immunolocalisation and they consist of two long chains (heavy or H chains) and two short chains (light or L chains) which are linked together by disulphide bridges. The constant region of the molecule contains the Fc fragment. This portion of the antibody may be cleaved from the remainder of the molecule by the enzyme pepsin. The remaining portion of the molecule in which the immunologically reactive regions reside is called the $F(ab)_2$ fragment. Further treatment with the enzyme papain will break the disulphide bridge between the two heavy chains yielding two fragments or Fab fragments. Immunoreactivity is preserved following such cleavage. The combination of an antibody with its corresponding antigen triggers a complex immunoloigical response which includes phagocytosis of the foreign antigen, complement fixation and cytokine release.

When labelling an antibody with a radionuclide it is fundamental that immunoreactivity must be preserved during the labelling procedure and antibodies have been successfully labelled with iodine-131 and yttrium-90 (Larsen et al. 1983).

Two facts remain clear in the field of immunolocalisation. The first is that this technique has tremendous potential in the management of patients with cancer both diagnostically and therapeutically. The second fact, however, is that the technique remains at present a research tool only, despite expenditure of significant time and money. Current problems that exist are the non-specific uptake of antibody which results from the fact that most currently available antibodies are tumour-associated rather than tumour-specific. Uptake by non-tumour tissue occurs as a result of a non-tumour expression of the antigen from which the antibody is derived. Non-specific uptake in the liver and spleen and bone marrow is a further problem which limits the doses that may be used in therapy. "Cocktails" of antibodies have been used in an attempt to increase sensitivity (Goodwin et al. 1990) and, more recently, specific antibodies have been produced with different specificities associated with the two arms of the Y (Shaw et al. 1988). Agents that might augment tumour uptake such as interferon are also being evaluated. The use of Fab fragments has already been shown to improve tumour to background ratios with some tumours.

The production of human antibodies as opposed to mouse antibodies has been attempted both to reduce the human antimouse antibody response (HAMA) and also in an attempt to increase specificity. Unfortunately, current experiences are disappointing as almost all isolated tumour monoclonal antibodies are specific for intracellular epitopes and most of the isolated human tumour monoclonal antibodies express the IgM isotype which is less suitable for in-vivo application. Also the problem of virus transmission necessitates vigorous screening of any antibody that is used.

During the past few years recombinant DNA technology has been used to address the problem of antigenicity of mouse antibodies. Recently an advanced molecular biological approach has been successful that reduces the mouse portion of the monoclonal antibody to the minimum essential part, the rest of the molecule being human (Seeman et al. 1987).

Radionuclide Therapy for Bone Metastases: Current Status

Iodine-131

As follicular carcinoma of the thyroid commonly metastasises to bone, the treatment of bone metastases with iodine-131 is well established. In 1967 Pochin demonstrated a 30% failure rate in 100 patients treated with iodine-131 for metastases. Charbord et al. (1977) followed 60 patients with bone metastases. In these patients with positive uptake of iodine-131 the survival rate was 25% at 10 years and 10% at 15 years. At 10 years the survival rate in those patients whose bone metastases did not take up iodine-131 was 8% and no survivors were reported at 15 years. Although some dramatic responses are now observed in patients with bone metastases after therapy with iodine-131 with slow resolution over a number of years, patients with bone metastases are generally older and this may partially explain the poor results of [131]I- therapy for bone metastases when compared with the results for treating lung metastases. Survival of patients with bone metastases in the sternum or base of the skull is better than that of patients with metastases at other bony sites (Tubiana et al. 1975).

Therapy with iodine-131 is reserved for those patients who require minimal nursing care in view of the radiation risk to staff. Doses of 3.7 to 7.4 GBq are given orally and patients are isolated for 4–5 days post-therapy. Thyroxine therapy is discontinued for 1 month prior to treatment to allow TSH levels to rise and to maximise uptake into the metastases. Treatment may be repeated at 6-monthly intervals until uptake in the metastases is no longer detected on the diagnostic tracer scan (Fig. 10.1).

Treatment is generally well tolerated although some patients may develop radiation sialitis after treatment. Long-term side-effects of leukaemia have been reported but the incidence is low at 1%–2% (Pochin 1969).

[131]I-mIBG

Neuroblastomas, together with some other neuroectodermally derived tumours, frequently metastasise to bone. Cumulative imaging experience of ^{131}I-mIBG in patients with neuroblastomas yields a sensitivity of over 90%. ^{131}I-mIBG has now been used to treat many children with metastatic neuroblastoma in whom

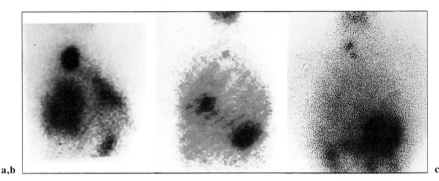

a,b   c

Fig. 10.1a–c. A 69-year-old female with a history of follicular carcinoma of the thyroid. **a** She was imaged with iodine-131 after incomplete removal of her primary tumour and uptake in the neck and lungs bilaterally was observed. She was treated with 3700 MBq of iodine-131 and re-imaged 8 months later. **b** Partial resolution of the disease in her neck and lungs. She received a second dose of 3700 MBq of iodine-131. **c** A further scan 1 year later showed further resolution of lung disease with persistent disease in the neck.

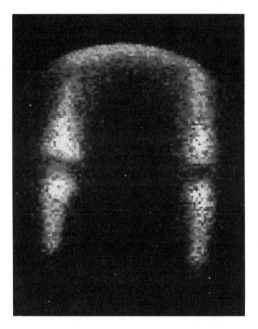

Fig. 10.2. A 5-year-old boy with a history of neuroblastoma treated with conventional therapy and clinical evidence of relapse. ^{131}I-mIBG scan of legs shows significant uptake in both femora and tibiae at the sites of metastases. The patient was subsequently treated with a therapeutic dose of ^{131}I-mIBG. (Scan by kind permission of Prof. B. Ackery, Southampton General Hospital.)

other forms of therapy have failed. When the data are reviewed 5% of all patients treated have undergone complete remission, 40% have experienced partial remission and in 10% the disease progresses. Up to 7.5 GBq doses have been used and the usual treatment interval is 8–12 weeks. Since bone-marrow involvement is often extensive, anaemia, reduction in platelet counts and occasionally complete marrow supression have been reported. Marrow harvesting is now performed as a cautionary measure in patients with extensive bone metastases (Fig. 10.2).

Bone metastases in malignant phaeochromocytoma are common and ^{131}I-mIBG has been used therapeutically by a number of groups. Doses of 3.7–7.4 GBq have been infused slowly at 3–6-month intervals. Cumulative results show partial response in one-third of patients treated for malignant phaeochromocytoma and palliation in over 50% of patients. No complete cures have been reported. Treatment is well tolerated and reported side-effects are minimal (Hoefnagel 1989).

Experience in therapy for bone metastases in patients with MTC is limited. Cumulative experience in 9 patients has yielded complete responses in 2, partial responses in 3, palliation in 3 and no change in 1 patient (Fig. 10.3).

Small series of therapy with ^{131}I-mIBG have been reported for carcinoids and paragangliomas, with limited success (Hoefnagel 1989). Because of the high gamma emission of ^{131}I-mIBG, the patient must be admitted for therapy and standard precautions for ^{131}I therapy observed.

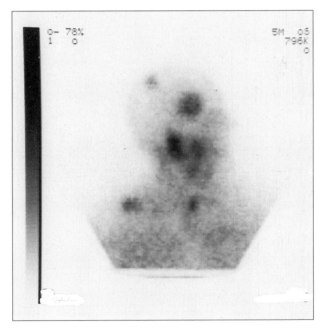

Fig. 10.3. A 67-year-old male with a history of medullary thyroid cancer and evidence of bone metastases following initial surgery. An ^{131}I-mIBG imaging study showed uptake at sites of metastatic disease. Patient received a therapeutic 5500 MBq does of ^{131}I-mIBG and the figure shows a post-therapy scan of uptake in skull, ribs and clavicle metastases. Patient experienced significant pain relief following therapy.

[131]I-mIBG has now been used therapeutically for 4 years. Experience is still limited but palliation of bone pain in patients with bone metastases has been widely reported. Studies are being undertaken to assess the optimal dose and the frequency of administration of ^{131}I-mIBG which should be used.

Strontium-89

Strontium-89 has been shown to localise at the sites of prostatic and breast bone metastases. The behaviour of intravenous strontium has been studied using strontium-85 which, unlike strontium-89, has a gamma emission convenient for imaging (Blake 1986). The study demonstrated that metastatic bone lesions accumulate strontium more avidly than does normal bone. It was also observed that the biological half life of strontium in metastases was long compared to the 50.5 days physical half life of strontium-89, whilst the turnover in normal trabecular bone was 14 days. Whole body retention of strontium-89 at 3 months ranged from 11% to 88% depending on the degree of skeletal involvement. The radiation dose to individual vertebral metastases from a single 150 MBq dose of strontium-89 has been shown to vary from 9 to 92 Gy depending on the extent of metastatic spread. The dose to the bone marrow has been estimated to be approximately one-tenth of the dose to the bone metastases (Blake et al. 1988) (Fig. 10.4).

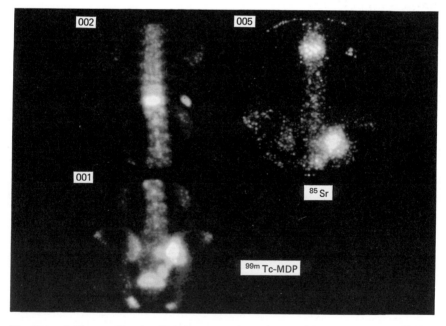

Fig. 10.4. A 64-year-old male with known prostatic carcinoma whose bone scan using ^{99m}Tc-MDP (*left images*) showed metastases at T12, right 11th rib and right sacro-iliac joint. A scan performed using strontium-85, a gamma-emitting radioisotope of strontium (*right images*), shows strontium accumulation at the site of metastatic disease. The patient was subsequently treated with strontium-89 with relief of bone pain. (Scan by kind permission of Prof. D. Akery, Southampton General Hospital.)

A number of studies have now been undertaken using strontium-89 to treat patients with severe bone pain, unresponsive to radiotherapy. The dose used is 1–2 MBq per kg. In all studies reported, 80% of patients have shown some response in terms of pain relief with up to 50% of patients reporting a significant improvement in pain and 10%–20% becoming pain-free (Robinson et al. 1987; Lewington et al. 1988).

A double-blind trial has also been undertaken to compare the effects of strontium-89 with strontium chloride in pain palliation. The data showed a pain-palliative effect of strontium-89 versus strontium chloride placebo with confidence levels of greater than 99%. The usual time of onset of pain relief was typically 10–20 days after injection and a plateau of improvement was reached by 5 weeks. The duration of response varied from 4 to 12 months (mean 6 months) (Amersham Int PLC, personal communication).

Patients with normal bone marrow have shown mild marrow toxicity which is dose-related. Pretreatment in 5% of patients with reduced marrow reserve showed a significant fall in platelet count and white count after treatment. A transient pain flare has been reported in some patients approximately 48 h after injection and this has been regarded as a good prognostic sign (Lewington et al. 1988). As strontium-89 does not emit gamma radiation, the patient does not need to be hospitalised for therapy. As strontium-89 is now commercially available, results from larger series of patients are awaited.

Samarium-153 EDTMP

Samarium-153 ethylene diamine tetramethylene phosphonic acid (EDTMP) has been developed at the University of Missouri for the treatment of bone metastases (Ketring 1987). The radiopharmaceutical is chemically and biologically stable and preferentially concentrates in skeletal metastases. The short half life (46.3 h) makes it suitable for repeated irradiations of a tumour.

A number of reports have now appeared indicating that samarium-153 EDTMP can be used successfully to palliate pain from bone metastases. Harvey Turner et al. (1989) reported that 79% of patients with bone metastases unresponsive to conventional treatment had experienced pain palliation within 14 days of treatment with samarium-153 EDTMP. The duration of response ranged from 4 to 35 weeks. The primary tumours included breast and prostate.

Reversible myelotoxicity was observed when the radiation absorbed dose to the bone marrow exceeded 270 cGy. Carichner et al. (1989) have treated patients with prostatic bone metastases and reported resolution of focal disease in some patients. The doses administered are currently 2–2.5 mCi/kg patient bodyweight. The patients are admitted for therapy for 24–48 h and the dose is infused intravenously.

The Future

Despite decades of experience of iodine-131 in therapy, the therapeutic use of other radiopharmaceuticals has only recently begun to be explored. In the past 5 years new radiopharmaceuticals have been produced which localise in bone metastases and can be labelled with beta-emitting radionuclides for therapeutic purposes. At the present time new agents have been used mainly in patients who have failed conventional therapy and who have widespread disease. The encouraging palliative results in a significant number of patients treated have encouraged some groups to consider using these new agents earlier in the disease in an attempt to treat rather than palliate the metastases. Iodine-131 mIBG neuroblastoma therapy is one such agent. Much remains to be learnt about the doses that can be tolerated and the frequency with which treatment should be repeated. It is now known that doses of 11 GBq (300 mCi) may be tolerated by patients treated with ^{131}I-mIBG although marrow toxicity may be a significant problem in some patients. It may be postulated that in the future patients may receive courses of therapy similar to those undertaken using chemotherapeutic agents.

The cost of beta-emitting radiopharmaceuticals (apart from iodine-131) remains a problem and single treatment doses range in cost from £600 for strontium-89 to over £2000 for a therapeutic dose of ^{131}I-mIBG. The high cost of these agents severely limits the research that can be undertaken at the present time.

While most of the current therapy work is being undertaken using beta-emitting radiopharmaceuticals, the use of alpha emitters and electron capture and internal conversion decaying radionuclides has significant therapeutic potential if the radionuclides can be targeted within the tumour cell, close, if not bound, to the tumour cell DNA. The production of such radiopharmaceuticals will require a multidisciplinary approach with tumour biochemists and radiobiologists.

Therapy using radiolabelled antibodies, whilst having theoretical potential, is at present in its infancy. Uptake in non-target tissue is hampering the development of antibodies for therapy but it is hoped that molecular engineering and the production of chimeric antibodies may reduce non-target tissue accumulation.

Targeted radiotherapy using tumour-specific radiopharmaceuticals is no longer only a theoretical possibility but is rapidly becoming established in clinical practice. Although only palliation of terminal disease is being achieved at present, it may be predicted that within a decade adjuvant therapy using radiopharmaceuticals will be an established practice.

References

Allen SJ, Blake GM, McKeeney DB, Lazarus CR, Blower P, Singh J, Page C, Clarke SEM (1990) Rh-186-v-DMSA: dosimetry of a new radiopharmaceutical for therapy of medullary carcinoma of the thyroid. Nucl Med Commun 11:220–221

Andres R, Blattman H, Pfeiffer G, Schubiger PA, Vogt M, Weinreich R, Wernli C (1986) Radionuclides for therapy: a review. In: Schubiger P, Hasler PH (eds) Radionuclides for therapy. Proceedings of the 4th Bottstein Colloquium. Hoffman la Roche, Basle, pp 9–20

Baulieu JL, Guilloteau D, Baulieu F, Le Floch O, Chambon C, Pourcelot L, Besnard JL (1988) Therapeutic effectiveness of Iodine-131 MIBG for metastases of a non-secreting paraganglioma. J Nucl Med 29:2008–2013

Beer HF, Blauenstein P, Andres R, Hasler PH, Schubiger P (1986) How to get the radionuclide to the right site. In Schubiger P, Hasler PH (eds) Radionuclides for therapy, Proc of 4th Bottstein Colloquium. Hoffman la Roche, Basle, pp 60–74

Blake G (1986) Strontium-89 therapy: strontium kinetics in disseminated carcinoma of the prostate. Eur J Nucl Med 12:447–454

Blake GM, Zivanovic MA, Blaquere RM, Fine DR, McEwan EJ, Ackery DM (1988) Sr-89 therapy – measurement of observed dose to skeletal metastases. J Nucl Med 29:549–557

Blower PJ, Clarke SEM, Bisuriadan MM, Singh J, West MJ (1990) Preparation and characterisation of pentavalent Rh-186 DMSA. A possible tumour therapy agent. Nucl Med Commun 11: 212–213

Boniface G, Izard M, Walker K, McKay D, Sorby P, Harvey Turner J, Morris J (1989) Labelling of monoclonal antibodies with Sm-153 for combined radioimmunoscintigraphy and radioimmunotherapy. J Nucl Med 30:683–691

Bowen BM, Darracott J, Garnett ES, Tomlinson RH (1975) Yttrium-90 citrate colloid for radioisotope synovectomy. Am J Hosp Pharm 32:1027–1030

Carichner S, Eary J, Collins C, Nemiroff K, Richter D, Lewis D, Applebaum F (1989) Samarium-153 EDTMP. Technical aspects of imaging and treatment. Clin Nucl Med 14:B1,11

Carrelta R, Martin P, Malekian T (1989) Strontium-89 therapy for metastatic prostate and breast carcinoma: a community hospital experience. Clin Nucl Med 14:A5, 11

Charbord P, L'heritier C, Cukerstein W, Lumbroso J, Tubiana M (1977) Radio-iodine treatment in differentiated thyroid carcinomas. Treatment of first local recurrences and of bone and lung metastases. Ann Radiol 20:783–786

Clarke SEM, Lazarus CR, Edwards S, Murby B, Clarke DG, Roden T, Fogelman I, Maisey MN (1987) Scintigraphy and treatment of MCT with ^{131}I-MIBG. J Nucl Med 28:1820

Dunscombe PB, Ramsey NW (1980) Radioactivity studies on two synovectomy specimens after radiation synovectomy with Yttrium-90-silicate. Ann Rheum Dis 39:87–89

Ehrlich P (1906) Collected studies of immunity. John Wiley and Sons, Chichester

Ehrlich P (1960) The collected papers of Paul Ehrlich. Pergamon Press, New York, pp 505–518

Fischer M, Kamanabroo D, Sonderkarys H (1984) Scintigraphic imaging of carcinoid tumours with ^{131}I-MIBG. Lancet ii:165

Fisher DR (1985) The microdosimetry of monoclonal antibodies labelled with alpha particles. Fourth International Radiopharmaceutical Symposium. CONF – 851113, 446–457, Oakridge, Tennessee

Francis MD, Slough CL, Tofe AJ (1976) Distribution and effect of P32 EHDP in normal and bone tumour bearing dogs. J Nucl Med 17:548

Goodhead DT (1985) Saturable repair models of radiation action in mammalian cells. Radiat Res 104:S58–S67

Goodwin D, Meares C, Diamonti C, McCall M, Lai C, Torti F, McTigue M, Martin B (1990) Use of specific antibody for rapid clearance of circulating blood background from tumour imaging proteins. Eur J Nucl Med 9:209–215

Gorckler WF, Edwards B, Volkert WA (1987) Skeletal localisation of Sm-153 chelates, potential therapeutic bone agents. J Nucl Med 28:495–504

Griffiths MH, York ED, Wessels BW, Denardo GL, Neacy WP (1988) Direct dose confirmation of quantitative autoradiography with micro TLD measurements for radioimmunotherapy. J Nucl Med 29:1795–1809

Hall N, Tokars RP, O'Mara RE (1975) P32 diphosphonate: a potential therapeutic agent. J Nucl Med 16:532

Harvey Turner J, Martindale A, Sorby P, Hetherington E, Fleay R, Hoffman R, Caringbold P (1989) Samarium-153 EDTMP therapy of disseminated skeletal metastases. Eur J Nucl Med 15:784–795

Hill JM, Lobe E, Spear RJ (1962) IV colloidal zirconyl phosphate P-32. Clinical studies of over 250 cases. J Nucl Med 3:196

Hisada K, Ando (1973) Radiolanthides as promising tumour scanning agents. J Nucl Med 14:615–617

Hoefnagel CA (1989) The clinical use of ^{131}I metaiodobenzylguanidine for the diagnosis and treatment of neural crest tumours. Academisch Proef Schrift

Hoefnagel CA, DeKraker J, Marcuse HR, Voute PA (1986) Detection and treatment of neural crest tumours using ^{131}I-MIBG. In: Schmidt HAE, Ell PJ, Britton KE (eds) Nuklearmedizin – nuclear medicine in research and practice. Schattauer Verlag, Stuttgart, pp 473–476

Hoefnagel CA, Voute PA, DeKraker J, Marcuse HR (1987) Radionuclide diagnosis and therapy of neural crest tumours using iodine-131 MIBG. J Nucl Med 28:308–314

Humm JL, Cobb LM (1990) Non-uniformity of tumour dose in radioimmunotherapy. J Nucl Med 31:75–83

Ketring A (1987) Sm-153-EHDP and rhenium-186 HEDP as bone therapeutic radiopharmaceuticals. Int J Rad Appl Instrum [B] 14:223–232

Kohler G, Milstein C (1975) Continuous cultures of fused cells secreting antibody of predefined specificity. Nature 256:495–496

Larsen SM, Carrasquillo JA, Krohn KA, Brown JP, McGuffin RW, Ferens JM, Graham MM, Hill LD, Beaumier PL, Helstrom KE, Helstrom I (1983) Localization of ^{131}I labelled P97 specific Fab fragments in human melanoma as a basis for radiotherapy. J Clin Invest 72:2101–2114

Lewington VJ, Zivanovic MA, Blake GB, Buchanan RB, Akery DM (1988) Treatment of bone pain in disseminated prostatic cancer using strontium-89. Nucl Med Commun 9:179–186 (abstr)

Marchandise X, Brendel AJ, Caudry M, Charbonnel B, Chatal JF, Lanheche B, Lumsioso J, Marnex R, Schlumberger M, Werneaun JL (1985) Treatment of malignant phaeochromocytomas with I-131 MIBG. Results of a French multicenter study. Nucl Med 26:51–52

McCardle RJ, Harper P, Spar I, Bale W, Andros G, Jiminez F (1966) Studies with ^{131}I-labeled antibody to human fibrinogen for diagnosis and therapy of tumours. J Nucl Med 7:837–847

McEwan AJ, Catz A, Fields AL, Lewington V, Harbara D, Fine D, Ackery DM (1987) ^{131}I-MIBG in the diagnosis and treatment of carcinoid syndrome. J Nucl Med 28:658

Milstein C (1980) Monoclonal antibodies. Sci Am 243:66–74

O'Mara RE (1978) In: RP Spencer (ed) Therapy in nuclear medicine. Grune and Stratton, New York, p 257

Pecker C (1942) Biological investigations with radioactive calcium and strontium: preliminary report on the use of radioactive strontium in the treatment of metastatic bone cancer. Pharmacology, 1:117–139

Peng TX, Moya A, Ayala FJ (1986) Irradiation resistance conferred by super oxide dismutase: possible adaptive role of a natural polymorphism in Drosophila melanogaster. Proc Natl Acad Sci USA 83:684–687

Pochin EE (1967). Prospects from the treatment of thyroid carcinoma with radio-iodine. Clin Radiol 18:113–125

Pochin EE (1969) Long term hazards of radio-iodine treatment of thyroid carcinoma. In: Hedinger CE (ed). Thyroid cancer. UICC Monograph Series, vol 12. Springer Verlag, Berlin Heidelberg New York p 293

Poston GJ, Thomas H, MacDonald DW, Lynn JA, Lavender JP (1985) ^{131}I-MIBG uptake by medullary carcinoma of the thyroid. Lancet ii:560

Potsaid M, Irwin F, Castronovo G, Prout G, Harvey W, Francis M, Tofe A (1976) Phophorus-32 EHDP clinical study of patients with prostatic carcinoma bone metastases. J Nucl Med 17:548

Robinson R, Spicer JA, Preston DF, Wegst AV, Martin NL (1987) Treatment of metastatic bone pain with strontium-89. Nucl Med Biol 14:219–222

Seeman G, Bosslet K, Sedlacek HA (1987) Human anti-tumour antibodies: problems, opportunities, immunotherapy and scintigraphy of tumours with monoclonal antibodies. Aktuel Onkol 41:21–25

Seidlin SM, Marinelle LD, Oshry E (1946) Radioactive iodine therapy: effect on functioning metastases of adenocarcinoma of the thyroid. JAMA 132:838

Shapiro B, Sisson JC, Lloyd R, Nakajo M, Satterlee W, Bierwalters WH (1984) Malignant phaeochromocytoma: clinical, biochemical and scintigraphic characterisation. Clin Endocrinol 20:189–203

Shapiro B, Andrews J, Figg L, Carey J, Walker-Andrews S, Smith J, Ensminger W (1989) Therapeutic intraarterial administration of yttrium-90 glass microspheres for hepatic tumours. Eur J Nucl Med 8:401

Shaw DR, Khazaeli MB, Lobuglio AF (1988) Mouse/human chimeric antibodies to a tumour associated antigen; biological activity of the four human IgG subclasses. J Natl Cancer Inst 80:1553–1559

Stewart JSW, Griffiths M, Munro AJ, Lambert JO, Coutter C, Epenetos A (1987) Intraperitoneal radioimmunotherapy for ovarian cancer. Aktuel Onkol 41:65–73

Todd P, Wood JCS, Walker JT, Weiss St J (1985) Lethal, potential lethal and non-lethal damage induction by heavy ions in cultured human cells. Radiat Res 104:S5–S12

Tubiana M, Lacour T, Marnier J, Bergiron C, Gerard Marchant R, Roujean J, Bok B, Parmentier C (1975) External radiotherapy and radio-iodine in the treatment of 359 thyroid cancers. Br J Radiol 49:894–907

Van Gils APG, Van Der May AGL, Hoogma RPJM, Falke TITM, Moolenaar AJ, Pauwels EKJ, Van Kroonen Burgh MJPG (1989) Iodium-123 MIBG scintigrafie bij chemodactomen een

oprallend resultaat. Nucl Geneeskd Bull II:61
Wieland DM, Brown LE, Mangner TJ, Swanscombe DP, Bierwaters W (1980) Radiolabeled
    adrenergic neuro blocking agents: Adreno-medullary imaging with ^{131}I-iodobenzylguanidine. J
    Nucl Med 21:349–353

11   The Role of the Orthopaedic Surgeon in the Treatment of Skeletal Metastases

C.S.B. Galasko

Introduction

Skeletal metastases may present with pain, hypercalcaemia, impending fractures, pathological fractures, spinal instability or compression of the spinal cord or cauda equina. Furthermore, patients with metastatic cancer may present with pain from benign conditions that require treatment.

Skeletal metastases most frequently present with pain, which occurs in approximately two thirds of patients with radiographically detectable lesions (Galasko 1972), although pain may and frequently does develop before the lesion becomes detectable on radiographs. Unless a further complication arises, the orthopaedic surgeon is not usually involved in the treatment of painful skeletal metastases. The treatment of pain is covered in Chap. 12.

Bone pain may be the presenting feature of hypercalcaemia and an increase in bone pain was the commonest symptom of this condition in one series (Galasko and Burn 1971). The treatment of hypercalcaemia is described in Chap. 8. Its recognition is important and the serum calcium must be measured in all patients presenting with the complications of skeletal metastases. The hypercalcaemia may be secondary to the bone destruction consequent upon skeletal metastases, humoral factors secreted by the tumour, or a combination of these causes. In the former it appears as if the development of hypercalcaemia is related more to the rapidity of bone destruction than to the extent of metastatic involvement.

Impending Fractures

Large lytic metastases present with pain and are evident on plain radiographs. By the time a large lytic metastasis has developed there is considerable destruction and the cortex has been involved. Edelstyn et al. (1967) showed that at least 50% of the bone must be destroyed in the beam axis of the x-ray before a lytic lesion, arising in the medulla, will be evident on a plain radiograph. The mechanism of pain in these lesions is not fully understood, but may be associated with infractions of the surrounding bone. The risk of fracture is high. Fidler (1981) found that the risk of fracture correlated with the degree of cortical destruction. If less than 25% of the cortex was destroyed the risk of fracture was virtually negligible. He reported a fracture incidence of 3.7% when 25%–50% of the cortex was involved, 61% when the degree of involvement ranged between 50% and 75%, and 79% if more than 75% of the cortex was involved.

Although most fractures are associated with large lytic metastases, they can also occur in other types of metastases (Fig.11.1). There basically are three types of bone destruction consequent upon skeletal metastases (Lodwick 1964, 1965).

1. Geographic. These are large, solitary, well-defined lytic areas more than 1 cm in diameter and usually with a sharply demarcated edge.
2. "Moth-eaten". There are multiple, smaller lytic areas (2–5 mm) which may coalesce to form larger confluent areas. The margins are usually ill-defined.

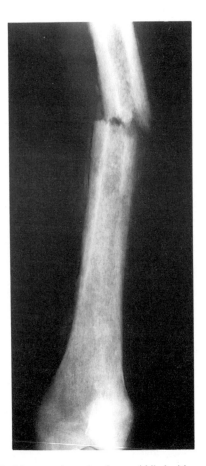

Fig. 11.1. Pathological fracture through a femur riddled with permeative metastases.

3. Permeative. There are multiple, tiny lytic areas (usually 1 mm or less) seen principally in cortical bone. The bone is weakened and such lesions predispose to pathological fracture even though a large lytic metastasis cannot be seen on the radiograph (Fig.11.1).

Geographic destruction is usually found in the slowest developing metastases, whereas permeative destruction occurs in the most aggressive lesions. A patient with multiple metastases usually shows one of the three principal patterns.

Radiotherapy relieves pain, but temporarily weakens the bone, probably owing to the associated transient osteoporosis and, as a result, may increase the risk of pathological fracture. Biopsy of a lytic lesion may also predispose to fracture.

Primary internal stabilisation of the weakened bone, followed by irradiation, is the treatment of choice. It is easier to fix the bone while it is still intact and the rehabilitation and convalescence are much shorter and easier. If the patient is not fit for surgery then radiotherapy alone is indicated. Prior to treatment scintigrams and radiographs are obtained of the entire length of the affected bone so that any other metastases, which may subsequently develop into a pathological fracture, are stabilised and are included in the radiotherapy field. A pathological fracture at the edge of a plate or intramedullary nail, particularly if the implant has also been fixed with methylmethacrylate, is more difficult to treat than if there was no implant in the bone, and it is extremely difficult to irradiate a metastasis if part of the lesion has been included in a previous field.

The type of internal stabilisation depends on the site of the lesion. Where feasible, closed intramedullary nailing is preferred, and if indicated, a biopsy specimen can be taken using bronchial biopsy forceps or through a separate incision. However, at the end of the long bones intramedullary nailing alone provides inadequate stabilisation. It is often possible to stabilise the ends of a long bone by the use of an interlocking nail but alternative techniques might be required. Care must be taken to avoid producing a fracture when positioning the patient or when stabilising the lesion.

It is essential that the internal stabilisation of the lesion provides sufficient strength to allow unsupported use of the limb, including weight bearing in the lower limb. If the implant alone is not likely to provide this, the stabilisation should be supplemented with methylmethacrylate. The tumour is removed, the cavity filled with methylmethacrylate, and the implant fixed across the methylmethacrylate whilst still soft, as well as bridging normal bone above and below the lesion.

Irradiation is an essential part of treatment to inhibit further tumour growth, since the latter will result in progressive bone destruction, resultant loosening of the stabilisation, and an increased risk of fracture. Depending on the primary lesion the patient may also require endocrine treatment or chemotherapy.

Surgery carries the theoretical risk of disseminating tumour cells both locally and into the circulation. However, this has never been proved, providing the lesion is irradiated. Furthermore, there is no evidence that the combined effect of surgical intervention and general anaesthesia has affected the overall prognosis in these patients. On the contrary, there is some experimental evidence that pathological fractures are associated with an increased incidence of pulmonary metastases, and that prophylactic stabilisation of an impending pathological fracture decreases the incidence of pulmonary metastases (Bouma et al. 1983).

Table 11.1. Pathological fractures

Primary tumour	No. of patients	No. of fractures
Breast	102	117
Lung	24	25
Prostate	21	22
Kidney	7	7
Rectum	6	6
Stomach	4	4
Bladder	3	3
Melanoma	2	2
Uterus	2	2
Thyroid	1	1
Colon	1	1
Oesophagus	1	1
Bile duct	1	1
Cervix	1	1
Ovary	1	1
Penis	1	1
Squamous cell	1	1
Lymphoma	4	5
Leukaemia	6	6
Myeloma	24	34
Not known	5	5
Total	218	246

Pathological Fractures

Although virtually every malignant tumour can metastasise to bone and may be associated with a pathological fracture, almost half are secondary to mammary carcinoma (Table 11.1), probably because skeletal metastases occur more commonly from mammary carcinoma than with any other tumour. The commonest site of pathological fracture is in the femur (Table 11.2), particularly at its upper end, but virtually any long bone is at risk.

The development of a pathological fracture is not necessarily a terminal event. With improvement in chemotherapy and endocrine therapy there has been an increase in survival over the years. In 1974 Galasko reported an average survival of 10.1 months. Fifty-four per cent of patients survived for more than 3 months and 23% for more than 1 year. The survival was related to the primary tumour; none of the patients with bronchial carcinoma survived more than 6 months, but several of the patients with carcinoma of the breast lived for more than 1 year and some for 6 or 7 years. By 1981 the survival had increased to 19 months (Harrington 1981). Patients with metastatic prostatic carcinoma had the longest survival (29.3 months) compared with mammary carcinoma (22.6 months), renal carcinoma (11.8 months) and bronchial carcinoma (3.6 months). Gainor and Buchert (1983) also reported that none of their patients with fractures from metastatic bronchial carcinoma lived for more than 6 months.

Table 11.2. Pathological fractures

Site	Number
Pelvis	2
Femur	
Transcervical	59
Intertrochanteric	25
Subtrochanteric	29
Shaft	41
Distal	10
Humerus	
Proximal	19
Shaft	48
Distal	3
Tibia	
Proximal	2
Shaft	1
Radius	
Shaft	2
Ulna	
Shaft	1
Clavicle	3
Mandible	1
Total	246

Management of Pathological Fracture

There are three aspects to the management of pathological fractures.

1. The orthopaedic management
2. Localised irradiation
3. The treatment of the causative tumour

The orthopaedic management will be discussed in this chapter. Localised irradiation is an essential part of treatment in an attempt to control the underlying tumour, prevent further osteolysis and loosening of the implant. It can be delayed until the wound has healed but this is not essential. The implant dose not appear to affect the radiation, providing megavoltage is used. Orthovoltage should not be used when there is a metal implant in the bone, because of dose enhancement in the immediate vicinity of the metal and the shielding of tumour cells in the shadow of the implant. The causative tumour should be treated by chemo or endocrine therapy depending on its sensitivity.

The evaluation of a patient with a pathological fracture or impending fracture includes an assessment of the general fitness of the patient, the degree of dissemination of the tumour, the diagnosis of the primary tumour, if not already known, and the presence of other complications. In addition to a careful clinical examination the evaluation includes appropriate blood films, radiographs, skeletal scintigrams and other forms of radiographic imaging as required. Skeletal scintigrams and radiographs of the entire bone are a prerequisite to internal fixation of a pathological fracture. As indicated for impending fractures it is essential that the implant stabilises all metastases in the affected bone and not just the pathological fracture. If the primary lesion is not known, or if there is any uncertainty about the origin of the pathological fracture, a biopsy of the lesion is essential. This can be carried out at the time of surgical stabilisation. Biopsy is not an essential part of every internal stabilisation, particularly if a closed method of intramedullary fixation is used. If the patient is not fit for surgery, he or she must be made comfortable and allowed to die with dignity.

Transcervical Femoral Fractures

Pathological transcervical femoral fractures do not unite irrespective of the method of orthopaedic treatment and irrespective of the degree of displacement (Galasko 1974), probably due to the effect of irradiation on an area where fractures are associated with impaired vascularity. Replacement arthroplasty gives the best results, the type of arthroplasty depending on the degree of tumour involvement. This can only be assessed from plain radiographs and a skeletal scintigram of the pelvis and femora. CT scanning or MRI may also be helpful. If there is no metastatic involvement of the acetabulum a hemiarthroplasty may be all that is required. It should be cemented into the femoral shaft with methylmethacrylate. If the acetabulum is involved, a total replacement arthroplasty is indicated, the tumour being curetted from the acetabulum and the defect filled with methylmethacrylate. If there is more extensive involvement of the acetabulum pelvic reconstruction may be required (Harrington 1981). If more distal metastases are found in the femur a long stemmed femoral component is used. It is reasonable to treat all fractures with a long stemmed total replacement arthroplasty in case there are acetabular or distal femoral metastases. At the time of surgery the tumour is curetted from the femoral neck and the defect filled with methylmethacrylate.

Other Femoral and Tibial Fractures

Unlike transcervical femoral fractures the majority of pathological fractures involving the rest of the femur or tibia united with bone in patients who survived for more than three months, irrespective of the type of orthopaedic treatment (Galasko 1980). However, internal fixation provided definite advantages over external support. It gave the patient greater and much more rapid relief of pain; it was associated with easier nursing and more comfortable turning of the patient and prevention of pressure sores; and it allowed much earlier mobilisation of the patient and discharge from hospital. It is also thought to increase the prospects of union. As with impending fractures it is essential to stabilise the bone adequately, sufficient for weight-bearing, at the time of surgery. If necessary the internal fixation must be supplemented by methylmethacrylate, even though this may interfere with callus formation. However, methylmethacrylate will not compensate for inadequate mechanical stability due to a poorly positioned implant. The method of internal stabilisation depends on the site of fracture, and the presence and site of other metastases in the same bone. In general terms fractures of the shaft of a long bone should be fixed by an intramedullary nail, or a locking nail if there is further metastatic involvement near the extremities of the bone; whereas fractures in the metaphysis may require fixation with a plate, blade plate or locked nail. The method of fixation must also stabilise other metastases in the affected bone to avoid the risk of subsequent fracture adjacent to the implant.

Closed intramedullary rodding can be supplemented by methylmethacrylate but pressure injection of the latter carries the risk of fat embolism (Kunec and Lewis 1984). Gainor and Buchert (1983) reported that 67% of pathological fractures from myeloma united, compared with 44% secondary to metastatic hypernephroma, 37% in mammary carcinoma and none in bronchial carcinoma. They also reported that internal fixation improved the rate of fracture union by 23% compared with cast immobilisation.

Humeral Fractures

Internal fixation is also of benefit, in that it provides the patients with much greater mobility and earlier use of the limb and more rapid and greater pain relief, but the advantages over conservative treatment are not as marked as with pathological fractures of the lower limb (Galasko 1980). McCormack et al. (1985) suggested that a functional cast brace was indicated if the patient had a limited life expectancy, but for those patients expected to survive longer than 3 months, internal fixation was the method of choice to ensure pain relief, restoration of function and avoid later re-fracture.

Fractures of the proximal humerus may require replacement arthroplasty if they cannot be stabilised. The indication for replacement arthroplasty is different from transcervical femoral fractures. In the humerus, replacement is indicated if it is not possible to stabilise the fracture because of its site or degree of bone destruction, whereas in the femur replacement is indicated because pathological fractures of the femoral neck do not unite irrespective of the method of treatment.

The vast majority of pathological fractures of the humerus, radius or ulna can be treated by intramedullary nailing. Fractures around the metaphysis may require plate fixation. Where necessary, the implant must be supplemented with methylmethacrylate.

Multiple Fractures

Some patients present with several pathological fractures and each must be treated on its merit (Fig.11.2).

Fracture through an Isolated Metastasis

Occasionally patients present with an isolated skeletal metastasis. They usually present with pain, may present with an impending fracture and occasionally with a pathological fracture. The commonest primary is renal carcinoma and providing there is no other evidence of dissemination of the tumour, resection of the lesion should be considered either in the form of local resection and prosthetic replacement or amputation. It is easier to excise and replace a

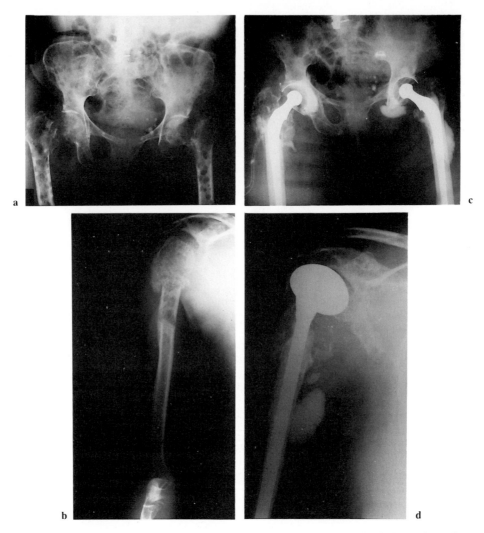

Fig. 11.2.a–d. Patient with multiple myeloma. Two years previously she had had her spine stabilised for spinal instability. She presented with multiple pathological fractures. **a** Bilateral femoral transcervical fractures. **b** Fracture of the neck of her right humerus. **c,d** She was treated with bilateral long stemmed total hip replacement arthroplasties **c** and a right shoulder hemiarthroplasty **d**. Part of the Banks' rod, used to stabilise her spine, can be seen in **a** and **c**. Following these procedures the patient was mobilised, and returned home. She was re-admitted 18 months later for terminal care.

metastasis with impending fracture than one that has already fractured. The haematoma consequent upon the latter may have caused widespread local dissemination of the tumour which makes it impossible to carry out a local resection with adequate margins.

Highly Vascular Lesions

Occasional metastases, particularly those from renal carcinoma, may be highly vascular and surgery may be associated with massive blood loss. Pre-operative angiography may be indicated in metastases from renal carcinoma and if the lesion is highly vascular pre-operative embolisation may be required.

Post-operative Irradiation

Local irradiation is an essential part of treatment for the reasons given above. It does not interfere with fracture healing, providing the fracture is adequately immobilised (Bonarigo and Rubin 1967; Gainor and Buchert 1983). Fractures of the humeral shaft treated by intramedullary nailing and post-operative radiotherapy healed more rapidly than non-pathological, traumatic fractures at the same site and with greater amounts of bone (Galasko 1980).

Non-Pathological Fracture in a Patient with Malignant Disease

Patients with an underlying malignancy may develop a fracture like any other individual, without a metastasis at the site of fracture. However, if the patient has a past history of malignancy a biopsy should be taken from the fracture. In some instances this may be the first manifestation of dissemination of the disease, even though there has been a long disease-free interval.

Non-pathological fractures must be treated on their merits, as should other non-metastatic orthopaedic fractures (Galasko 1986, see below).

The development of a non-pathological fracture in a patient with a previous history of cancer may subsequently be associated with dissemination of the cancer. The author has experience of 2 patients with mammary carcinoma, one of whom developed a transcervical femoral fracture 16 years following mastectomy, and the second a fracture/dislocation of her hip 22 years following mastectomy. In both patients there was no evidence of dissemination at the time of fracture and histological examination of biopsies taken from the fracture showed no tumour yet both patients developed multiple metastases affecting lung and bone within 3 months.

Spinal Instability

Back pain is a frequent symptom in patients with disseminated carcinoma and in 10% is due to spinal instability (Galasko and Sylvester 1978). Spinal instability can be associated with excruciating pain, which is mechanical in nature. In the severe form the patient is only comfortable when lying absolutely still. Any

Table 11.3.   Spinal instability

Primary tumour	No. of patients
Breast	31 + 1[a]
Myeloma	8
Prostate	2
Melanoma	2
Bronchus	1
Kidney	1
Bladder	1
Colon	1
Uterus	1
Cervix	1
Vagina	1
Stomach	1
Parotid	1
Lymphoma	1
Chondrosarcoma	1
Histiocytoma	1
Cordoma	1
Total	56 + 1[a]

[a] Lumbar stabilisation 22 months after successful dorsal stabilisation.
One patient's metastatic destruction was too extensive for surgical stabilisation.

Table 11.4. Spinal instability

Destruction too extensive for surgical reconstruction	1
Infection resulting in removal of implant	1
Loosening of implant	2
Relief of pain	
Complete	51
Partial	2
Complications in the 53 patients with relief of pain	
Infection: successfully treated	1
Wound dehiscence: successful secondary suture	1
Fracture L rod: successful anterior fusion	1
Fracture Hartshill rectangle at 5 years	1

movement, including log rolling by 2 or 3 trained nurses, is associated with severe pain and the patient may not be able to sit, stand or walk because of the pain even with the use of a spinal orthosis.

In the milder form the patient may be relatively free from pain when wearing a rigid spinal orthosis, but any movement of the back, for example, turning in bed, sitting or standing, may be impossible without the support. Radiographs show destruction of bone with vertebral collapse of a greater or lesser extent. Spinal instability should be considered the equivalent of a pathological fracture in a long bone, because the pain is due to the instability and not the metastasis. Radiotherapy or chemotherapy will not alleviate the pain. As with pathological fractures of the long bones stabilisation is required for pain relief.

We have treated 56 patients with spinal instability secondary to spinal metastases. The primary tumours are shown in Table 11.3, the commonest being mammary carcinoma. The survival is similar to that following pathological fractures of the long bones, several of our patients being alive 4, 5 and 6 years following their stabilisation.

The results are shown in Table 11.4. Several methods of spinal stabilisation are available. It is essential that the method chosen adequately stabilises the spine. A posterior stabilisation, using an implant that can be fixed to the spine at multiple levels, either with screws or sublaminal wires, such as the Banks' rod or Hartshill rectangle, has the great advantage that it can stabilise a large area of the spine. The implants must be fixed to at least 2 and preferably 3 vertebrae above and 2 or 3 vertebrae below the unstable segment. In the lower dorsal and lumbar spine a pedicular screw system can be used. Pre-operative radiographs and skeletal scintigrams are important and if there are two areas of instability the stabilisation should support both areas. If posterior stabilisation is not likely to provide adequate support, for example instability at the 5th lumbar level, it must be combined with an anterior stabilisation. If the stabilisation extends to the sacrum, a lumbar lordosis must be moulded into the implant to prevent a post-operative flat back which will interfere with sitting (Fig. 11.3). If the disease is localised to 1 or 2 vertebrae anterior stabilisation might be indicated, particularly if the patient presents with marked neurological symptoms and anterior decompression is required.

Spinal instability can affect the cervical spine, as well as the dorsal or lumbar spine and anterior and/or posterior spinal stabilisation may be required for the cervical spine (Fidler 1987). Minor degrees of cervical instability can usually be controlled by a surgical collar.

Twenty-nine of our patients with instability of their dorsal or lumbar spine had an associated neurological deficit. These patients did not present because of the spinal cord or cauda equina compression. They presented with pain due to spinal instability, but evidence of cord or cauda equina compression was found on clinical examination. We routinely carry out a radiculogram prior to spinal stabilisation, and this is usually accompanied by CT scanning. MRI is an alternative form of investigation. Irrespective of any clinical evidence of cord/cauda equina compression, the cord/cauda equina is decompressed at the time of stabilisation if there is any evidence of compression on the pre-operative radiological investigations. Both laminae and the spinous process are removed as the Banks' rod or Hartshill rectangle provides sufficient stability. Twenty of the patients obtained significant recovery (Fig. 11.4), 2 of whom developed recurrent signs of cord compression months later. Eleven of the 17 patients reported by DeWald et al. (1985) had an associated neurological deficit. Five of these obtained significant recovery following spinal decompression and stabilisation.

As with pathological fractures of the long bones, post-operative irradiation is an essential part of treatment. Pre-operative irradiation is to be avoided, as it may be associated with delayed wound healing, wound breakdown and infection. The sensitivity of the spinal cord to radiation limits the amount of radiotherapy that can be given to the spinal column and if the patient has had previous radiotherapy further treatment might not be possible, because of the risk of post-irradiation transverse myelitis.

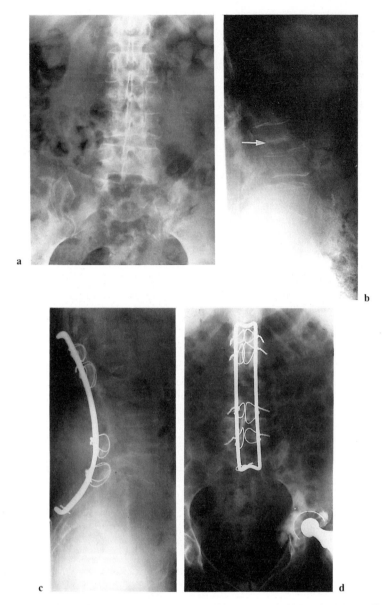

Fig. 11.3.a–d. Patient with mammary carcinoma who presented with spinal instability. She previously had had a left total hip replacement for a transcervical fracture. **a,b** AP and lateral radiographs of her lumbar spine showing complete destruction of L3. (arrow) **c,d** She has been stabilised with a Hartshill rectangle fixed to two vertebrae above, and L4, L5 and the sacrum below. Note the lordosis which has been moulded into the Hartshill rectangle to allow her sitting balance.

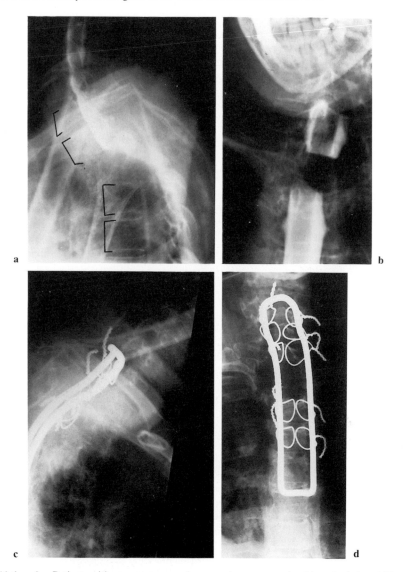

Fig. 11.4.a–d. Patient with mammary carcinoma who presented with spinal instability. On admission to hospital she was paraplegic and had urinary retention of 8-h duration. **a** Lateral radiograph. D3 is destroyed and D2 is subluxed forwards. The anterior borders of the vertebral bodies have been inked in. **b** A myelogram showing a complete block at the level of the lesion. **c,d** She was treated by posterior decompression and stabilisation using a Hartshill rectangle. The subluxation of the spine has been corrected. The patient regained bladder control and most of her motor function, such that she was able to walk out of hospital 6 weeks after surgery.

Compression of the Spinal Cord or Cauda Equina

Compression of the spinal cord or cauda equina may occur in association with spinal instability (where the treatment of choice is decompression, spinal stabilisation and post-operative radiotherapy) or in isolation. In the latter circumstance the choice of treatment (surgical decompression or radiotherapy, combined with high dosage steroids) depends on the duration of the symptoms. The early symptoms include weakness, disturbance of gait, paraesthesiae, urinary hesitancy or precipitancy and constipation or spurious diarrhoea. Persisting and increasing back pain may herald spinal cord compression. The sequence of events is often pain, motor dysfunction, paraesthesiae and sensory loss. Pin prick and deep pain sensation may be retained until late. Schaberg and Gainor (1985) reported that cord compression occurred in 20% of patients with vertebral metastases.

Decompression is urgent. Surgical decompression is indicated in patients with recent onset of symptoms, particularly a developing paraplegia, or a urinary retention of less than 24–30-h duration; a block (shown on the pre-operative radiculogram) localised to no more than 2 or 3 segments; and in a patient with a life expectancy of at least several weeks. Once the paraplegia has been established for several days, or urinary retention has been present for more than 30 hours, surgical decompression is often associated with some return of sensation and pain relief, but recovery of bladder and motor function is rare. Under these circumstances irradiation is indicated as is the case with more extensive blocks, but if the patient has associated spinal instability (see above), spinal stabilisation is essential to ease the pain from the latter. Because of the risk of subsequent instability the spine must be stabilised at the time of decompression (Johnson et al. 1983; Kostuik 1983; Siegal and Siegal 1985; Galasko 1986).

It has been suggested that surgical decompression has no advantage over radiotherapy. Findlay (1984) found that radiotherapy and steroids were at least as effective as laminectomy and Cobb et al. (1977) found no significant difference in outcome between patients treated initially by laminectomy and those treated by radiotherapy. In order to minimise the oedema high dosage corticosteroids should be given, the dose being gradually decreased (Merrin et al. 1976; Johnson et al. 1983; Kostuik 1983; Siegal and Siegal 1985; Galasko 1986).

The result of treatment seems also to be related to the rapidity of onset of the neurological symptoms. Patients with slowly developing weakness and bladder dysfunction usually obtain a better result than patients whose paraplegia and loss of bladder function has occurred over a matter of hours.

Non-metastatic Orthopaedic Conditions in Patients with Malignant Disease

Patients with malignant disease may develop benign disorders of the skeleton which may mimic metastases, must be differentiated from metastatic disease and should be treated on their merits. Like any individual they may sustain a traumatic fracture (see above). Galasko and Sylvester (1978) found that a benign lesion was responsible for the back pain that developed in 11 of 31 consecutive patients with an underlying malignant disease. The benign conditions included spondylolisthesis, prolapsed disc, pyogenic spondylitis, degenerative spondylosis, and osteoporotic fractures. I have treated 4 patients with a prolapsed intervertebral disc confirmed by radiculography, and a history of malignancy. In 1 patient the symptoms settled with conservative treatment; 3 patients required surgical excision of the disc. In 3 patients (including the patient who responded to conservative treatment) there was no evidence of metastatic disease and 2 years after treatment the patients were still free from metastases, whereas the fourth patient had disseminated carcinoma. Nevertheless, it was felt that surgical excision of the disc was warranted in view of her severe symptoms to improve the quality of her remaining life. This patient was alive and asymptomatic 1 year later.

Painful osteoarthritis may occur in patients with malignancy. In some patients it may be secondary to avascular necrosis of the femoral or humeral head as a result of irradiation and steroids. If the symptoms warrant it, replacement arthroplasty is indicated even in the presence of disseminated carcinoma (Galasko 1986).

References

Bonarigo BC, Rubin P (1967) Non-union of pathologic fracture after radiation therapy. Radiology 88:889–898

Bouma WH, Mulder JH, Hop WCJ (1983) The influence of intramedullary nailing upon the development of metastases in the treatment of an impending pathological fracture: an experimental study. Clin Exp Metastasis 1:205–212

Cobb CA III, Leavens ME, Eckles N (1977) Indications for nonoperative treatment of spinal cord compression due to breast cancer. J Neurosurg 47:653–658

DeWald RL, Bridwell KH, Prodromas C, Rodts MF (1985) Reconstructive spinal surgery as palliation for metastatic malignancies. Spine 10:21–26

Edelstyn GA, Gillespie PJ, Grebbel FS (1967) The radiological demonstration of osseous metastases. Experimental observations. Clin Radiol 18:158–162

Fidler M (1981) Incidence of fracture through metastases in long bones. Acta Orthop Scand 52:623–627

Fidler MW (1987) Pathological fractures of the spine including those causing anterior spinal cord compression: surgical management. In: Noble J, Galasko CSB (eds). Recent developments in orthopaedic surgery: Festschrift to Sir Harry Platt. Manchester University Press, Manchester, pp 94–103

Findlay GFG (1984) Adverse effects of the management of malignant spinal cord compression. J Neurol Neurosurg Psychiatry 47:761–768

Gainor BJ, Buchert P (1983) Fracture healing in metastatic bone disease. Clin Orthop 178:297–302

Galasko CSB (1972) Skeletal metastases and mammary cancer. Ann R Coll Surg Engl 50:3–28

Galasko CSB (1974) Pathological fractures secondary to metastatic cancer. J R Coll Surg Edinb 19:351–362

Galasko CSB (1980) The management of skeletal metastases. J R Coll Surg Edinb 25:143–161

Galasko CSB (1986) Skeletal metastases. Butterworths, London

Galasko CSB, Burn JI (1971) Hypercalcaemia in patients with advanced mammary cancer. Br Med J iii:573–577

Galasko CSB, Sylvester BS (1978) Back pain in patients treated for malignant tumours. Clin Oncol 4:273–283

Harrington KD (1981) The management of acetabular insufficiency secondary to metastatic malignant disease. J Bone Joint Surg [Am] 63:653–684

Johnson JR, Leatherman KD, Holt RT (1983) Anterior decompression of the spinal cord for neurological deficit. Spine 8:396–405

Kostuik JP (1983) Anterior spinal cord decompression for lesions of the thoracic and lumbar spine, techniques, new methods of internal fixation results. Spine 8:512–531

Kunec JR, Lewis RJ (1984) Closed intramedullary rodding of pathologic fractures with supplemental cement. Clin Orthop 188:183–186

Lodwick GS (1964) Reactive response to local injury in bone. Radiol Clin North Am 2:209–219

Lodwick GS (1965) A systematic approach to the roentgen diagnosis of bone tumours. In: Tumours of bone and soft tissue, Year Book Pub, Chicago, pp 49–68

McCormack RR Jr, Glass DB, Lane JM (1985) Functional cast bracing of metastatic humeral shaft lesion. Orthop Trans 9:50–51

Merrin C, Avellanosa A, West C, Wajsman Z, Baumgartner G (1976) The value of palliative spinal surgery in metastatic urogenital tumours. J Urol 115:712–713

Schaberg J, Gainor BJ (1985) A profile of metastatic carcinoma of the spine. Spine 10:19–20

Siegal T, Siegal T (1985) Vertebral body resection for epidural compression by malignant tumours. Results of forty-seven consecutive operative procedures. J Bone Joint Surg [Am] 67:375–382

12 Symptomatic and Supportive Care

C. Terrell and J.R. Wedley

Introduction

Some symptoms, such as general weakness, poor appetite and weight loss, that patients experience when they have widespread cancer with soft tissue spread will also be present in patients who have bone metastases. In this chapter, however, the main focus will be on those symptoms more particularly caused by the bone involvement itself such as bone pain, poor mobility or anaemia, and the psychological support needed by such patients.

The treatment of bone pain is discussed in depth as there are very particular measures which can be taken for its control in addition to the biochemical or hormonal means covered in previous chapters.

The control of pain from bone metastases presents two major clinical problems. The pain from widespread metastatic disease requires the systemic administration of analgesic drugs, whereas a solitary metastasis may lead to collapse of bone and instability giving rise to excruciating pain on movement, "incident pain", which will require specific treatment.

The hospice movement has not only taught the value of treating the patients' symptoms in the context of their psychological, physical, social and economic consequences, but has also taught two major lessons in the use of drugs to control malignant pain. The first is that analgesic agents are most effective when given regularly to maintain a constant blood level and the second is that for the vast majority of patients the oral route of administration is the simplest and most convenient.

The Use of Drugs to Control Pain from Bone Metastases

Opiate Analgesia

In 90% of patients the pain due to cancer can be adequately controlled by the regular use of oral morphine or its analogues. Despite this, pain was found to be uncontrolled in 35% of patients dying of cancer in the United Kingdom (Wilkes 1984).

The World Health Organization (WHO) regards cancer pain relief as a priority area (Stjernswärd 1985). It has advocated an analgesic ladder where specific analgesic drugs with or without adjuvants are given in increasing strength. Step 1 requires the administration of simple non-opioid analgesic such as aspirin or paracetamol; in Step 2 weak opioids such as codeine or dextropropoxyphene are administered and Step 3 requires the use of morphine or another strong opioid. The efficacy of these guidelines has been demonstrated worldwide (Walker et al. 1988; Toscani and Carini 1989; Vijayaram et al. 1989; Schug et al. 1990).

The administrative framework does not always exist in developing countries to make morphine legally available; however, problems of availability can also arise in Western urban environments where pharmacists may be reluctant to stock opiates for security reasons (Kanner and Portenoy 1986). Side-effects from regular oral opiate administration (e.g., nausea, vomiting and drowsiness) are only common when blood levels are changing, but once a constant level is reached they usually settle down in 48 h. Good analgesia with minimal side-effects can, however, only be achieved where there is an accurate titration of dosage (Ventafridda et al. 1987; McGuire et al. 1987).

The oral route obviates the need for injections, is cheaper and enhances patient independance (Twycross 1988). The local effect on opiate receptors in the gut, however, decreases mobility causing constipation and a laxative is, therefore, almost always necessary. Oral morphine is usually given as an aqueous preparation of morphine sulphate. In Britain, a commercial preparation (Oramorph oral solution produced by Boehringer Ingelheim) is available in two concentrations (10 mg/5 ml and 20 mg/ml). Diamorphine is also available in Britain as a small 10 mg tablet. Diamorphine is essentially a pro-drug for morphine (Twycross and Lack 1983). It is rapidly degraded to 6-monoacetylmorphine and thence to morphine itself. It therefore has no pharmacological advantage over morphine, but the tablets may be more convenient to store and transport than heavy bottles of liquid. Diamorphine is extremely soluble and large numbers of tablets can be dissolved in small volumes of water immediately prior to administration.

Most patients with bone pain will respond well to conventional analgesics titrating from paracetamol, to coproxamol and to morphine (Hanks 1988). There are frequent suggestions in the literature that morphine and related drugs are ineffective in bone pain: this is not true. Fears of respiratory depression or addiction with oral morphine are unfounded. Nausea and vomiting are not uncommon and are usually easily controlled with a suitable anti-emetic. When control is difficult, hypercalcaemia should be considered (see Chap. 8). Where no other cause can be found and nausea and vomiting are intractable another route of administration may be necessary (Rogers 1988). Drowsiness may be a problem at the start of treatment but usually resolves within a few days. Occasionally a small dose of amphetamine may be useful when drowsiness persists (Bruera et al. 1989).

The dose of oral morphine or diamorphine must be adjusted to the needs of each individual patient. Doses of 5–200 mg 4 hourly are common and higher doses may be required. There is no arbitrary maximum (Hanks 1988). There are other mu-agonists which provide suitable alternatives to oral morphine and diamorphine. Oral preparations of oxycodone and hydromorphone are available in the USA. In Britain, phenazocine and methadone are available as oral preparations: phenazocine 5 mg $\equiv$ 20–25 mg morphine (Twycross 1988); methadone 1mg $\equiv$ 4–9 mg morphine (Ventafridda et al. 1986a).

Dextromoramide is a short-acting mu-agonist. Its duration of action is only 2 h and this makes it unsuitable for maintenance therapy; however, because of its rapid onset of action it can be extremely useful for breakthrough pain, prior to painful procedures and for incident pain.

Oral pethidine has no place in the treatment of chronic pain. It is only weakly effective when taken by mouth due to the fact that 50% of it is eliminated pre-systemically on first pass through the liver and converted to norpethidine. Norpethidine is an active metabolite which causes central nervous system excitation and is cumulative due to its long plasma half-life, 14–21 h; whereas the short plasma half-life of pethidine (3–7 h) means that orally it only provides weak analgesia for approximately 3 h. The danger of CNS toxicity from norpethidine is increased in patients with poor renal function (Inturrisi and Umans 1983).

In the last decade the availability of a controlled release form of oral morphine (MST Continus in the UK and MS Contin in the USA) has proven to be valuable. It is usually easier and quicker to stabilise patients who present with severe pain on a 4-hourly oral liquid morphine regimen and transfer to a 12-hourly regimen of controlled release morphine at a similar daily dose. Controlled release morphine has proven to be equally effective as liquid morphine with few side-effects (Brescia et al. 1987; Savarese et al. 1987; Ventafridda et al. 1989). A small proportion of patients (5%–10%) may require an 8-hourly regimen. Slow-release morphine has less appeal than liquid morphine as a drug of abuse and is more willingly stocked by inner-city pharmacists.

Buprenorphine is a partial agonist at the mu-receptor. The powerful agonist effects are almost balanced by its powerful antagonist characteristics (Budd 1983). It has self-limiting opiate effects showing an analgesic plateau at less than maximum effect. It only rarely causes psychotomimetic side-effects and has a very low dependence liability. It has considerably less respiratory depressant effect than morphine and can be used to reverse the respiratory depressant effects of opiate overdose without reversing all of the analgesia. The antagonistic effects to morphine are only seen in very high doses and, in the therapeutic range (0.2 mg tds–0.9 mg qds), the analgesic effects are summative. Because of its high first-pass metabolism it needs to be given sublingually or parenterally. Sublingual absorption is slow and despite its high lipid solubility it has sluggish receptor kinetics with high affinity to the receptor site. When given sublingually, therefore, it has a slow onset but long duration of action (6–8 h). This makes the sublingual route unsuitable for breakthrough pain, but it is useful in patients who cannot swallow or who vomit oral drugs. It is little appreciated by clinicians that all of the opiates, including morphine itself, are well absorbed by the sublingual and buccal mucosa. They are also well absorbed by the respiratory mucosa and nebulised opiates can be used clinically to relieve cancer pain (Masters et al. 1985).

Another route of administration, avoiding injections in patients who cannot take oral drugs, is rectal administration. In Britain morphine suppositories (15 mg) and oxycodone suppositories (30 mg) are available. In the USA morphine

(5, 10 and 20 mg), hydromorphone (3 mg) and oxymorphone (5 mg) suppositories are available (Rogers 1986).

The development of small, battery-driven infusion pumps has allowed the continuous infusion of opiates in ambulant patients who cannot take oral therapy. Subcutaneous infusion is safer than intravenous infusion and just as effective (Miser et al. 1986; Ventafridda et al. 1986b; Rogers 1987). Morphine and diamorphine are the commonest drugs to be given by this route, but buprenorphine has also been used successfully (Noda et al. 1989). In the UK diamorphine is considered the narcotic of choice for subcutaneous infusions because of its solubility; 1 g dissolving in 1.6 ml of water to give a final volume of 2.4 ml (Hanks and Hoskin 1987). In comparison, 1 g of morphine sulphate cannot be dissolved in less than 20–25 ml. In the USA, where diamorphine is not available, hydromorphine 10 mg/ml (Dilaudid-HP) can be used instead of morphine if the volume to be administered becomes too large (Twycross 1988). Metoclopramide, methotrimeprazine or haloperidol may be added to the pump to control both pain and nausea (Storey et al. 1990). Seizures can be controlled by the addition of phenobarbitone or midazolam. Atropine or hyoscine can be added to control bronchial secretions and intestinal colic. Mixing of drugs in this way can lead to precipitation, with subsequent chemical irritation and inflammation. Problems may arise even when opiates alone are used (Adams et al. 1989).

Programmable infusion pumps are now available which enable patients to control their own analgesia within pre-set limits with or without a background infusion (Barkas and Duafala 1988). In their most sophisticated form these pumps are completely implantable; however, in this form they are extremely expensive and their use is usually reserved to deliver opiates either epidurally or intrathecally. The rationale for this is to deliver the drug directly to the opiate receptors in the dorsal horn. The opiate receptor block so produced will be segmental. It can be seen, therefore, that this mode of delivery is for the treatment of pain which is intractable and confined to a few segments. The more segments involved the greater the volume required to produce adequate spread in the epidural space and the less suitable this method becomes for a continuous portable infusion pump where the capacity is limited. This problem may be overcome in two ways, either by injecting a larger volume bolus into a subcutaneous epidural implantable reservoir once or twice daily or by placing the catheter intrathecally and injecting the same amount of drug in a small volume into the cerebrospinal fluid where it can spread more easily to reach the required area. Only preservative-free opiates must be used for epidural and intrathecal injection. Once again, diamorphine which is presented as a preservative-free powder, has an advantage over the usual commercial preparations of morphine, which contain preservative. The more lypophylic opiates such as diamorphine, buprenorphine and fentanyl will reach the receptor sites in the spinal cord more easily (the commercial preparations of buprenorphine and fentanyl do not contain preservative and are safe to use). The long-term use of epidural implantable reservoirs (Waldman et al. 1986) and the safety of epidural morphine in the treatment of cancer pain is well established (Driessen et al. 1989; Chabal et al. 1989). The dose of opiate required intrathecally is about 10% of that required epidurally for the same analgesic response (Nitescu et al. 1986). If tolerance occurs, sensitivity can be restored by producing a local anaesthetic epidural or spinal block for 48 h. The permanent addition of a local anaesthetic to the opiate spinal infusion may lower the opioid requirement and retard the development of tolerance. It may produce adequate analgesia where epidural opiates alone have failed (Ullman and Quarmby 1989; Nitescu et al. 1990).

The addition of noradrenaline to epidural morphine will reduce the dose requirement where tolerance has occurred (Stein and Brechner 1987). Noradrenaline binds on to the alpha$_2$-receptors in the spinal cord producing spinal analgesia, as will clonidine which may also be useful in this context. The long-term use of intrathecal morphine has been shown to be safe and effective (Madrid et al. 1988) and special fine catheters with low volume subcutaneously implantable reservoirs are now commercially available for this purpose. Hardy and Wells (1990) have used a patient-controlled on-demand delivery system to determine patients' 24-h requirement and subsequent bolus doses.

Steroids and Non-steroidal Anti-inflammatory Drugs

Pain caused by bone metastases is often only partially opioid-responsive. Response to non-steroidal anti-inflammatory drugs (NSAIDs) is variable. They sometimes work very well either alone or together with an opioid for metastatic bone pain; sufficiently well to justify their routine use. Rapidly growing tumours in bone cause distension of the periosteum and an increase in interosseous pressure, activating pressure-sensitive nerves and giving rise to pain. Radiotherapy and chemotherapy may shrink the tumours and relieve pain, but when it persists (or before treatments take effect) both steroids and NSAIDs may give symptomatic relief.

The margins of rapidly growing tumours show inflammatory activity. This involves the release of chemical mediators which provoke pain directly and the breakdown of arachidonic acid to prostaglandins and leukotrienes. Prostaglandins (in particular E_2 and I_2) cause vasodilatation and oedema and further increase pressure in the tissue. The extravasated oedema fluid contains the chemical mediators (histamine, 5-hydroxyhistamine, acetylcholine, bradykinin, angiotensin and potassium ions), all of which produce pain by acting directly on afferent nerve endings, which are sensitised to these mediators by prostaglandins. The formation of prostaglandins is, in turn, stimulated by bradykinin, Prostaglandins also have a central role in pain perception, facilitating the passage of noxious afferent stimuli in both the brain and the dorsal horn. Arachidonic acid is stored bound to cell membrane phospholipids. It is released by the enzyme phospholipase A_2. Cycloxygenase breaks down arachidonic acid to form prostaglandins and 5-lipoxygenase breaks it down to form the leukotrienes. Leukotrienes are also involved in pain perception, causing hyperalgesia when they interact with polymorphonuclear leucocytes, but the complete role is far from clearly understood. Apart from the prostaglandins and leukotrienes, other hydroperoxides are formed, which also mediate pain.

Corticosteroids block phospholipase A_2 and inhibit the production of arachidonic acid, whereas NSAIDs block cyclo-oxygenase and only inhibit the production of prostaglandins. The effects of corticosteroids are, therefore, more widespread. Prednisolone is often used as a primary therapeutic agent as part of a chemotherapy regimen. Patients with severe bone pain or nerve compression pain may respond dramatically to corticosteroids in high doses (prednisolone up to 20 mg qds or dexamethasone up to 4 mg qds). Dexamethasone has less mineralocorticoid effect and, therefore, less tendency to cause salt and water retention leading to oedema and weight gain (Hanks et al. 1983). The analgesic effects of corticosteroids in prolonged administration are often no greater than those of NSAIDs. The reason for this is unclear, but there is some controversy about the extent to which corticosteroids inhibit phospholipase A_2 in vivo (Bennett et al. 1987).

NSAIDs, similarly, sometimes work very well either alone or together with an opiate for metastatic bone pain, but often do not. The reason for this variation in response is uncertain. Perhaps the stimulation by pain mediators may be so great that potentiation by prostaglandins is not possible. Alternatively, the inhibition of prostaglandin formation may divert the metabolism of prostaglandin precursors into analgesic lipoxygenase products (leukotrienes). A trial of NSAIDs is, however, always worth while, changing once or twice to alternative agents if no response is obtained.

NSAIDs can damage gastrointestinal mucosa and impair renal function in some patients. Both effects are mainly related to prostaglandin synthesis. Prostaglandins have a gastric mucosal "cytoprotective" effect which may be impaired by inhibition of prostaglandin synthesis, and inhibition of prostacyclin production may lead to some degree of gastric mucosal ischaemia (Hanks 1988).

Misoprostol (Cytotec) is a synthetic analogue of prostaglandin E_1 (alprostadil) which inhibits gastric acid secretion. It has been newly introduced for the treatment of gastric and duodenal ulceration and for the prophylaxis of NSAID-induced ulcers. Its success in this respect is still to be evaluated.

Rectal administration of NSAIDs avoids the direct irritant effect on gastro-duodenal mucosa, but does not reduce the systemic effects on the gastrointestinal tract. The co-prescription of an H_2-receptor blocker (cimetidine or ranitidine) may be beneficial, particularly in patients with a history of peptic ulceration.

The toxicity of NSAIDs with a long plasma elimination half-life (for the drug and active metabolite) is greater (Drug and Therapeutics Bulletin 1987). Half-lives vary widely between patients and tend to be longer in the elderly. Prolonged high concentrations of a drug in the tissues are likely to exacerbate any toxic effects. Short-acting drugs may allow some recovery between doses from the potentially damaging inhibition of prostaglandin synthesis at vulnerable sites. Sustained-release forms of NSAIDs may, therefore, present a greater risk but are useful in patients who require multiple drug therapy. The concomitant use of corticosteroids and NSAIDs raises the specific risk of "silent", painless gastric perforation.

Calcitonin

Calcitonin is a non-opioid peptide which is secreted by the parafollicular cells of the thyroid and has a hormonal role in the control of blood calcium levels, but also shows anti-nociceptive action. There are species differences in the structure of calcitonin and the anti-nociceptive action is most marked in salmon calcitonin (Candeletti and Terri 1990). It is claimed to have a specific analgesic effect against bone pain (Schiraldi et al. 1985) and to benefit especially those patients who experience pain on weight bearing (Hunton 1989). Its mode of analgesic action is poorly understood. Gennari et al. (1985a) suggested that the relief of bone pain was related to an increase in circulating β-endorphin levels. However, the analgesic effect is not reversible by naloxone at normal therapeutic dosage (Braga et al. 1978). Salmon calcitonin receptors have been demonstrated in the hypothalamus, brainstem and dorsal horns of the spinal cord (Candeletti and Terri 1990). Its effects are variable whatever route of administration is used. It crosses the blood–brain barrier poorly and does not easily enter the dura when given epidurally (Blanchard et al. 1990). Its central analgesic action when injected intracisternally is blocked by the simultaneous injection of calcium through the same route (Satoh et al. 1979). Its central analgesic effect may, therefore, be due to its lowering extracellular calcium. The lowering of calcium-ion concentrations may modify the sensitivity of some pain mediator–receptor interactions. A central analgesic action independent of opioid systems and possibly related to catecholaminergic pathways is supported by the use of salmon calcitonin to relieve phantom limb pain (Kessel and Wörz 1987).

However, Blanchard et al. (1990) have shown that its anti-nociceptive activity at spinal cord level is not related to substance P or calcium-ion movement. Pecile et al. (1975) ascribed the analgesic effect of calcitonin to the inhibition of the prostaglandin system at the level of cyclo-oxygenase, but Gennari (1983) failed to show any relationship between analgesia and serum calcium or circulating prostaglandin E levels.

Salmon calcitonin requires parenteral administration and there is a very high incidence of nausea and vomiting. It may be useful in patients with widespread bony metastases whose pain has failed to respond to opiates and NSAIDs, particularly if the serum calcium is raised.

Different dosage regimens have been tried. In Britain and Ireland a 2-day treatment pack is marketed by Rorer Pharmaceuticals (Calsynar).

Bisphosphonates

Etidronate disodium can be taken by mouth. It inhibits bone resorption and may offer benefit in pain from bone metastases. The effects of clodronate on bone pain have been compared to calcitonin (Gennari et al. 1985b) and it has been shown to relieve metastatic bone pain effectively in breast cancer (Elomaa et al. 1983). Doubts about its safety have, however, delayed its general release (see Chap. 7)

Dopamine Agonists and Antagonists

Phenothiazines are dopamine antagonists. They are sedative and anti-emetic. Only methotrimeprazine has been shown to have analgesic activity (Hanks 1984). It is a useful adjuvant in opioid-intolerant patients, but sedation and orthostatic hypotension are limiting side-effects.

Levodopa has been reported to relieve metastatic bone pain (Dickey and Minton 1972; Minton et al. 1976). Prolactin is a major hormonal stimulant to the development of breast or prostatic cancer and levodopa suppresses prolactin release. Subsequent studies, however, have failed to show any benefit (Sjolin and Trykker 1985; Engelsman et al. 1975) and the case for dopamine agonists remains unproven.

Tricyclic Antidepressants

Tricyclic antidepressants block the re-uptake of serotonin (5-hydrox-ytryptamine, 5HT) and noradrenaline. They activate serotoninergic inhibitory pathways and potentiate opiate analgesia. They are widely used for non-malignant pain, particularly neuropathic pain. Amitriptyline has the best-documented analgesic actions (Couch et al. 1976; Watson et al. 1982; Max et al. 1987) but is also the least tolerated because of its anticholinergic effects (dry mouth, urinary retention). The analgesic effect seems to be independent of the effect on mood. It is seen at lower doses (25–150 mg/day for amitriptyline) and pain relief may occur in 48 h, whereas relief of depression takes 2–3 weeks. Amitriptyline produces sedation which is most marked in the first few days of administration. This can be used to advantage by giving a single dose at night, improving sleep and relieving anxiety. The potentiation of morphine can be utilised by prescribing amitriptyline in combination with an opiate (Richlin et al. 1987). Antidepressants which block serotonin re-uptake (clomipramine and amitriptyline) potentiate morphine-induced analgesia and relieve deafferenta-tion pain but those that block noradrenaline re-uptake (nortriptyline and trazadone) do not (Panerai et al. 1990). Serotonin re-uptake blockers increase β-endorphin concentrations in the brain areas of normal or deafferentated animals. They are particularly effective in the burning dysaesthetic or hyper-aesthetic pain associated with nerve destruction (e.g., brachial plexopathy) or post-herpetic neuralgia, which is common in immunosuppressed patients (Walsh 1989).

Anticonvulsants

Anticonvulsants are valuable in neuropathic and deafferentation pain (Swerd-low 1986). Carbamazepine, clonazepam, phenytoin and valproate have all been used successfully. The combination of an anticonvulsant and a tricyclic antidepressant is particularly effective.

Orthopaedic Surgical Treatment

Incident pain due to instability and neuropathic pain due to compression require orthopaedic intervention which is dealt with in the previous chapter. Supportive orthotic devices are useful to patients with movement-related or incident pain.

Radiotherapy

Radiotherapy remains the treatment of choice if there is a well-localised bony lesion which is painful, where fracture is likely or has occurred and been fixed, or if there is imminent or recent collapse of vertebrae causing symptoms or signs of spinal cord compression. Hemibody irradiation for multiple metastases has also been covered in the chapter on radiotherapy. Unfortunately, access to a radiotherapy centre at a long distance from an ill person may make hemibody irradiation impractical, but the use of single or few fractions of treatment involving fewer journeys can make it more tolerable for patients and should always be considered.

Transcutaneous Nerve Stimulation

Radicular or neuropathic pain can occur as a result of direct tumour invasion of nervous tissue, as a result of compression due to vertebral collapse or bony fracture, or secondary to chemotherapy or radiotherapy. Transcutaneous nerve stimulation (TNS or TCNS) may be helpful when the pain is confined to the distribution of one or two discrete nerve roots or groups of nerves. Originally devised after the theories of Melzack and Wall (1965) to stimulate large myelinated fibres and close the "gate" in the dorsal horn to noxious C-fibre input, it is now known to produce complex biochemical changes and to activate the long loop inhibitory serotoninergic pathways depending on the frequency and pattern of stimulation used (Thompson 1988). It is not possible to place electrodes on skin where radiotherapy is concurrently taking place or has recently done so, but relief may be obtained by placing electrodes above or below the segmental level on the same side or at the same segmental level on the opposite side of the body.

Acupuncture

Many physiotherapists now use acupuncture as a standard technique and it may be helpful in metastatic bone pain. Filshie (1988) has reviewed the sparse literature on its use for pain of malignant origin.

Intercostal Nerve Block

Chemical neurolysis of peripheral somatic nerves does not usually provide long-lasting relief in cancer patients (Swerdlow 1990). Intercostal nerve blocks, however, are useful in pain due to rib metastases (Wedley 1989). A diagnostic block with the long-acting local anaesthetic bupivacaine should be performed first to establish the level and effectiveness of the block. A "permanent" block can be performed by injecting phenol (5% in glycerine or 6% in water). If nerve destruction is incomplete neuritis may develop weeks to months after the block, and, even if complete, anaesthesia dolorosa (deafferentation pain in a numb area) may subsequently develop. Neurolytic block should, therefore, be confined to patients with a limited life expectancy.

Paravertebral Block

The advantage of this block is its simplicity as it only requires the skill to perform a lumbar puncture. In the past, neurolytic procedures were performed in patients with cancer and a limited life expectancy in a manner that is no longer considered acceptable. The same standards of care should apply to all patients. Dr. Sampson Lipton no longer considers that this block should be done without x-ray screening and the use of contrast medium to determine the spread of the neurolytic solution (personal communication). This block is useful for pain confined to a single or few dermatomes where numbness is acceptable in exchange for pain relief. The patient is positioned so that the neurolytic solution is deposited on the posterior spinal sensory root at the level of the painful dermatome. This can be done most accurately with a hyperbaric solution of phenol (5% in glycerine). A lumbar puncture is performed at the appropriate level with a 19-gauge spinal needle. The patient is positioned painful-side down and rolled 45° toward the supine position. Injection should only take place when there is free flow of cerebrospinal fluid and only small volumes (0.5–1 ml) are used. If the patient is unable to lie on the painful side, alcohol (95%) may be injected with the painful side uppermost and the patient rolled 45% towards the prone position. The alcohol will float on the cerebrospinal fluid and tends to spread more than phenol in glycerine. The patient should be kept in the position in which the injection was performed for at least 30 min afterwards. Pain involving the lower sacral roots will involve the risk of neurolytic damage resulting in urinary and faecal incontinence. If bladder and bowel function are intact at the time of injection every effort should be made to localise the block to one side by appropriate positioning (Maher and Mehta 1977).

Dorsal Root Ganglion Rhizolysis

A radiofrequency temperature-controlled lesion to destroy only the sensory fibres in the dorsal root ganglion may be employed where vertebral collapse causes compression of a single root; however, the distortion of anatomy so produced can make the procedure technically difficult.

Percutaneous Cervical Cordotomy

The elegant technique of percutaneous cervical cordotomy involves a radiofrequency lesion of the antero-lateral tract in the upper cervical region. The awake cooperation of the patient is essential. Analgesia is produced in the opposite side of the body to the lesion. Dysaesthetic deafferentation pain will develop some months after the lesion in the distribution affected. The complication rate (sphincter disturbance, motor weakness and damage to the respiratory centre) is much higher following bilateral cordotomy. Ideally, then, this procedure is most useful in patients with unilateral pain in the lower half of the body who have a limited life expectancy. This restricts its usefulness in patients with widespread bony metastases who may live for many years.

Pituitary Alcohol Injection

Alcohol injection of the pituitary was originally performed to produce chemical hypophysectomy in women with carcinoma of the breast and bony metastases. It was quickly realised that excellent analgesia was produced which was not related to the loss of pituitary function. The high success rate (75%–90%) has been confirmed in several studies (Morrica 1977; Miles 1984; Waldman et al. 1987) in many cancers, with breast and prostate being the most common. The reason for the analgesia produced in unclear. It is not related to loss of hormonal function nor does it appear to be due to spread of the alcohol to the hypothalamus. Both freezing (Duthie 1983) and electrically stimulating the pituitary (Yanagida et al. 1988) seem to relieve cancer pain effectively. The risk of alcohol injection is that spread to the adjacent optic chiasma may result in visual field impairment. In order to eliminate this risk we have measured visual evoked responses during pituitary alcohol injection at Guy's Hospital since 1984. We have restricted the volume injected to 1 ml and have stopped if there was any change in latency or amplitude of the visual evoked response which did not recover within a few minutes. We have seen no optic sequelae but in such a small personal series it is impossible to claim effective elimination of risk, which is only 2 out of 250 cases in the Liverpool series reported by Miles (1984). Despite the presence of the Hedley Atkins Breast Unit at Guy's Hospital we are only called upon to perform pituitary alcohol injection 2 or 3 times a year for patients whose pain cannot be controlled by other means. Dr. Sampson Lipton reports (personal communication) that since the drug Zoladex (an LHRH analogue) became available very few pituitary alcohol injections are performed in Liverpool.

The Place of the Support Team

Analgesic drugs are the foundation of management in active patients with cancer although it can still be argued that the early use of nerve blocks improves the quality of life. (Baines 1989; Lipton 1989). The fact that so few patients require nerve blocks is a reflection of the success of both hospital- and community-based support teams who are able to advise on treatment, and support the patients with cancer and their families.

Much of the treatment and support needed will depend on the prognosis. Most treatment should be palliative where the prognosis is poor. The outlook for patients once bone involvement is detected will differ considerably for those with carcinoma of the bronchus, who will have a very limited life span, to those with spread in carcinoma of the breast or prostate where either hormonal manipulation or chemotherapy may be well justified as their outlook may be measured in years.

In most of these situations much of the patient's time will be spent outside the hospital, at home or even at work, before the onset of the terminal phase of their disease. The multidisciplinary support teams are in a good position to enhance the quality of life for both patient and carers in collaboration with the primary health care team, and to form a bridge of communication between them and the hospital. Ideally they will then already know the patient and family when life is nearing its end, and can continue to give support and enable death to take place at home, if appropriate, or arrange admission to hospital or hospice in a planned way. This final phase, including the preparation for bereavement of the patient's relatives, will not be emphasised in this chapter as terminal care will not be substantially different for patients with bone metastases from those with other forms of cancer.

There are various members who make up a multidisciplinary support team depending on location, financial support and attitudes, to advise the patient, family and professional carers over their stress and symptoms, whether in hospital or at home. All members offer specific practical help according to their own discipline, but the aim of all is the same, to ensure the patient is pain-free and independent, in order to retain self-respect and self-care and to feel a worthwhile member of society for as long as possible. They often enable the patient to stay at home for a longer time.

The psychological help given to patients and their relatives is not the prerogative of any one discipline but tends to overlap considerably between members of a team. Many people who specialise in this work see this side as the more interesting and it is, therefore, important to have regular team meetings to share this information and to allow those members who are particularly gifted in their communicative skills to contribute. Although it is often regarded as the field of the social worker it can frequently happen that the physiotherapist or the nurse who visits regularly may be the person to whom many anxieties are confided, and it is important that they should be in a position to give support.

Practical Support Offered in the UK by Individual Members of a Team for Patients with Bone Metastases

The Clinical Nurse Specialist

This member of the team is likely to be the person who has most contact with the patient and is, therefore, in a good position to monitor the effectiveness of analgesia for bone pain. With use of pain charts and diagrams as well as by direct questioning about the pain and observation of the patient's expression and activity, it should be possible to determine an optimal level of analgesia. Initially a daily visit may be necessary to titrate drug effectiveness and dose, but quite often visits can become less frequent unless the patient is obviously going down-hill in other ways. The nurse will enquire about other symptoms; nausea, if the patient is suspected of being hypercalcaemic; constipation, if the intake of opioids is rising; indigestion if the patient is on non-steroidal drugs; and, in regard to general well-being, other symptoms relevant to that particular cancer. The nurse is in regular contact with relatives and carers and has the opportunity to educate them about the disease and the causes of pain as well as encouraging a suitable diet. Sadly, relatives often feel that large meals will strengthen bones and muscles, and these may be rejected by the patient. Smaller, more attractive snacks or high calorie foods may often be more appropriate. Another practical duty of the clinical nurse specialist is to be in regular contact with the General Practitioner in order to discuss alterations or make suggestions about the drugs being used, and with the district nurses if they are also visiting.

The Doctor

The doctor will also monitor the analgesia and may suggest alterations in the drugs used or the route by which they are given. Regular medical examination is as vital where palliative treatment may be indicated as at other times during the more active phase of treatment. When bone metastases are known to be present a keen eye must be kept open to pick up a potential fracture or an imminent vertebral collapse so that immediate treatment can be instituted (Closs and Bates 1987). To allow a patient to become wheelchair or bed-bound unnecessarily adds a burden of great magnitude to both patient and relatives.

Anaemia is common when bone metastases are extensive. However, if a patient is inactive it may not produce symptoms, and in this case should not be treated by transfusion. But if symptoms, such as drowsiness or palpitations, appear to be due directly to low haemoglobin then transfusion may be beneficial, particularly if the level is below 8 g (Doyle 1987). An initial transfusion may improve matters, but repeated transfusions may become less effective. Patients and relatives may become distressed when what they regard as their "lifeline" is withheld, and it is on these occasions that careful explanation and discussion can prevent unnecessary upset and admission to hospital.

Nausea may occur in some patients with hypercalcaemia but is not necessarily related to the calcium level. Similarly there is no clear relationship between the extent of bone involvement and the occurrence of hypercalcaemia (Regnard 1985). If nausea is due to a raised calcium level, specific treatment as outlined in the chapter on hypercalcaemia can be undertaken (Chap. 8). As this may lead to repeated admissions to hospital for intravenous therapy it may become unacceptable, and symptomatic treatment will be needed. Encouraging a high intake of fluids and administering regular steroids, once the calcium is normal, may reduce the nausea. Routine anti-emetics are often given but are of limited value.

The Physiotherapist

Once bone metastases are present physiotherapy has to be undertaken with a realistic goal in mind. It relies on good pain control having been achieved before it can be initiated, as there is no place in this situation for a pain barrier to be overcome (O'Gorman B (1987) unpublished paper, Physiotherapy in a hospice setting. Presented at the Physiotherapy conference, St Christopher's Hospice, London). If a patient is in bed, passive exercises should start as soon as possible in order to prevent deformities; joints should be mobilised to avoid increasing stiffness, while massage can relieve muscle spasm. Nurses and relatives can be taught to continue these procedures when the physiotherapist is not there. Positioning in bed or in a chair is also important, and such aids as collars, slings, bed cradles and transfer aids may be of assistance.

When mobilisation is possible, following the pinning of a fracture or radiotherapy, active exercises should be started and gradually increased. With most patients it is better to allow them to discover their own capabilities rather then to impose restrictions. When a patient is starting to walk again parallel bars allow limited weight-bearing, and rollator walking frames are helpful for weak patients or where there are metastases causing pain in the upper limbs or back with difficulty in lifting. Where there are multiple rib metastases causing difficulty in expectorating postural drainage may be possible rather than more active methods.

The physiotherapist is also well placed to monitor the effectiveness of pain control, being able to see patients on a regular basis and to watch their increasing activities. At times it may be necessary for short-acting analgesics, such as palfium, to be given before activities involving walking or bathing. In addition a physiotherapist involved in this sort of work with a team will usually teach general relaxation which relieves anxiety and raises the pain threshold.

The Occupational Therapist

Although rehabilitation is the skill associated with occupational therapists, re-adaptation is possibly a wiser term to apply when assisting patients who are restricted by their bone disease and are unlikely to be cured. It eliminates misconceptions and unrealistic expectations of returning to former levels of function. The occupational therapist teaches the patient to develop strategies to cope with new situations as they arise and to tolerate advancing disease more easily (A. Rix, 1989, personal communication). The home visits to assess whether the patient and family are going to cope, and the practical aids that can be rapidly obtained when an occupational therapist is attached to a support team, are invaluable. Feeding aids, hand grips on walls, raised lavatory seats, bath seats, walking frames and, if necessary, wheelchairs, can increase the patient's independence and comfort both within the hospital and at home. In addition, an important part of the occupational therapist's role, particularly in the home, is to teach relatives how to move and wash patients with weakened bones who may also be in pain.

Treatment which includes purposeful activities, guided imagery, meditation and other forms of distraction, has been shown to increase pain tolerance in healthy subjects, and has also been successfully used with cancer patients in pain. Relaxation, using tapes if appropriate, also raises the pain threshold.

The Social Worker

This member of the support team is employed by the local authority, and is usually seconded either part- or full-time to work with the multidisciplinary team. The input from social workers is highly valued by patients and their carers and can enable some patients to remain at home with more security. Examples of the type of service which they organise are the installation of telephones with money provided from charitable sources, home helps to do the shopping and cleaning, and "meals on wheels" arranged through the local authority.

The social worker's knowledge of the statutory and voluntary services allow financial assistance to be sought. Two allowances in particular are likely to be appropriate for patients with increasing bone involvement. Firstly, the mobility allowance, which is available for patients who have difficulty in walking which has lasted for a year and need extra help with transport. Secondly, the attendance allowance where regular care is needed at home but which is payable only after six months' illness. The obligatory delays for payment of these allowances is at present (1989) under scrutiny by the Government as often, if the patient is terminally ill, the allowance is not available until the need for it has passed. Advice on making a will or settling personal affairs such as mortgage payments will relieve extra burdens from the patient and his family and reduce anxiety. Quite a high proportion of patients will be living alone, or being looked after by a single relative who may even be caring for young children at the same time (Lamerton 1980). The social worker can assist in these situations to a great extent by knowing the lines of contact for financial or practical help.

Psychological Morbidity

For the patient, the psychological impact of knowing the disease has spread to bones will vary depending on the symptoms produced, the pace of the disease with consequent prognosis, and the possibility, or otherwise, of future palliative treatment. In some patients with breast cancer many years may have elapsed since the primary cancer was treated, or the patient may be under active curative treatment at the time the metastases appear. In other cancers bone metastases may be detected at presentation, or the primary site may remain obscure even after investigation.

The impact of these situations is different. Cameron and Parkes showed that time was a mode of adjustment. If there is no prospect of curative treatment the future can be hard to face; if, however, hormone or chemotherapy can be offered for palliative management there is a prospect of longer survival and time for the patient to become adjusted to a possible fatal outcome. For families, too, the implication of bone spread is that the prognosis is limited and that they may have to face a bereavement. Awaiting results of bone scans can thus particularly enhance anxiety.

The question of prognosis is, therefore, one which is relevant and frequently requested. The accuracy of prediction of survival in later stages of cancer has been studied (Parkes 1972) where it was shown that 83% of professional carers were optimistic as regards prognosis when patients were admitted to a hospice; and it made no difference whether they were general practitioners, hospice doctors or ward sisters. Fifteen years later a further study was made after it was believed doctors had become more experienced in palliative care. This showed that there was no improvement in accuracy of estimation by any of the professionals and that over-optimism was still alive (Heyse-Moore and Johnson-Bell 1987).

Depression and anxiety have been studied in cases of advanced cancer although not specifically in those who have bone metastases; but as a high proportion of patients dying with cancer have bone involvement these studies will obviously include many such patients. However, it is important to recognise that depression can be helped by treatment. Many patients with advanced disease have somatic symptoms which mimic depression, such as anorexia, weight loss and fatigue. Their mood may vary during the course of the illness, and different methods have been used to assess the depression in different studies. These problems make interpretation and comparability difficult.

In Hinton's study (1972), carried out in hospital, about half the patients with cancer had suffered a depression of mood which increased as the illness lengthened and if physical discomfort persisted. Significantly, those patients free from physical discomfort were rarely depressed. His nursing staff observed that 13% of patients were obviously anxious, but Hinton himself found that the figure for those who had frequent periods of distressing fear was nearer 25%. This was enhanced in patients with difficulty in breathing.

A study by Plumb and Holland (1977) tried to differentiate between the somatic and psychological functions in hospitalised patients with cancer and to compare them with healthy, caring relatives and with patients who were physically well but had recently attempted suicide. By using the Beck Depression Inventory it appeared that very few cancer patients and no next-of-kin were severely depressed in comparison to 13% of the attempted suicide group, and that over three-quarters of the cancer patients and their next-of-kin were not in the depressed group at all.

For assessment of the symptoms which could have a physical origin, such as weight loss, insomnia or anorexia, cancer patients and suicide patients were nearly identical. It was also shown that depression symptoms in cancer patients did not increase with nearness to death. Psychiatric referral was recommended for those cancer patients who develop a negative self image.

Derogatis et al. (1983) found that although two-thirds of the patients seen in three cancer centres had reactive types of adjustment disorders when specifically interviewed, 13% had major depressive disorders which could be treated by pharmacological intervention.

When the liaison psychiatry service for the breast cancer unit at Guy's Hospital was established, the first 50 patients referred with anxiety and depression were analysed. Half had severe psychological reactions which benefited from formal treatment, whereas the other half had more transient psychological disturbances and were distressed rather than ill (Ramirez 1989).

All these studies indicate that although staff sensitivity, support and common sense help the majority of patients, it is essential to be aware of those patients who may have a major psychiatric disturbance which can be treated by active antidepressant treatment.

Conclusion

The physical and emotional support of those patients with bone metastases is a challenge, but awareness of the possible problems and the appropriate treatment for them can do much to enhance the quality of life remaining to a patient and can help to lessen the grief of relatives and carers.

References

Adams F, Cruz L, Deachman MJ, Zamora E (1989) Focal subdermal toxicity with subcutaneous opioid infusion in patients with cancer pain. J Pain Symptom Management 4:31–33

Baines M (1989) Pain relief in active patients with cancer: analgesic drugs are the foundation of management. Br Med J 298:36–38

Barkas G, Duafala ME (1988) Advances in cancer pain management: a review of patient-controlled analgesia. J Pain Symptom Management 3:150–160

Bennett A, Melhuish PB, Patel S, Randles H, Stamford IF (1987) Cancer in mice; effects of prednisolone on mepacrine alone and with cytotoxic drugs. Br J Cancer 55:385–388

Blanchard J, Menk E, Ramamurthy S, Hoffman J (1990) Subarachnoid and epidural calcitonin in patients with pain due to metastatic cancer. J Pain Symptom Management 5:42–45

Braga P, Ferri S, Santagostino A et al. (1978) Lack of opiate receptor involvement in centrally induced calcitonin analgesia. Life Sci 22:971–978

Brescia FJ Sr, Walsh M, Savarese JJ, Kaiko RF (1987) A study of controlled-release oral morphine (MS Cortin) in an advanced cancer hospital. J Pain Symptom Management 2:193–198

Bruera E, Brenneis C, Paterson AH (1989) Use of methylphenidate as an adjuvant to narcotic analgesics in patients with advanced cancer. J Pain Symtom Management 4:3–6

Budd K (1983) Buprenorphine. Clin Anaesthesiol 1:147–152

Candeletti S, Ferri S (1990) Calcitonin-related peptides in the modulation of nociceptive stimuli. In: Lipton S, Tunks E, Zoppi M (eds) Advances in pain research and therapy, vol 13. Raven Press, New York, pp 45–53

Chabal C, Buckley P, Jacobsen L, Butler S, Murphy T (1989) Long-term epidural morphine in the treatment of cancer pain. Pain Clinic 3:1–23

Closs S, Bates T (1987) The management of malignant spinal cord compression. In: Bates T (ed) Contemporary palliation of difficult symptoms. Baillière's clinical oncology, vol 1, no. 4, pp 431–441

Couch JR, Ziegler DK, Hassanein R (1976) Amitriptyline in the prophylaxis of migraine. Effectiveness and relationship of anti-migraine and anti-depressant drugs. Neurology 26: 121–127

Derogatis LR, Morrow GR, Fetting J et al. (1983) The prevalence of psychiatric disorders among cancer patients. J A M A 249:751–757

Dickey RP, Minton JP (1972) Levodopa relief of bone pain from breast cancer. New Engl J Med 286:843

Doyle D (1987) Symptom control in domiciliary terminal care. Churchill Livingstone, Edinburgh, London, Melbourne, New York, pp 22–51

Driessen JJ, de Molder PHM, Claessen JJL, van Diejen D, Wobbes TL (1989) Epidural administration of morphine for control of cancer pain. Long-term efficacy and complications. Clin J Pain 5:217–222

Drug and Therapeutics Bulletin (1987) Which NSAID? (19 Oct, p 81). A Postcript and a correction; 25:103

Duthie AM (1983) Pituitary cryoablation. Anaesthesia 38:495–497

Engelsman E, Heuson JC, Blonk-Van Der Wijst J et al. (1975) Controlled clinical trial of L-dopa and nafoxidine in advanced breast cancer: an EORTC study. Br Med J 2:714–715

Filshie J (1988) The non-drug treatment of neuralgic and neuropathic pain of malignancy. Cancer Surv 7:161–193

Gennari C (1983) Clinical aspects of calcitonin in pain. Triangle 22:157–163

Gennari C, Chierichetti SM, Piolini M et al. (1985a) Analgesic activity of salmon and human calcitonin against cancer pain: A double-blind, placebo-controlled clinical study. Curr Ther Res 38:298–308

Gennari C, Francini G, Gommelli B, Bigazzi S (1985b) Treatment of bone metastasis with antiresorption drugs. In Garrattini S (ed). Bone resorption, metastasis and diphosphonates. Raven Press, New York, pp 127–136

Hanks GW (1984) Psychotrophic drugs. Clin Oncol 3:135–151

Hanks GW (1988) The pharmacological treatment of bone pain. Cancer Surv 7:87–101

Hanks GW, Hoskin PJ (1987) Opioid analgesics in the management of patients with cancer: a review. Pall Med 1:1–25

Hanks GW, Trueman T, Twycross RG (1983) Corticosteroids in terminal cancer – a prospective analysis of current practice. Postgrad Med J 59:702–706

Hardy PAJ, Wells JCD (1990) Patient controlled intrathecal morphine for cancer pain: a method used to assess morphine requirements and bolus doses. Clin J Pain 6:57–59

Heyse-Moore L, Johnson-Bell VG (1987) Can doctors accurately predict the expectancy of patients with terminal cancer? Pall Med 1:165–166

Hinton J (1972) Dying. Penguin Books, Harmondsworth, Middx, pp 79–93

Hunton J (1989) Metastatic bone pain. Mediq Ltd, London

Inturrisi CE, Umans JG (1983) Pethidine and its active metabolite, norpethidine. Clin Anaesthesiol 1:123–138

Kanner RM, Portenoy RK (1986) Unavailability of narcotic analgesics for ambulatory cancer patients in New York City. J Pain Symptom Management 1:87–89

Kessel C, Wörz R (1987) Immediate response of phantom limb pain to calcitonin. Pain 30:79–87

Lamerton R (1980) Care of the dying. Penguin Books, Harmondsworth, Middx, pp 63–92

Lipton S (1989) Pain relief in active patients with cancer: the early use of nerve blocks improves the quality of life. Br Med J 298:37–38

Madrid Jose L, Fatela LV, Alcorta J, Guillen F, Lobato RD (1988) Intermittent intrathecal morphine by means of an implantable reservoir: a survey of 100 cases. J Pain Symptom Management 3:67–71

Maher R, Mehta M (1977) Spinal (intrathecal) and extradural analgesia. In: Lipton S (ed) Persistent pain: modern methods of treatment, vol 1. Academic Press, London, pp 61–99

Masters NJ, Bennett MRD, Wedley JR (1985) Nebulised morphine: a new delivery method for pain relief. Practitioner 229:649–653

Max MB, Culnane M, Schafer SC et al. (1987) Amitriptyline relieves diabetic neuropathy pain in patients with normal or depressed mood. Neurology 37:589–596

McGuire DB, Barbour L, Boxler J et al. (1987) Fixed-interval v as-needed analgesics in cancer outpatients. J Pain Symptom Management 2:199–205

Melzack R, Wall PD (1965) Pain mechanisms: a new theory. Science 150:971–979

Miles J (1984) Pituitary destruction. In: Wall PD, Melzack R (eds) Textbook of pain. Churchill Livingstone, London, pp 656–665

Minton JP, Bronn DG, Kibbey WE (1976) L-dopa effect in painful bony metastases. N Engl J Med 294:340

Miser AW, Moore L, Greene R, Gracely RH, Miser JS (1986) Prospective study of continuous intravenous and subcutaneous morphine infusions for therapy-related or cancer-related pain in children and young adults with cancer. Clin J Pain 2:101–106

Morrica G (1977) Pituitary adenolysis in the treatment of intractable pain from cancer. In: Lipton S (ed). Persistent pain: modern methods of treatment, vol 1. Academic Press, London, pp 149–174

Nitescu P, Moulin DE, Coyle N (1986) Spinal opioid analgesics and local anaesthetics in the management of chronic cancer pain. J Pain Symptom Management 1:79–86

Nitescu P, Appelgren L, Linder LE, Sjöberg M, Hultman E, Curelaru I (1990) Epidural versus intrathecal morphine-bupivacaine; assessment of consecutive treatment in advanced cancer pain. J Pain Symptom Management 5:18–26

Noda J, Umeda S, Arai T, Harima A, Mori K (1989) Continuous subcutaneous infusion of buprenorphine for cancer pain control. Clin J Pain 5:147–152

Panerai AE, Sacerdote P, Bianchi M et al. (1990) Neuropharmacological approach to nociception. In: Lipton S, Janks E, Zoppi M (eds) Advances in pain research and therapy, vol 13. Raven Press, New York, pp 41–44

Parkes CM (1972) Accuracy in predictions of survival in later stages of cancer. Br Med J ii:29–31

Pecile A, Ferri S, Braga PC et al. (1975) Effects of intracerebroventricular calcitonin in the conscious rabbit. Experientia 31:322–333

Plumb M, Holland J (1977) Comparative studies of psychological function in patients with advanced cancer. I. Self reported depressive symptoms. Psychosom Med 39:264–276

Ramirez A (1989) Liaison psychiatry in a breast cancer unit. J R Soci Med 82:15–17

Regnard C (1985) A guide to symptom relief in advanced cancer. Haigh and Hochland, Manchester, pp 19–40

Richlin DM, Jamron LM, Novick NL (1987) Cancer pain control with a combination of methadone, amitriptyline, and non-narcotic analgesic therapy: a case series analysis. J Pain Symptom Management 2:89–94

Rogers AG (1986) The use and availability of rectal narcotics. J Pain Symptom Management 1:229–230

Rogers AG (1987) The use of continuous subcutaneous infusion of narcotics in chronic cancer pain. J Pain Symptom Management 2:167–168

Rogers AG (1988) When all oral opioids cause nausea and vomiting. J Pain Symptom Management 3:114

Satoh M, Amano H, Takahiro N et al. (1979) Inhibition by calcium of analgesia induced by intracisternal injection of porcine calcitonin in mice. Res Commun Chem Pathol Pharmacol 26:213–216

Savarese JJ, Shepherd L, Krant MJ (1987) Long acting morphine in cancer pain analgesia. Clin J pain 3:177–181

Schiraldi GF, Scoccia S, Soresi E (1985) Analgesic activity of high doses of salmon calcitonin in lung cancer. Curr Ther Res 38:592

Schug SA, Zech D, Dörr U (1990) Cancer pain management according to WHO analgesic guidelines. J Pain Symptom Management 5:27–32

Sjolin SU, Trykker H (1985) Unsuccessful treatment of severe pain from bone metastases with sinemet, 25/100. N Engl J Med 312:650–651

Stein C, Brechner T (1987) Epidural morphine tolerance: use of norepinephrine. Clin J Pain 2:267–269

Stjernsward J (1985) Cancer pain relief: an important global public health issue. Clin J Pain 1:95–97

Storey P, Hill HH Jr, St Louis RH, Tarver EE (1990) Subcutaneous infusion for control of cancer symptoms. J Pain Symptom Management 5:33–41

Swerdlow M (1986) Anticonvulsants in the therapy of neuralgic pain. Pain Clin 1:9–19

Swerdlow M (1990) The role of chemical neurolysis. In: Lipton S, Tunks E, Zoppi M (eds) Advances in pain research and therapy, vol 13. Raven Press, New York, pp 315–317

Thompson JW (1988) Pharmacology of transcutaneous electrical nerve stimulation (TENS). J Intract Pain Soc 7:33–40

Toscani F, Carini M (1989) The implementation of WHO guidelines for the treatment of advanced cancer pain at a district general hospital in Italy. Pain Clin 3:37–48

Twycross RG (1988) Opioid analgesics in cancer pain: current practice and controversies. Cancer Surv 7:29–53

Twycross RG, Lack SA (1983) Symptom control in far-advanced cancer: pain relief. Pitman, London

Ullman DA, Quarmby R (1989) Epidural administration of bupivacaine and morphine in chronic cancer pain. Pain Clin 3:25–29

Ventafridda V, Ripamonti C, Bianchi M, Sbanotto A, Deconno F (1986a) A randomized study on oral administration of morphine and methadone in the treatment of cancer pain. J Pain Symptom Management 1:203–207

Ventafridda V, Spoldi E, Caraceni A, Tamburini M, De Conno F (1986b) The importance of continuous subcutaneous morphine administration for cancer pain control. Pain Clin 1:47–55

Ventafridda V, Oliveri E, Caraceni A, Spoldi E, De Conno F, Saita L, Ripamonti C (1987) A retrospective study on the use of oral morphine in cancer pain. J Pain Symptom Management 2:77–81

Ventafridda V, Saita L, Barletta L, Sbanotto A, De Conno F (1989) Clinical observations in controlled-release morphine in cancer pain. J Pain Symptom Management 4:124–129

Vijayaram S, Bhargava K, Ramamani, Chandrasekhar, Sudharshan, Heranjal R, Lobo B (1989) Experience of oral morphine for cancer pain relief. J Pain Symptom Management 4:130–134

Waldman SD, Feldstein GS, Allen ML (1986) A trouble-shooting guide to the subcutaneous epidural implantable reservoir. J Pain Symptom Management 2:217–222

Waldman SD, Feldstein GS, Allen ML (1987) Neuroadenolysis of the pituitary: Description of a modified technique. J Pain Symptom Management 2:45–49

Walker VA, Hoskin PJ, Hanks GW, White ID (1988) Evaluation of WHO analgesic guidelines for cancer pain in a hospital-based palliative care unit. J Pain Symptom Management 3:145–149

Walsh TD (1989) Cancer pain. In: Walsh TD (ed) Symptom control. Blackwell Scientific Publications, Inc., Boston, pp 329–343

Watson CP, Evans RJ, Reed K, Merskey H, Goldsmith L, Warsh J. (1982) Amitriptyline versus placebo in post-herpetic neuralgia. Neurology 32:671–673

Wedley JR (1989) Nerve blocks. In: Walsh TD (ed) Symptom control. Blackwell Scientific Publications, Inc., Boston, pp 365–377

Wilkes E (1984) Dying now. Lancet i:950–952

Yanagida H, Suwa K, Trouwborst A, Erdmann W, Corssen G (1988) Electrical stimulation of the pituitary: its use in the treatment of cancer pain. Pain Clin 2:225–228

Subject Index